国家卫生和计划生育委员会"十三五"英文版规划教材
全国高等学校教材

供临床医学专业及来华留学生（MBBS）双语教学用

Dermatovenereology

皮肤性病学　改编教学版
Annotated Edition

David J. Gawkrodger　Michael R. Ardern-Jones

主　审　陈洪铎
Chief Examiner and Reviewer　Hongduo Chen

主　编　高兴华
Chief Editor　Xinghua Gao

副主编　徐金华　　晋红中　　陶　娟
Vice Chief Editor　Jinhua Xu　Hongzhong Jin　Juan Tao

人民卫生出版社

图书在版编目（CIP）数据

皮肤性病学：英、汉 /（英）戴维·J. 高柯罗哲
（David J. Gawkrodger）原著；高兴华主编. —北京：
人民卫生出版社，2020

ISBN 978-7-117-29555-0

Ⅰ. ①皮… Ⅱ. ①戴…②高… Ⅲ. ①皮肤病学－医
学院校－教材－汉、英②性病学－医学院校－教材－汉、
英 Ⅳ. ①R75

中国版本图书馆 CIP 数据核字（2020）第 023235 号

人卫智网	www.ipmph.com	医学教育、学术、考试、健康，购书智慧智能综合服务平台
人卫官网	www.pmph.com	人卫官方资讯发布平台

皮肤性病学

主　　编：高兴华
出版发行：人民卫生出版社（中继线 010-59780011）
地　　址：北京市朝阳区潘家园南里 19 号
邮　　编：100021
E - mail：pmph @ pmph.com
购书热线：010-59787592　010-59787584　010-65264830
印　　刷：北京盛通印刷股份有限公司
经　　销：新华书店
开　　本：889×1194　1/16　　印张：18
字　　数：532 千字
版　　次：2020 年 5 月第 1 版　2020 年 5 月第 1 版第 1 次印刷
标准书号：ISBN 978-7-117-29555-0
定　　价：88.00 元

打击盗版举报电话：010-59787491　E-mail：WQ @ pmph.com
质量问题联系电话：010-59787234　E-mail：zhiliang @ pmph.com

编者（按姓氏笔画排序）

王秀丽　同济大学医学院
Xiuli Wang　School of Medicine, Tongji University

王亮春　中山大学孙逸仙纪念医院
Liangchun Wang　Sun Yat-sen Memorial Hospital, Sun Yat-sen University

方　红　浙江大学医学院附属第一医院
Hong Fang　The First Affiliated Hospital of Zhejiang University School of Medicine

孙　青　山东大学齐鲁医院
Qing Sun　Qilu Hospital, Shandong University

李珊山　吉林大学第一医院
Shanshan Li　The First Hospital of Jilin University

李厚敏　北京大学人民医院
Houmin Li　Peking University People's Hospital

李晓东　沈阳医学院附属中心医院
Xiaodong Li　Central Hospital Affiliated to Shenyang Medical College

杨永生　复旦大学附属华山医院
Yongsheng Yang　Huashan Hospital, Fudan University

何　威　陆军军医大学
Wei He　Army Medical University

宋智琦　大连医科大学附属第一医院
Zhiqi Song　The First Affiliated Hospital of Dalian Medical University

赵　邑　清华大学附属北京清华长庚医院
Yi Zhao　Beijing Tsinghua Changgung Hospital, Tsinghua University

柏冰雪　哈尔滨医科大学附属第二医院
Bingxue Bai　The Second Affiliated Hospital of Harbin Medical University

施伟民　上海交通大学附属第一人民医院
Weimin Shi　Shanghai General Hospital, Shanghai Jiao Tong University School of Medicine

晋红中　中国医学科学院北京协和医学院
Hongzhong Jin　Chinese Academy of Medical Sciences & Peking Union Medical College

夏育民　西安交通大学第二附属医院
Yumin Xia　The Second Affiliated Hospital of Xi'an Jiaotong University

徐金华　复旦大学附属华山医院
Jinhua Xu　Huashan Hospital, Fudan University

高　敏　安徽医科大学
Min Gao　Anhui Medical University

高兴华　中国医科大学附属第一医院
XingHua Gao　The First Hospital of China Medical University

陶　娟　华中科技大学同济医学院
Juan Tao　Tongji Medical College of HUST

蒋　献　四川大学华西临床医学院
Xian Jiang　West China School of Medicine, Sichuan University

喻　楠　宁夏医科大学总医院
Nan Yu　General Hospital of Ningxia Medical University

鲁建云　中南大学湘雅三医院
Jianyun Lu　The Third Xiangya Hospital, Central South University

满孝勇　浙江大学医学院附属第二医院
XiaoYong Man　The Second Affiliated Hospital of Zhejiang University School of Medicine

潘　萌　上海交通大学医学院附属瑞金医院
Meng Pan　Rui Jin Hospital, Shanghai Jiao Tong University School of Medicine

潘炜华　第二军医大学附属长征医院
Weihua Pan　Changzheng Hospital, The Second Military Medical University

ELSEVIER

Elsevier (Singapore) Pte Ltd.

3 Killiney Road, #08-01 Winsland House I, Singapore 239519

Tel: (65) 6349-0200; Fax: (65) 6733-1817

This English Adaptation of Dermatology: An Illustrated Colour Text, 6/E by David J. Gawkrodger and Michael R. Ardern-Jones was undertaken by People's Medical Publishing House and is published by arrangement with Elsevier (Singapore) Pte Ltd.

Dermatology: An Illustrated Colour Text, 6/E by David J. Gawkrodger and Michael R. Ardern-Jones 由人民卫生出版社进行改编影印，并根据人民卫生出版社与爱思唯尔（新加坡）私人有限公司的协议约定出版。

皮肤性病学 Dermatovenerology，改编教学版，（高兴华 改编）

ISBN: 978-7-117-29555-0

图字号：01-2018-0684

1995 年，我国首次招收全英文授课医学留学生，到 2015 年，接收临床医学专业 MBBS（Bachelor of Medicine & Bachelor of Surgery）留学生的院校达到了 40 余家，MBBS 院校数量、规模不断扩张；同时，医学院校在临床医学专业五年制、长学制教学中陆续开展不同规模和范围的双语或全英文授课，使得对一套符合我国教学实际、成体系、高质量英文教材的需求日益增长。

为了满足教学需求，进一步落实教育部《关于加强高等学校本科教学工作提高教学质量的若干意见（教高 [2001]4 号）》和《来华留学生医学本科教育（英文授课）质量控制标准暂行规定（教外来 [2007]39 号）》等相关文件的要求，规范和提高我国高等医学院校临床医学专业五年制、长学制和来华留学生（MBBS）双语教学及全英文教学的质量，推进医学双语教学和留学生教育的健康有序发展，完善和规范临床医学专业英文版教材的体系，人民卫生出版社在充分调研的基础上，于 2015 年召开了全国高等学校临床医学专业英文版规划教材的编写论证会，经过会上及会后的反复论证，最终确定组织编写一套全国规划的、适合我国高等医学院校教学实际的临床医学专业英文版教材，并计划作为 2017 年春季和秋季教材在全国出版发行。

本套英文版教材的编写结合国家卫生和计划生育委员会、教育部的总体要求，坚持"三基、五性、三特定"的原则，组织全国各大医学院校、教学医院的专家编写，主要特点如下：

1. 教材编写应教学之需启动，在全国范围进行了广泛、深入调研和论证，借鉴国内外医学人才培养模式和教材建设经验，对主要读者对象、编写模式、编写科目、编者遴选条件等进行了科学设计。

2. 坚持"三基、五性、三特定"和"多级论证"的教材编写原则，组织全国各大医学院校及教学医院有丰富英语教学经验的专家一起编写，以保证高质量出版。

3. 为保证英语表达的准确性和规范性，大部分教材以国外英文原版教科书为蓝本，根据我国教学大纲和人民卫生出版社临床医学专业第八轮规划教材主要内容进行改编，充分体现科学性、权威性、适用性和实用性。

4. 教材内部各环节合理设置，根据读者对象的特点，在英文原版教材的基础上结合需要，增加本章小结、关键术语（英中对照）、思考题、推荐阅读等模块，促进学生自主学习。

本套临床医学专业英文版规划教材共 38 种，均为国家卫生和计划生育委员会"十三五"规划教材，计划于 2017 年全部出版发行。

In 1995, China recruited overseas medical students of full English teaching for the first time. Up to 2015, more than 40 institutions enrolled overseas MBBS (Bachelor of Medicine & Bachelor of Surgery) students. The number of MBBS institutions and overseas students are continuously increasing. At the meantime, medical colleges' application for bilingual or full English teaching in different size and range in five-year and long-term professional clinical medicine teaching results to increasingly demand for a set of practical, systematic and high-qualified English teaching material.

In order to meet the teaching needs and to implement the regulations of relevant documents issued by Ministry of Education including "Some Suggestions to Strengthen the Undergraduate Teaching and to Improve the Teaching Quality" and "Interim Provisions on Quality Control Standards of International Medical Undergraduate Education (English teaching)", as well as to standardize and improve the quality of the bilingual teaching and English teaching of the five-year, long-term and international students (MBBS) of clinical medicine in China's higher medical colleges so as to promote the healthy and orderly development of medical bilingual teaching and international students education and to improve and standardize the system of English clinical medicine textbooks, after full investigation, People's Medical Publishing House (PMPH) held the writing discussion meeting of English textbook for clinical medicine department of national colleges and universities in 2015. After the repeated demonstration in and after the meeting, PMPH ultimately determined to organize the compilation of a set of national planning English textbooks which are suitable for China's actual clinical medicine teaching of medical colleges and universities. This set will be published as spring and autumn textbooks of 2017.

This set of English textbooks meets the overall requirements of the Ministry of Education and National Health and Family Planning Commission, the editorial committee includes the experts from major medical colleges and universities as well as teaching hospitals, the main features are as follows:

1. Textbooks compilation is started to meet the teaching needs, extensive and deep research and demonstration are conducted across the country, the main target readers, the model and subject of compilation and selection conditions of authors are scientifically designed in accordance with the reference of domestic and foreign medical personnel training model and experience in teaching materials.

2. Adhere to the teaching materials compiling principles of "three foundations, five characteristics, and three specialties" and "multi-level demonstration", the organization of English teaching experts with rich experience from major medical schools and teaching hospitals ensures the high quality of publication.

3. In order to ensure the accuracy and standardization of English expression, most of the textbooks are modeled on original English textbooks, and adapted based on national syllabus and main content of the eighth round of clinical medicine textbooks which were published by PMPH, fully reflecting the scientificity, authority, applicability and practicality.

4. All aspects of teaching materials are arranged reasonably, based on original textbooks,the chapter summary, key terms (English and Chinese), review questions, and recommended readings are added to promote students' independent learning in accordance with teaching needs and the characteristics of the target readers.

This set of English textbooks for clinical medicine includes 38 species which are among "13th Five-Year" planning textbooks of National Health and Family Planning Commission, and will be all published in 2017.

全国高等学校临床医学专业第一轮英文版规划教材 · 教材目录

教材名称		主 审	主编	
1 人体解剖学	Human Anatomy		刘学政	
2 生理学	Physiology		闫剑群	
3 医学免疫学	Medical Immunology		储以微	
4 生物化学	Biochemistry		张晓伟	
5 组织学与胚胎学	Histology and Embryology		李 和	
6 医学微生物学	Medical Microbiology		郭晓奎	
7 病理学	Pathology		陈 杰	
8 医学分子生物学	Medical Molecular Biology		吕社民	
9 医学遗传学	Medical Genetics		傅松滨	
10 医学细胞生物学	Medical Cell Biology		刘 佳	
11 病理生理学	Pathophysiology		王建枝	
12 药理学	Pharmacology		杨宝峰	
13 临床药理学	Clinical Pharmacology		李 俊	
14 人体寄生虫学	Human Parasitology		李学荣	
15 流行病学	Epidemiology		沈洪兵	
16 医学统计学	Medical Statistics		郝元涛	
17 核医学	Nuclear Medicine		黄 钢	李 方
18 医学影像学	Medical Imaging		申宝忠	龚启勇
19 临床诊断学	Clinical Diagnostics		万学红	
20 实验诊断学	Laboratory Diagnostics		胡翊群	王 琳
21 内科学	Internal Medicine		文富强	汪道文
22 外科学	Surgery		陈孝平	田 伟
23 妇产科学	Obstetrics and Gynecology	郎景和	狄 文	曹云霞
24 儿科学	Pediatrics		黄国英	罗小平
25 神经病学	Neurology		张黎明	
26 精神病学	Psychiatry		赵靖平	
27 传染病学	Infectious Diseases		高志良	任 红

全国高等学校临床医学专业第一轮英文版规划教材 · 教材目录

	教材名称		主 审	主编
28	皮肤性病学	Dermatovenereology	陈洪铎	高兴华
29	肿瘤学	Oncology		石远凯
30	眼科学	Ophthalmology		杨培增　刘奕志
31	康复医学	Rehabilitation Medicine		虞乐华
32	医学心理学	Medical Psychology		赵旭东
33	耳鼻咽喉头颈外科学	Otorhinolaryngology-Head and Neck Surgery		孔维佳
34	急诊医学	Emergency Medicine		陈玉国
35	法医学	Forensic Medicine		赵　虎
36	全球健康学	Global Health		吴群红
37	中医学	Chinese Medicine		王新华
38	医学汉语	Medical Chinese		李　骢

Preface to the sixth edition

There has been a near revolution in how a published medical text is handled by its users since we wrote the fifth edition of this work in 2011. For this type of book, there will be considerable usage online. The content and presentation of the sixth edition of this book has been developed to accommodate readers' likely use in the smartphone age. Our publishers, Elsevier, have been of considerable assistance in this task, providing the platform for the delivery of an interactive, searchable and well illustrated text.

In order to make use of the opportunities offered by online publication, we have increased the flexibility of the educational level of the text. Previously we aimed to write and illustrate a book that was suitable for medical students and general practitioners but which would also appeal to the early trainee in dermatology. This is still the case, and the printed version has been fully updated, but online publication has given us the chance to broaden the scope of the book. We have added some material at a higher level that can be accessed by those that opt to use it, whilst bolstering the basic strengths of the text through the use of additional illustrations.

Online publishing has allowed us, for each topic covered, to introduce innovations. These include selfassessment questions, flashcards, a picture gallery of dermatological diseases and direct Internet links to other sources of information and reference. It has also been possible to highlight throughout the text, new treatments and dermatological emergencies.

We are aware that the specialty of dermatology is constantly changing. There is presently a greater emphasis than ever before on skin cancer, its recognition and management, and we have reflected this in our content. Other areas that have developed into subspecialisms, which have required additional text, include genital dermatoses, psychodermatology, cosmetic procedures, and advances in dermatologic surgery. We trust that our target audience of medical students, family doctors, hospital residents, specialty registrars in dermatology or internal medicine, and specialist nurses will continue to find our book helpful in the diagnosis and management of patients with skin diseases.

David J. Gawkrodger and
Michael R. Ardern-Jones
Sheffield and Southampton, 2015

Preface to the first edition

Recent advances in publishing technology and book presentation demand that a modern text be attractively and concisely presented, in colour and at an affordable price. This is essential for success in a very competitive market. In writing this book, I have attempted to present an introductory dermatology text for the 1990s, using a format of individually designed double-page spreads, generously illustrated with colour photographs, line drawings, tables, bulleted items and 'key point' summaries. This unique approach, which deals with each topic as an educational unit, allows the reader better accessibility to the facts and greater ease in revision than is possible with a conventional textbook.

The book is aimed at medical students but contains sufficient detail to be of use to family practitioners, physicians in internal medicine, registrars or residents in dermatology and dermatological nurses. The contents are divided into three sections. The first presents a scientific basis for the understanding of and clinical approach to skin disease. The second details the major dermatological conditions, and the third outlines special topics, such as photoageing and dermatological surgery, that are of current importance or that are poorly dealt with in other textbooks.

David J. Gawkrodger
Sheffield 1992

Acknowledgements

In the production of the sixth edition of this book it is a pleasure to acknowledge the contribution of the publishing staff at Elsevier, notably Jeremy Bowes, Alisa Laing and Kim Benson. We are grateful to colleagues who have advised on various aspects of the book, especially to Dr Louise Ardern-Jones for her detailed review.

We thank colleagues who have generously provided figures for this and previous editions, including Dr E.C. Benton of Edinburgh, Dr J.E. Bothwell of Doncaster, Dr J.S.C. English of Nottingham, Dr J. Bowling of Oxford (dermoscopy images), the late Dr S.M. Morley of Dundee, Dr M. Shah of Burnley, Dr H.S. Ghura of Salford, and Dr A.J.G. McDonagh, Dr A.G. Messenger, Dr C. Yeoman, Mr D. Dobbs, Professor S.S. Bleehen and Dr C.I. Harrington of Sheffield, and also Dr Efrem Eren, for provision of autoantibody fluorescence images.

We are grateful to the following for advice or for the provision of illustrations: Professor R.StC. Barnetson, Dr G.W. Beveridge, Professor Chris Bunker (University College Hospital, London), Dr P.K. Buxton, Dr G.B. Colver, the late Professor F.J.G. Ebling, Dr M.E. Kesseler, Dr Fiona Lewis (St Thomas Hospital, London), Dr C. McGibbon, Dr A. McMillan, Mrs E. McVittie, Dr C.StJ. O'Doherty, Dr Glenda Sobey (Sheffield Children's Hospital), Miss M.J. Spencer, Dr M.D. Talbot and the late Dr A.E. Walker.

We also thank those patients who gave permission for their faces to be shown without eyebars.

Adaptation Preface

This book is intended to serve as a textbook for medical students in China whose dermatological curricula are taught in English and a quick reference for starters in practicing dermatology. The book covers the basic knowledge about skin physiology and pathology, as well as the general introduction to management of common skin diseases.

Our grateful thanks go to Elsevier Health that authorized our use of materials and beautiful illustration of the textbook. It would be impossible for us to send this textbook to the printer without permission and authorization from the publisher and the authors, Drs. David Gawkrodger and Michael R Ardern-Jones. We chose this textbook from among a host of English-language dermatology textbooks for its well-arranged content, concise manner and straightforward language for medical students. We made some adjustments to the text based on China's medical curricula, added a number of new illustrations, and appended quiz and take-home questions to each chapter. Our fantastic team of authors shared their knowledge, their clinical experience and expertise, and their creativity in and provided their own fresh ideas in compiling this book, endeavoring to tailor this textbook to Chinese readers or students from other nations who entered medical college in China. Lastly, I would like to give special thanks to Dr. Yuxiao Hong, serving as secretary of the team, has paid great efforts in the management for publication of the book.

Hopefully, this book will usher our readers into a fascinating clinical discipline of dermatology, serving as valuable resource for any medical students and practitioners.

Xinghua Gao MD, Ph.D.
Professor and Chair of Dermatology
The First Hospital of China Medical University
President elect, Chinese Society of Dermatology

Table of Contents

Diseases　　　　　　　　　　　　　　　　　　　53

Special topics in dermatology   213

Index · 265

Basic principles

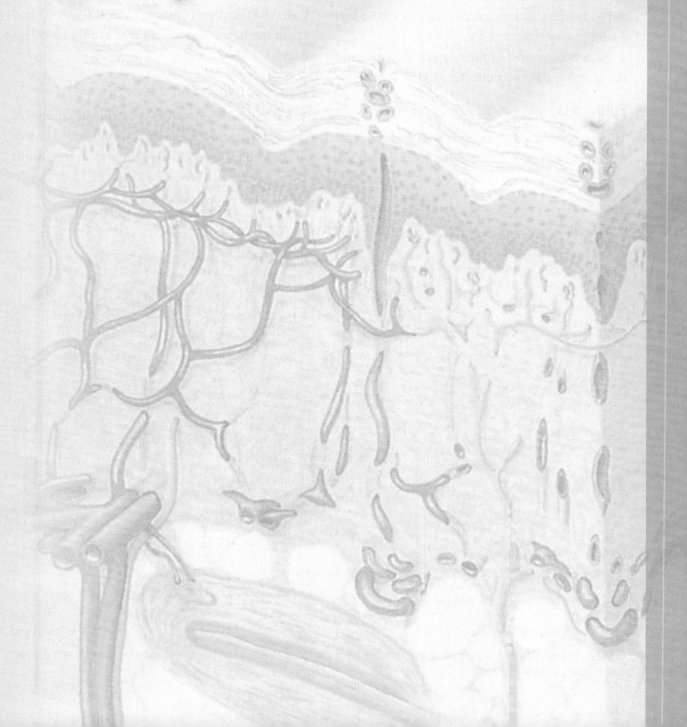

Chapter 1 Microanatomy of the skin

Introduction

The skin is one of the largest organs in the body, having a surface area of around 1.8m² and making up about 16% of body weight. It has many functions, the most important of which is as a barrier to protect the body from noxious external factors and to keep the internal systems intact.

Skin is composed of three layers: the epidermis, the dermis and the subcutis (Fig. 1-1).

Epidermis

The epidermis is a stratified squamous epithelium that is about 0.1mm thick, although the thickness is greater (0.8~1.4mm) on the palms and soles. Its prime function is to act as a protective barrier. The main cells of the epidermis are *keratinocytes*, which produce the protein keratin. Keratinocytes are squamous cells functionally similar to all other structural epithelial cells as found in the airways and gastrointestinal tract. The four layers of the epidermis (Fig. 1-2) represent the stages of maturation of keratin by keratinocytes.

Basal cell layer (stratum basale)

The basal cell layer of the epidermis is composed mostly of keratinocytes, which are either dividing or non-dividing. The cells contain keratin tonofibrils

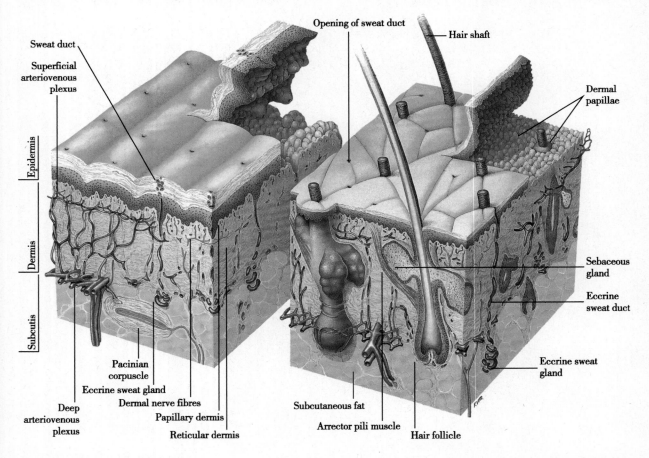

Thick (hairless) skin

Thin (hairy) skin

Fig. 1-1 **Structure of the skin.** The diagram shows a comparison between thick, hairless skin (plantar and palmar) and thinner, hirsute skin.

and are secured to the basement membrane (see Fig. 1-2) by hemidesmosomes. *Melanocytes* make up 5%~10% of the basal cell population. These cells synthesize melanin and transfer it via dendritic processes to neighbouring keratinocytes.

Melanocytes are most numerous on the face and other exposed sites, and are of neural crest origin. *Merkel cells* are also found, albeit infrequently, in the basal cell layer. These cells are closely associated with terminal filaments of cutaneous nerves and seem to have a role in sensation. Their cytoplasm contains neuropeptide granules, as well as neurofilaments and keratin. Basal keratinocytes synthesize antimicrobial peptides, important in defence against bacteria.

Prickle cell layer (stratum spinosum)

Daughter basal cells migrate upwards to form this layer of polyhedral cells, which are interconnected by desmosomes (the 'prickles' seen at light microscope

level). Keratin tonofibrils form a supportive mesh in the cytoplasm of these cells. *Langerhans cells* are mostly found in this layer.

Embryology of the skin

The epidermis (ectoderm) begins to develop at 4 weeks of life, and, by 7 weeks, flat cells overlying the basal layer form the periderm (which is eventually cast off). Nails start to take shape at 10 weeks. The dermis (mesoderm) develops at 11 weeks, and, by 12 weeks, indented basal buds of the epidermis form the hair bulbs, with dermal papillae supplying vessels and nerves. Fingerprint ridges are determined by 17 weeks' gestation. Maturation of the epidermis into a fully functional protective barrier continues throughout gestation and, because of this, pre-term infants are now frequently cared for with plastic occlusion to replicate this function.

Granular cell layer (stratum granulosum)

Cells become flattened and lose their nuclei in the granular cell layer. Keratohyalin granules are seen

Fig. 1-2 **Cross-sectional anatomy of the epidermis.(a)** Layers of the epidermis and other structures. **(b)** Detailed view of the basement membrane zone at the dermoepidermal junction. Components are arranged in three layers. The lamina lucida is traversed by filaments connecting the basal cells with the lamina densa, from which anchoring fibrils extend into the papillary dermis. These laminae are the sites of cleavage in certain bullous disorders).

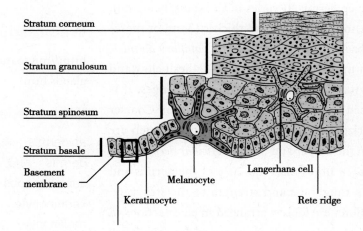

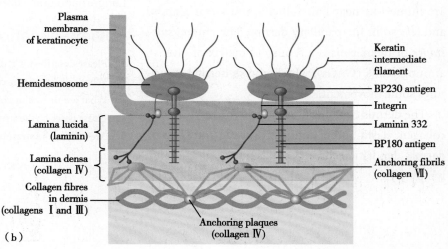

in the cytoplasm together with membrane-coating granules (which expel their lipid contents into the intercellular spaces).

Horny layer (stratum corneum)

The end result of keratinocyte maturation can be found in the horny layer, which is composed of sheets of overlapping polyhedral cornified cells with no nuclei (corneocytes). The layer is several cells thick on the palms and soles, but less thick elsewhere. The corneocyte cell envelope is broadened, and the cytoplasm is replaced by keratin tonofibrils in a matrix formed from the keratohyalin granules. Cells are stuck together by lipid glue that is partly derived from membrane-coating granules.

Dermis

The dermis is defined as a tough supportive connective tissue matrix, containing specialized structures, found immediately below and intimately connected with the epidermis. It varies in thickness, being thin (0.6mm) on the eyelids and thicker (3mm or more) on the back, palms and soles. The *papillary dermis* - the thin upper layer of the dermis - lies below and interdigitates with the epidermal rete ridges. It is composed of loosely interwoven collagen. Coarser and horizontally running bundles of collagen are found in the deeper and thicker *reticular dermis*.

Collagen fibres make up 70% of the dermis and impart a toughness and strength to the structure. *Elastin* fibres are loosely arranged in all directions in the dermis and provide elasticity to the skin. They are numerous near hair follicles and sweat glands, and less so in the papillary dermis. The *ground substance* of the dermis is a semisolid matrix of glycosaminoglycans (GAGs), which allows dermal structures some movement.

The dermis contains fibroblasts (which synthesize collagen, elastin, other connective tissue and GAGs), dermal dendritic cells, mast cells, macrophages and lymphocytes.

Subcutaneous ayer

The subcutis consists of loose connective tissue and fat (up to 3cm thick on the abdomen).

Microanatomy

- The skin constitutes 16% of body weight, with a surface area of about $1.8m^2$.
- Structure and thickness vary with site.
- The epidermis is the outer covering, mainly composed of keratinocytes arranged in four layers, namely stratum corneum, stratum granulosum, stratum spinosum and stratum basale.
- The epidermis also contains melanocytes and Langerhans cells.
- The thickness of the epidermis varies from 0.1mm to 0.8~1.4mm on the palms and soles.
- The dermis is supportive connective tissue, mainly collagen, elastin and glycosaminoglycans. The thickness varies between 0.6mm (e.g. eyelids) and 3mm (e.g. back and soles).
- The dermis contains fibroblasts that synthesize the collagen, elastic fibres and glycosaminoglycans. Dermal dendritic cells are also found together with other immunocompetent cells.

Web resource

http://microanatomy.net/skin/skin_and_mammary_glands.htm

Key words

epidermis   表皮
dermis   真皮
subcutaneous fat   皮下脂肪
keratinocyte   角质形成细胞
melanocyte   黑素细胞
Langerhans cell   朗格汉斯细胞

Review questions

1. Please describe the sturcture of the epidermis.
2. What cells are major constituents of the epidermis?
3. What are the major constituents of the dermis?
4. Please describe the structure of basement membrane zone.
5. Are cells in the stratum corneum of the epidermis viable?

(Xinghua Gao)

Chapter 2 Derivatives of the skin

Hair

Hairs are found over the entire surface of the skin, with the exception of the glabrous skin of the palms, soles, glans penis and vulval introitus. The density of follicles is greatest on the face. Embryologically, the hair follicle has an input from the epidermis, which is responsible for the matrix cells and the hair shaft, and the dermis, which contributes to the papilla, with its blood vessels and nerves.

There are three types of hair:

1. *Lanugo* hairs are fine and long, and are formed in the fetus at 20 weeks' gestation. They are normally shed before birth, but may be seen in premature babies.
2. *Vellus* hairs are the short, fine, light-coloured hairs that cover most body surfaces.
3. *Terminal* hairs are longer, thicker and darker, and are found on the scalp, eyebrows, eyelashes and also on the pubic, axillary and beard areas. They originate as vellus hair; differentiation is stimulated at puberty by androgens.

Structure

The hair follicle is an invagination of the epidermis containing a hair. The portion above the site of entry of the sebaceous duct is the infundibulum. The hair shaft consists of an *outer cuticle* that encloses a cortex of packed keratinocytes with (in terminal hairs) an *inner medulla* (Fig. 2-1). The germinative cells are in the hair bulb; associated with these cells are melanocytes, which synthesize pigment. The *arrector pili* muscle is vestigial in humans; it contracts with cold, fear and emotion to erect the hair, producing 'goose pimples'.

Nails

The nail is a phylogenetic remnant of the mammalian claw and consists of a plate of hardened and densely packed keratin. It protects the fingertip and facilitates grasping and tactile sensitivity in the finger pulp.

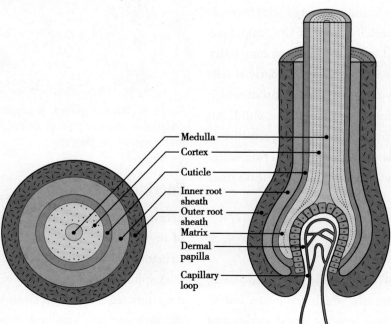

Medulla
Cortex
Cuticle
Inner root sheath
Outer root sheath
Matrix
Dermal papilla
Capillary loop

Fig. 2-1 **Structure of the hair follicle.**

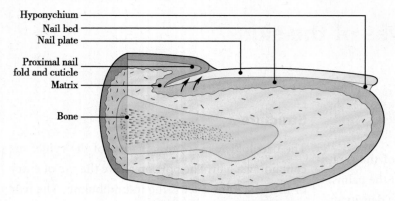

Hyponychium
Nail bed
Nail plate
Proximal nail fold and cuticle
Matrix
Bone

Fig. 2-2 **Structure of the fingernail.**

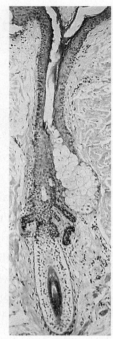

Structure

The *nail matrix* contains dividing cells which mature, keratinize and move forward to form the *nail plate* (Fig. 2-2). The nail plate has a thickness of 0.3~0.5mm and grows at a rate of 0.1mm/24h for the fingernail. Toenails grow more slowly. The *nail bed*, which produces small amounts of keratin, is adherent to the nail plate. The adjacent dermal capillaries produce the pink colour of the nail; the white lunula is the visible distal part of the matrix. The *hyponychium* is the thickened epidermis that underlies the free margin of the nail.

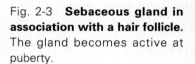

Fig. 2-3 **Sebaceous gland in association with a hair follicle.** The gland becomes active at puberty.

Sebaceous glands

Sebaceous glands are found associated with hair follicles (Fig. 2-3), especially those of the scalp, face, chest and back, and are not found on non-hairy skin. They are formed from epidermis-derived cells and produce an oily sebum, the function of which is uncertain. The glands are small in the child, but become large and active at puberty, being sensitive to androgens. Sebum is produced by holocrine secretion in which the cells disintegrate to release their lipid cytoplasm.

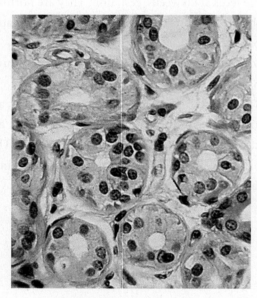

Fig. 2-4 **Sweat gland.** A cross-section through the coiled secretory portion of an eccrine sweat gland, situated deep in the dermis.

Sweat glands

Sweat glands (Fig. 2-4) are tube-like and coiled glands, located within the dermis, which produce a watery secretion. There are two separate types: eccrine and apocrine.

Eccrine

Eccrine sweat glands develop from downbudding of the epidermis. The secretory portion is a coiled structure in the deep reticular dermis; the excretory duct spirals upwards to open onto the skin surface. An estimated 2.5 million sweat ducts are present on the skin surface. They are universally distributed, but are most profuse on the palms, soles, axillae and forehead where the glands are under both psychological and thermal control (those elsewhere being under thermal control only). Eccrine sweat glands are innervated by sympathetic (cholinergic) nerve fibres.

Apocrine

Also derived from the epidermis, apocrine sweat glands open into hair follicles and are larger than eccrine glands. They are most numerous around the axillae, perineum and areolae. Their sweat is generated by 'decapitation' secretion of the gland's cells and is odourless when produced; an odour develops after skin bacteria have acted upon it. Sweating is controlled by sympathetic (adrenergic) innervation. The apocrine glands represent a phylogenetic remnant of the mammalian sexual scent gland.

Other structures in skin

Nerve supply

The skin is richly innervated (Fig. 2-5), with the highest density of nerves being found in areas such as the hands, face and genitalia. All nerves supplying the skin have their cell bodies in the dorsal root ganglia. Both myelinated and non-myelinated fibres are found. The nerves contain neuropeptides, e.g. substance P.

Free sensory nerve endings are seen in the dermis and also encroaching into the epidermis where they may abut onto *Merkel cells*. These nerve endings detect pain, itch and temperature. Specialized corpuscular receptors are distributed in the dermis, such as the *Pacinian corpuscle* (detecting pressure and vibration) and touch-sensitive *Meissner's corpuscles*, which are mainly seen in the dermal papillae of the feet and hands.

Autonomic nerves supply the blood vessels, sweat glands and arrector pili muscles. The nerve supply is dermatomal with some overlap.

Blood and lymphatic vessels

The skin also has a rich and adaptive blood supply. Arteries in the subcutis branch upwards, forming a superficial plexus at the papillary/reticular dermal boundary. Branches extend to the dermal papillae (Fig. 2-6), each of which has a single loop of capillary vessels, one arterial and one venous. Veins drain from

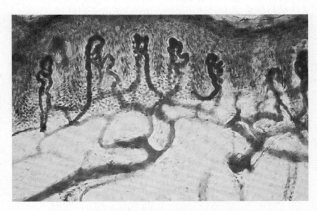

Fig. 2-6 **Superficial dermal blood vessels.** Capillary loops branch off the superficial vascular plexus and extend into each dermal papilla.

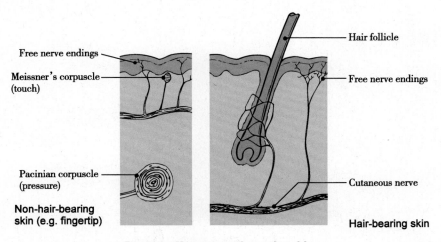

Fig. 2-5 **Nerve supply to the skin.**

the venous side of this loop to form the mid-dermal and subcutaneous venous networks. In the reticular and papillary dermis, there are arteriovenous anastomoses that are well innervated and concerned with thermoregulation.

The lymphatic drainage of the skin is important, and abundant meshes of lymphatics originate in the papillae and assemble into larger vessels that ultimately drain into the regional lymph nodes.

Derivatives
- Sebaceous glands, associated with hair follicles, are androgen sensitive.
- Vellus hairs cover most body surfaces; terminal hairs occur on the scalp, beard, axillary and pubic areas.
- Skin has extensive nerve networks with specialized nerve endings.
- Skin has a rich and adaptive blood supply; lymphatics drain to regional lymph nodes.
- Eccrine sweat glands, with sympathetic innervation, are under thermal/psychological control; apocrine glands are largely vestigial in humans.

Key words

hair　毛发

nail　甲

sebaceous gland　皮脂腺

sweat gland　汗腺

eccrine sweat gland　外泌汗腺

apocrine sweat gland　顶泌汗腺

blood vessel　血管

lymphatic vessel　淋巴管

Review question

What are the functions of the derivatives of the skin?

(Hong Fang)

Chapter 3   Physiology of the skin

The skin is a metabolically active organ with vital functions (Table 3-1), including the protection and homeostasis of the body.

Table 3-1   **Functions of skin**
Presents barrier to physical agents
Protects against mechanical injury
Antimicrobial peptides have a bactericidal effect
Prevents loss of body fluids
Reduces penetration of UV radiation
Helps to regulate body temperature
Acts as a sensory organ
Affords a surface for grip
Plays a role in vitamin D production
Acts as an outpost for immune surveillance
Cosmetic association

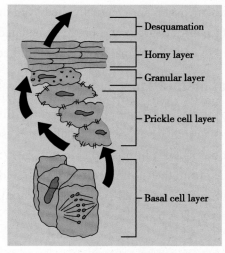

Fig. 3-1   **Keratinocyte maturation.**

Skin barrier function

The skin presents barrier to external harmful factors and prevents the body's fluids from getting out. The horny layer is important in preventing all manner of agents from entering the skin, including micro-organisms, water and particulate matter. Antimicrobial peptides of the defensin and cathelicidin classes, present on the epidermal surface, have bactericidal activity. The epidermis also protects against mechanical injury and reduces penetration of UV radiation.

Keratinocyte maturation

The differentiation of basal cells into dead, but functionally important, corneocytes is a unique feature of the skin. The horny layer is important in preventing all manner of agents from entering the skin, including micro-organisms, water and particulate matter. Antimicrobial peptides of the defensin and cathelicidin classes, present on the epidermal surface, have bactericidal activity.

Epidermal cells undergo the following sequence during keratinocyte maturation (Fig. 3-1):

1. Undifferentiated cells in the *basal layer* and the layer immediately above divide continuously. Half of these cells remain in place, and half progress upwards and differentiate.

2. In the *prickle cell layer*, cells change from being columnar to polygonal. Differentiating keratinocytes synthesize keratins, which aggregate to form tonofilaments. The *desmosomes* connecting keratinocytes are composed of the structural molecules cadherins, desmogleins and desmocollins. Desmosomes distribute structural stresses throughout the epidermis and maintain a distance of 20nm between adjacent cells.

3. In the *granular layer*, enzymes induce degradation of nuclei and organelles. Keratohyalin granules containing filaggrin mature the keratin and provide an amorphous protein matrix for the tonofilaments. Membrane-coating granules attach to the cell membrane and release an impervious lipid-containing cement, which contributes to cell adhesion and to the *horny layer* barrier.

4. In the *horny layer*, the dead, flattened corneocytes have developed thickened cornified envelopes containing involucrin that encase a matrix of keratin macrofibres aligned by filaggrin. The strong

disulphide bonds of the keratin provide strength to the stratum corneum, but the layer is also flexible and can absorb up to three times its own weight in water. However, if it dries out (i.e. water content falls below 10%), pliability fails.

5. The corneocytes are eventually shed from the skin surface after degradation of the lamellated lipid and loss of desmosomal intercellular connections.

Rate of maturation

Kinetic studies show that, on average, the dividing basal cells replicate every 200~400h. The resultant differentiating cells in normal skin take 52~75 days to be shed from the stratum corneum. The epidermal transit time is considerably reduced in keratinization disorders such as psoriasis.

Melanocyte function

Melanocytes (located in the basal layer) produce the pigment melanin in elongated, membrane-bound organelles known as melanosomes (Fig. 3-2). These are packaged into granules, which are moved down dendritic processes and transferred by phagocytosis to adjacent keratinocytes. Melanin granules form a protective cap over the outer part of keratinocyte nuclei in the inner layers of the epidermis. In the stratum corneum, they are uniformly distributed to form a UV-absorbing blanket, which reduces the amount of radiation penetrating the skin. Thickening of the epidermis also blocks UV.

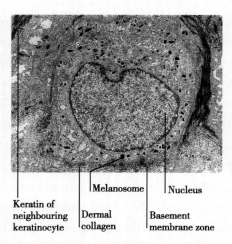

Fig. 3-2 **Electron micrograph of a melanocyte.**

UV radiation - mainly the wavelengths of 290~320nm (UVB) - darkens the skin first by immediate photo-oxidation of preformed melanin and second, over a period of days, by stimulating melanocytes to produce more melanin. UV radiation also induces keratinocyte proliferation, resulting in thickening of the epidermis.

Variations in racial pigmentation result not from differences in melanocyte numbers, but in the number and size of melanosomes produced.

Hair growth

The rate of hair growth differs depending on the body site. For example, eyebrow hair grows faster and has a shorter anagen (see below) than scalp hair. On average, there are about 100 000 hairs on the scalp, and the normal rate of hair growth is 0.4mm/24h. Hair growth is cyclical, with three phases, and is randomized for individual hairs, although synchronization does occur during pregnancy. The three phases of hair development (Fig. 3-3) are anagen, catagen and telogen.

1. *Anagen* is the growing phase. For scalp hair, this period lasts from 3 to 7 years, but for eyebrow hair, it lasts only 4 months. At any one time, 80%~90% of scalp hairs are in anagen, and about 50~100 scalp follicles switch to catagen per day.

2. *Catagen* is the resting phase and lasts 3~4 weeks. Hair protein synthesis stops, and the follicle retreats towards the surface. At any one time, 10%~20% of scalp hairs are in catagen.

3. *Telogen* is the shedding phase, distinguished by the presence of hairs with a short club root. Each day, 50~100 scalp hairs are shed, with less than 1% of hairs being in telogen at any one time.

Thermoregulation

The maintenance of a near-constant body core temperature of 37℃ is a great advantage to humans, allowing a constancy to many biochemical reactions that would otherwise fluctuate widely with temperature changes. Thermoregulation depends on several

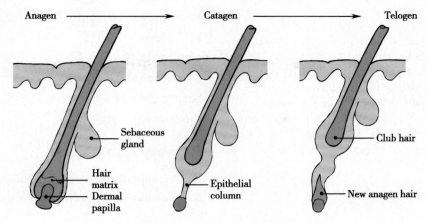

Fig. 3-3 **The three phases of hair development.**

factors, including metabolism and exercise, but the skin plays an important part in control through the evaporation of sweat and by direct heat loss from the surface.

Blood flow

Skin temperature is highly responsive to skin blood flow. Dilatation or contraction of the dermal blood vessels results in vast changes in blood flow, which can vary from 1 to 100ml/min per 100g of skin for the fingers and forearms. Arteriovenous anastomoses under the control of the sympathetic nervous system shunt blood to the superficial venous plexuses (Fig. 3-4), affecting skin temperature. Local factors, both chemical and physical, can also have an effect.

Sweat

The production of sweat cools the skin through evaporation. The minimum insensible perspiration per day is 0.5L. Maximum daily secretion is 10L, with a maximum output of about 2L/h. Men sweat more than women.

Watery isotonic sweat, produced in the sweat gland, is modified in the excretory portion of the duct so that the fluid delivered to the skin surface has:

■ a pH of between 4 and 6.8
■ a low concentration of Na^+ (30~70mEq/L) and Cl^- (30~70mEq/L)
■ a high concentration of K^+ (up to 5mEq/L), lactate (4~40mEq/L), urea, ammonia and some amino acids

Only small quantities of toxic substances are lost.

Sweating may also occur in response to emotion and after eating spicy food. In addition to thermoregulation, sweat also helps to maintain the hydration of the horny layer and improves grip on the palms and soles.

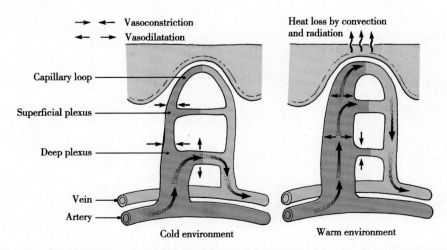

Fig. 3-4 **Variations in blood supply to the skin under cold and warm conditions.**

Physiology
- Basal cell replication rate: once every 200~400h.
- Transepidermal cycle time: 52~75 days.
- Growth rate for scalp hair: 0.4mm/24h.
- Normal hair fall (scalp): 50~100/24h.
- Fingernail growth: 0.1mm/24h (toenail is less).
- Skin blood flow is controlled by shunting at arteriovenous anastomoses.
- Minimum insensitive perspiration: 0.5L/24h.

Key words

epidermis　表皮

skin barrier function　表皮屏障功能

keratinocyte　角质形成细胞

horny layer　角质层

granular layer　颗粒层

prickle cell layer　棘层

basal layer　基底层

melanocyte　黑素细胞

Review questions

1. Please describe the process of keratinocyte maturation.
2. Please illustrate the three phases of hair development.

(Bingxue Bai)

Chapter 4   Biochemistry of the skin

The important molecules synthesized by the skin include keratin, melanin, collagen and glycosaminoglycans.

Keratins

Keratins are high-molecular-weight polypeptide chains produced by keratinocytes (Fig. 4-1). They

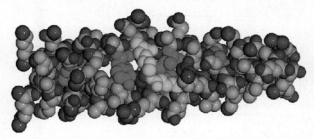

Fig. 4-1 **Molecular structure of alpha-keratin.** The molecule forms a helical coil which, if stretched, unwinds irreversibly to produce the beta form. The covalent bonds linking the cystine molecules provide extra strength. From *J Invest Dermatol* 2001: 116; 964-969, with permission of Blackwell Publishing.

are the major constituent of the stratum corneum, hair and nails. The stratum corneum comprises 65% keratin (along with 10% soluble protein, 10% amino acid, 10% lipid and 5% cell membrane).

Keratin proteins are of varying molecular weight (between 40 and 67kDa). Different keratins are found at each level of the epidermis, depending on the stage of differentiation. Epidermal keratin contains less cystine and more glycine than the harder hair keratin.

Melanins

Melanin is produced from tyrosine (Fig. 4-2) in melanocytes and takes two forms:
- *eumelanin*, which is more common and gives a brown-black colour.
- *phaeomelanin*, which is less common and produces a yellow or red colour.

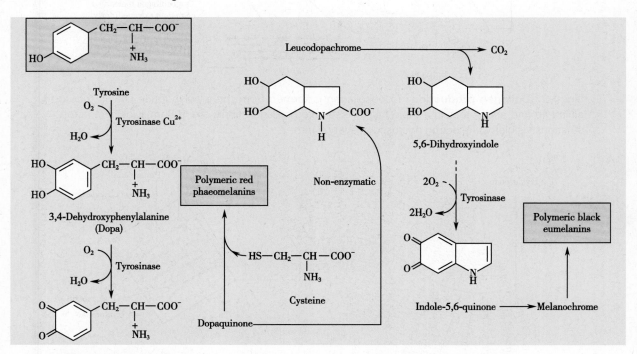

Fig. 4-2 **Biosynthesis of melanin.** Eumelanin is a high-molecular-weight polymer of complex structure formed by oxidative polymerization. The phaeomelanin polymer is synthesized from dopaquinone and cysteine (via cysteinyl DOPA).

Most natural melanins are mixtures of eumelanin and phaeomelanin. Melanins act as an energy sink and as free radical scavengers, and absorb the energy of ultraviolet (UV) radiation.

Collagens

Collagens are synthesized by fibroblasts (Fig. 4-3) and are the major structural proteins of the dermis, forming 70%~80% of its dry weight. The main amino acids in collagens are glycine, proline and hydroxyproline. Collagens are broken down, e.g. in wound healing, by collagenases, of which the matrix metalloproteinases are important. There are over 22 types of collagen; at least five are found in skin:

- type I - found in the reticular dermis
- type III - found in the papillary dermis
- types IV and VII - found in the basement membrane structures
- type VIII - found in endothelial cells.

Glycosaminoglycans (GAGs)

The 'ground substance' of skin is largely made up of GAGs, providing viscosity and hydration. In the dermis, chondroitin sulphate is the main GAG, along with dermatan sulphate and hyaluronan.

GAGs often exist as high-molecular-weight polymers with a protein core. These structures are known as *proteoglycans* (Fig. 4-4).

Skin surface secretions

The skin surface has a slightly acidic pH (between 6 and 7). Sebum (Table 4-1), sweat and the horny layer (including intercellular lipid) contribute to the sur-

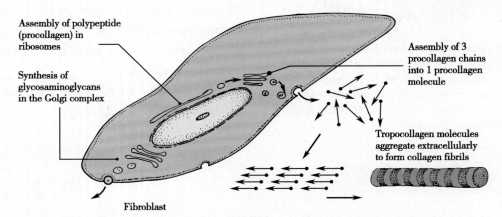

Fig. 4-3 **Collagen production.** Tropocollagen is formed from three polypeptide chains that are coiled around each other in a triple helix. Assembled collagen fibrils are 100nm wide, with cross-striations visible with electron microscopy every 64nm.

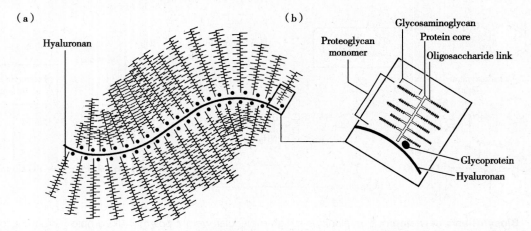

Fig. 4-4 **Proteoglycan. (a)** Proteoglycan aggregate with central filament of hyaluronan. **(b)** Detailed view of proteoglycan monomer with protein core.

face conditions, which generally discourage microbial proliferation.

Table 4-1 Sebum and epidermal lipid composition

Component	Sebum (%)	Epidermal lipid (%)
Glyceride/free fatty acid	58	65
Wax esters	26	0
Squalene	12	0
Cholesterol esters	3	15
Cholesterol	1	20

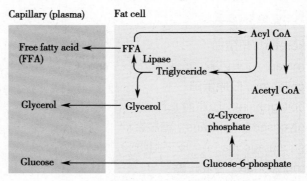

Fig. 4-5 Metabolism of subcutaneous fat.

Subcutaneous fat

Triglyceride is synthesized from α-glycerophosphate and acyl coenzyme A (CoA). Triglyceride is broken down by lipase to give free fatty acid (FFA) - an energy source - and glycerol (Fig. 4-5).

Hormones and the skin

The skin is the site of production of one hormone (vitamin D), but it is often a target organ for other hormones and is frequently affected in endocrine diseases (Table 4-2).

Table 4-2 Hormones and the skin

Hormone	Site of production	Effects
Vitamin D	Produced in the dermis from precursors though the action of UV radiation	Important for the absorption of calcium and for calcification
Corticosteroids	Adrenal cortex	Receptors on several cells in both epidermis and dermis Produce vasoconstriction Reduce mitosis by basal cells Generate anti-inflammatory effects on leucocytes Inhibit phospholipase A
Androgens	Adrenal cortex Gonads	Receptors on hair follicles and sebaceous glands Stimulate terminal hair growth and increased output of sebum
Melanocyte-stimulating hormone (MSH) Adrenocorticotrophic hormone (ACTH)	Pituitary gland	Stimulates melanogenesis
Oestrogens	Adrenal cortex Ovaries	Stimulate melanogenesis
Epidermal growth factor (EGF)	Skin (probably produced at several sites in, as well as outside, the skin)	Receptors found on keratinocytes, hair follicles, sebaceous glands and sweat duct cells Stimulates differentiation Alters calcium metabolism
Cytokines and eicosanoids	Cell membrane (may be produced by several skin cells, including keratinocytes and lymphocytes)	Effects on immune function, inflammation and cell proliferation

Key words

keratin　角蛋白

melanin　黑色素

collagen　胶原蛋白

collagenase　胶原酶

glycosaminoglycans　糖胺聚糖

subcutaneous fat　皮下脂肪

triglyceride　甘油三酯

free fatty acid　游离脂肪酸

androgen receptor　雄激素受体

Review questions

1. Please describe the main molecules synthesized by the skin.
2. Please explain why the epidermis can inhibit microbial proliferation.

(Bingxue Bai)

Chapter 5   Immunology of the skin

The immunological components of skin can be separated into structures, cells and immunogenetics.

Structures

The epidermal barrier is an important example of innate immunity, as most micro-organisms that have contact with the skin do not penetrate it. Equally, the generous blood and lymphatic supplies to the dermis are important channels through which immune cells can pass to or from their sites of action.

Cells

Professional antigen presenting cells

The Langerhans cells (epidermis) and dermal dendritic cells are the outermost sentinels of the cellular immune system (Fig. 5-1). They are dendritic, bone marrow-derived cells. Langerhans cells are characterized ultrastructurally by a unique cytoplasmic organelle known as the *Birbeck granule*. Langerhans cells are instrumental in recognizing, uptaking, processing, and presenting antigens to T lymphocytes for sensitization, and may induce (or suppress) the delayed-type sensitivity. Ultraviolet radiation plays

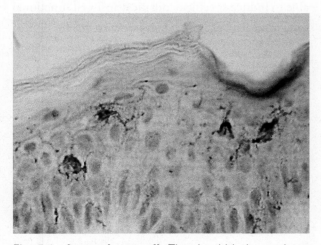

Fig. 5-1 **Langerhans cell.** The dendritic Langerhans cells form a network in the epidermis. In this section, the Langerhans cells have been stained with a monoclonal antibody to HLA-DR.

an important role in inducing photoimmunosuppression, which is mediated by effects on the skin dendritic cell population.

T lymphocytes

T cells are defined by expression of the T cell receptor (TCR), the structure of which determines the foreign antigens the T cell will recognize. Consequently, TCR specificity is closely regulated to prevent circulation of T cells strongly recognizing self-proteins. The TCR recognizes the antigen as presented by the major histocompatibility complex (MHC) and this interaction is stabilized by CD8+ (MHC class I) or CD4+ (MHC class II) molecules.

T lymphocyte circulation through normal skin for immunosurveillance is regulated by lymphocyte surface molecules that promote 'skin homing', including cutaneous leucocyte antigen (CLA), CCR4, CCR6 and CCR10. Epithelial danger signals induced by infection and inflammation increase cutaneous and endothelial expression of skin homing receptor ligands thereby enhancing the influx of lymphocytes into the cutaneous compartment.

Different types of T cell with differing functions are recognized in the skin, for example:

- CD4+ function is classified by cytokine production (Fig. 5-2), which also determines how they regulate class-switching of B cells to IgG (Th1) or IgE (Th2) production. Th cells also promote the function of Tc cells.
- CD8+ cells are capable of cytokine production (Tc1 and Tc2, etc.) and target cell killing mediated by granzyme B and perforin production as well as Fas/FasL signaling. The differentiation of Tc cells is based on the patterns of cytokine secretion.
- NKT (CD4+ or CD8+ or double or nil expressing) cells express a T cell receptor and NK cell surface markers. NKT cells are capable of high levels of

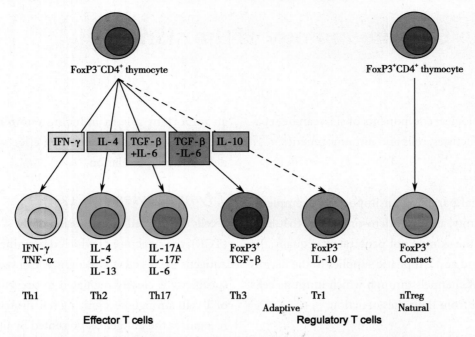

Fig. 5-2 **CD4⁺ T cell subsets.** The cytokine/function polarization of CD4⁺ T cells, which was until recently limited to the Th1/Th2 paradigm, has been expanded. Cytokines that are critical to lineage development are indicated in the arrow boxes. Below the cells are the effector or regulatory cytokine repertoires of each cell type (nTreg are contact dependent) and their abbreviated names.

cytokine production. NKT cells are supposed to have characteristics of both T cells and NK cells. It is also believed that NKT cells are involved in T-cell differentiation, autoimmunity control, and UV-induced downregulation of tumor immune responses.

Mast cells

Mast cells are principally known for their ability to degranulate and release histamine and other vasoactive molecules. This is very rapid because the granules are preformed. Degranulation arises in response to cross-linking of the high-affinity IgE receptor. Cross-linking arises when IgE molecules on the surface of the receptors bind the same protein antigen. Mast cells also synthesize a wide range of cytokines, and experimental models support the concept that mast cells play an important role in skin immune responses. Mast cells are normal residents of the dermis, and their circulating counterparts are basophils. Mast cell numbers increase during inflammatory reactions.

Keratinocytes

Keratinocytes synthesize antimicrobial peptides, produce proinflammatory cytokines (especially IL-1) and express immune reactive molecules such as major histocompatibility complex (MHC) class I and II molecules on their surface. They signal to cutaneous dendritic cells and have been shown to be able to induce specific dendritic cell: T cell functional outcomes. For example, keratinocyte production of thymic stromal lymphopoietin (TSLP) induces dendritic cells to drive T cells towards an inflammatory Th2 phenotype.

Eosinophils

Eosinophils are richly packed with potent mediators of inflammation and cytokines important in regulation of Th2-type immune responses.

Complement

Activation of the complement cascade down either the classical or the alternative pathways results in molecules that have powerful effects. These include opsonization, lysis, mast cell degranulation, smooth muscle contraction and chemotaxis for neutrophils and macrophages.

Immunogenetics

The tissue-type antigens of an individual are found in the MHC, located in humans on the human leucocyte antigen (HLA) gene cluster on chromosome 6. The classical HLA genes are HLA-A, B and C (MHC class I) and DP, DQ and DR (MHC class II). The MHC class I complexes (CD8$^+$ restricted) are ubiquitously expressed but MHC class II (CD4$^+$ restricted) is confined to professional antigen presenting cells (including B lymphocytes, Langerhans cells, dermal dendritic cells and macrophages). During inflammation, other cell types such as endothelial cells and keratinocytes can express MHC class II. There are specific HLA genes associated with an increased likelihood of certain diseases, some of which are 'autoimmune' in nature (Table 5-1).

Table 5-1	**Skin disease associations of HLA antigens**	
Disease	**HLA antigen**	**Relative risk**
Behçet's disease	B5	10
Dermatitis herpetiformis	B8 DRw3	15>15
Pemphigus	DRw4	10
Psoriasis	B13 Dw7 Cw6	4 10 12
Psoriatic arthropathy	B27	10
	Bw38	9
Reiter's disease	B27	35

Hypersensitivity reactions and the skin

Hypersensitivity is the term applied when an adaptive immune response is inappropriate or exaggerated to the degree that tissue damage results. The skin can exhibit all the main types of hypersensitivity response.

Type I (immediate)

Allergen-specific immunoglobulin (Ig) E bound to the surface of mast cells causes degranulation on antigen exposure (as discussed above). The result in the skin is urticaria, although massive histamine release can cause anaphylaxis. The response occurs within minutes, although a delayed component is recognized. Factors other than IgE can cause mast cell degranulation.

Type II (antibody-dependent cytotoxicity)

IgG antibodies directed against an antigen on target skin cells or structures induce cytotoxicity by killer T cells or by complement activation. For example, IgG pemphigus antibodies directed against desmoglein on the keratinocyte surface result in activation of complement, attraction of effector cells and lysis of the keratinocytes. Intraepidermal blisters result.

Type III (immune complex disease)

Immune complexes formed by the combination of antigen and IgG or IgM antibodies in the blood are deposited in the walls of small vessels, often those of the skin. Complement activation, platelet aggregation and the release of lysosomal enzymes from polymorphs cause vascular damage. This *leucocytoclastic vasculitis* is seen, for example, with systemic lupus erythematosus and dermatomyositis, but also occurs with microbial infections such as infective endocarditis.

Type IV (cell mediated or delayed)

Lymphocytes sensitized by cutaneous dendritic cells in the draining lymph node proliferate and undertake immunosurveillance of the tissues. On re-encounter with their cognate antigen-MHC complex, they become activated and induce inflammation and/or cell killing. From antigen exposure to sensitization takes 7~14 days. However, long-lived memory cells are able to undertake rapid expansion at a subsequent exposure and provide lasting immunity. Allergic contact dermatitis and the tuberculin reaction to intradermally administered antigen are both forms of type IV reaction. The responses to skin infections such as leprosy or tuberculosis are granulomatous variants of the reaction.

Immunology

■ Skin provides a physical barrier to infection and possesses antimicrobial peptides.

■ Dendritic cells in the skin, including epidermal Langerhans cells, form outposts of the cellular immune system and can present antigens to immunocompetent cells, e.g. T lymphocytes.

■ T cells circulate through normal skin and form part of the skin-associated lymphoid tissue. They are localized by adhesion molecules.

■ Keratinocytes can be immunologically active cells.

■ All four types of hypersensitivity reaction occur in the skin.

■ Genetic factors modulate immunological responses. Certain HLA antigens are associated with increased risk of skin disease, e.g. HLA-DRw4 with pemphigus.

Summary

The epidermal barrier is an important example of innate immunity, protecting skin from infection and injuries. The Langerhans cells, T lymphocytes, mast cells, eosinophils, and keratinocytes are main immune cells responsible for hypersensitivity reactions in the skin.

Key words

epidermal barrier   皮肤屏障

antigen presenting cell   抗原呈递细胞

Birbeck granule   伯贝克颗粒

major histocompatibility complex (MHC)   主要组织相容性复合体

human leucocyte antigen (HLA)   人类白细胞抗原

cytokine   细胞因子

hypersensitivity / hypersensitivity reactions   超敏反应

anaphylaxis   过敏反应

Review questions

1. What are the major components and their functions of skin immune system?

2. What else do you know about the components of skin immune system that haven't been described above?

3. How much do you know about the cytokines involved in skin immune system?

(Yumin Xia)

Chapter 6   Molecular genetics and the skin

Recent and rapid advances in genetics have had an impact on our understanding of skin diseases. The Human Genome Project has now mapped all human genes, of which there are about 35 000. Genetics has been found to be more complicated than the original Mendelian concept, and common conditions such as atopy occur as a result of a complex interaction between multiple susceptibility genes and the environment. An average pregnancy carries a 1% risk of a single gene disease and a 0.5% risk of a chromosome disorder, but genetically influenced traits, e.g. atopy, are much more common.

The human chromosomes

The human genome comprises 23 pairs of chromosomes that are numbered by size (Fig. 6-1). Chromosomes are packets of genes with support proteins in a large complex. The karyotype is an individual's number of chromosomes plus their sex chromosome constitution, i.e. 46XX for females and 46XY for males. The phenotype is the expression at a biological level of the genotype, e.g. blue eyes or atopy.

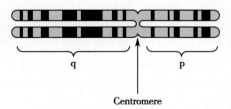

q   p

Centromere

Fig. 6-1   **Chromosome 2.** Divided by the centromere into the shorter (p) and the longer (q) arms, showing banding with the Giemsa stain.

Genes and DNA

Common variations in DNA sequence found in a population are called genetic polymorphisms and are inherited and not maintained by recurrent mutation. These polymorphisms may be functional (affect biological processes) or nonfunctional ('silent'). A new change or inherited alteration in DNA sequence that causes pathology (disease) is a mutation. Investigation of genetic causation of disease can be undertaken from a population/phenotype level down (genome screen - statistical association of gene sequence alterations in disease versus control group) or gene level up (candidate gene analysis - sequencing genes of interest in families or populations with disease versus control populations).

Molecular methods

DNA sequence variations can be identified by the consequent change in polymerase chain reaction (PCR) amplification product size (Fig.6-2), loss or gain of restriction endonuclease cutting, or sequence analysis. In recent years, DNA sequencing has become a high-throughput technology that has led to the concept of 'whole genome sequencing' studies of healthy versus controls. As this technique is so powerful, smaller numbers are required.

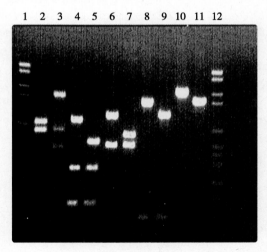

Fig. 6-2   **Agarose gel electrophoresis, showing migration of DNA after cutting with enzymes, screening for mutations in a keratin gene.**

To establish which molecular pathways may be important in disease pathogenesis, gene chip arrays and 'next generation sequencing' allow detailed and quantitative analysis of the transcribed genes in a diseased tissue (transcriptome). The transcribed genes are subject to further regulation by RNA degradation, silencing and inhibition. Thus, study of the protein repertoire in the diseased tissue (proteomics) may also be undertaken.

Molecular techniques can be used to:

- detect small amounts of DNA, e.g. of human papilloma virus within a skin cancer
- sequence DNA from a 'candidate' section of an individual's chromosome and compare the base sequences with family members similarly affected by a disorder, thus mapping a specific gene polymorphism characteristic for that disease (Table 6-1)
- sequence the entire genome of an individual

Table 6-1 **Skin conditions or characteristics with definite or probable gene localities on the chromosomes**	
Chromosome site	**Disease or characteristic**
1p34	Porphyria cutanea tarda: enzyme
2q31	Ehlers-Danlos syndrome: collagen III
3p21.3	Dystrophic epidermolysis bullosa: collagen VII
4, 4p	Red hair colour, psoriasis (Psors3 gene)
6p21.3	Psoriasis (Psors1 gene: 30% of susceptibility)
9p21	Familial malignant melanoma: kinase inhibitor
9q22.3	Xeroderma pigmentosum
9q34	Tuberous sclerosis: hamartin 11q12 Atopy: asthma and rhinitis: IgE response
12q13	Epidermolysis bullosa simplex: keratin 5
12q23	Darier's disease: adenosine triphosphatase
14q11.2	Ichthyosis: transglutaminase
15q11.2	Oculocutaneous albinism: homologue
17q11.2, 17q25	Neurofibromatosis NF1, psoriasis (Psors2)
17q21.31	Ehlers-Danlos syndrome: collagen I
19	Green/blue eye colour, brown hair colour
21 trisomy	Down syndrome
Xq28	Incontinentia pigmenti: nuclear factor (NF)-κB modulator
Xq22.32	X-linked ichthyosis: steroid sulphatase

- identify the repertoire of genes that have been transcribed as a measure of the protein profile of the cell.

Forms of inheritance

An individual with two different genes (alleles) at a particular locus is heterozygous, and one who has identical alleles is homozygous. Genes borne on chromosomes other than X and Y are autosomal, whereas those on X and Y are sex linked. Factors governing genetic penetrance are unclear.

- *Dominant.* Affected individuals (both sexes) are heterozygous for the gene, will have an affected parent (except for new mutations) and have a 50% chance of passing it to their children (Fig. 6-3).

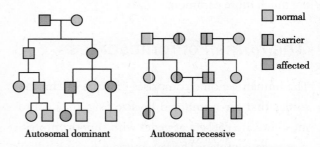

Autosomal dominant　　　Autosomal recessive

☐ normal
⊟ carrier
■ affected

Fig. 6-3 **Autosomal dominant and recessive patterns of inheritance.**

- *Recessive.* An affected individual (of either sex) is homozygous for the gene, and both parents will be carriers and healthy. Consanguinity increases the risk. Recessive disorders are often severe. There is a 25% chance of heterozygotes passing the gene to the next generation.
- *X-linked recessive.* Only affects males, as females are healthy carriers.
- *X-linked dominant.* Affects males and females, although some disorders, e.g. incontinentia pigmenti, are lethal in males.
- *Mosaicism.* In mosaicism, an individual has two or more genetically different cell lines. The somatic (postconceptional) mutation of a single cell in an embryo results in a clone of subtly distinct cells. In the skin, this is revealed by the developmental growth pattern of Blaschko's lines (Fig. 6-4). Certain dermatoses, e.g. naevi and

incontinentia pigmenti (Fig. 6-5), follow these lines, resulting in streaky or whorled patterns where the abnormal clone meets normal cells. A dermatomal distribution (Fig. 6-6) suggests nerve involvement.

■ *Imprinting.* Imprinting involves the differential switching off of genes according to whether they have come from the father or the mother. It may be caused by methylation of DNA.

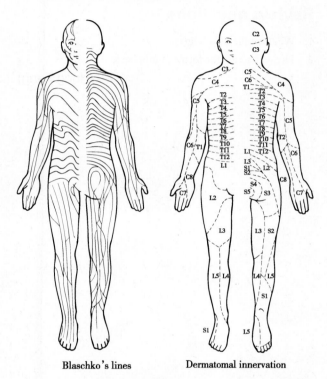

Blaschko's lines   Dermatomal innervation

Fig. 6-4   Blaschko's lines represent the growth trends of embryonic tissue, whereas the dermatomes map out areas of skin innervation.

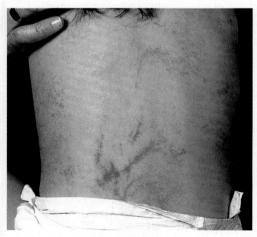

Fig. 6-5   Incontinentia pigmenti. Streaks and whorls follow the lines of Blaschko.

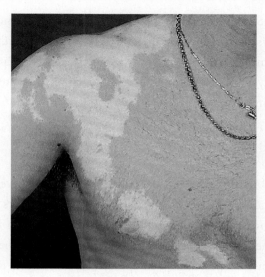

Fig. 6-6   Segmental vitiligo. Rather than follow Blaschko's lines, this occurs in a dermatomal distribution, suggesting a relationship with skin innervation.

Inheritance of specific skin disorders

In psoriasis and atopic eczema, a family history is common, but the exact mode of inheritance is unclear. Psoriasis may be inherited polygenically or by an autosomal dominant gene with incomplete penetrance. Atopic eczema has recently been shown to be strongly associated with chromosome 1q21 mutations in the gene encoding the epidermal protein, filaggrin. Inheritance patterns in the rarer conditions are often clearer (Table 6-2). Epidermolysis bullosa simplex and dystrophica, the porphyrias, the Ehlers-Danlos syndromes and some other conditions may be dominantly or recessively inherited.

Table 6-2	The inheritance of selected skin disorders
Inheritance	**Disorder**
Autosomal dominant	Darier's disease Dysplastic naevus syndrome Ichthyosis vulgaris Neurofibromatosis NF1 Palmoplantar keratoderma Peutz-Jeghers syndrome Tuberous sclerosis
Autosomal recessive	Acrodermatitis enteropathica Non-bullous ichthyosiform Erythroderma Phenylketonuria Pseudoxanthoma elasticum Xeroderma pigmentosum
X-linked recessive	X-linked ichthyosis
X-linked	Incontinentia pigmenti

Some dermatoses are associated with polymorphisms in the human leucocyte antigen (HLA) complex on chromosome 6. These tend to show polygenic inheritance and an association with auto-immunity.

Gene therapy

DNA-based prenatal diagnosis is possible in several genodermatoses. Although recessive disorders in which there is a single gene defect offer scope for genetic treatment and gene therapy, which has been shown to be possible in epidermolysis bullosa, this remains a highly complicated and expensive process with potentially severe complications including haematological malignancy.

Molecular genetics and the skin

- The human genome of 23 chromosomes (karyotype 46XY or 46XX) contains 35 000 genes, all of which have been mapped. Additionally, mitochondria encode 37 genes for oxidative enzymes.
- DNA segments can be amplified by PCR and demonstrated by gel electrophoresis.
- Whole genome sequencing and microarray technology have advanced the molecular approach to studying disease pathogenesis.
- Dominant, recessive and X-linked inheritances are seen, but heredity is still unclear in several disorders.
- A dermatosis caused by mosaicism, due to a mutation producing more than one cell line, may appear in Blaschko's lines.
- Gene therapy should be possible for some recessive single gene disorders.

Key words

dominant　显性
recessive　隐性
X-linked recessive　X-联锁隐性
X-linked dominant　X-联锁显性
mosaicism　镶嵌现象
Blaschko's lines　Blaschko 线
imprinting　印记

Review questions

1. What are Blaschko's lines?
2. Please describe the forms of inherence.

(Hong Fang)

Chapter 7   Terminology of skin lesions

Dermatology has a vocabulary that is quite distinct from that of other medical specialties and without which it is impossible to describe skin disorders. A *lesion* is a general term for an area of disease, usually small. An *eruption* (or *rash*) is a more widespread skin involvement, normally composed of several lesions, which may be the primary lesion (e.g. papules, vesicles or pustules) or secondary lesion (e.g. scales or crusts). Secondary lesion is due to secondary factors such as scratching or infection. Below is a selection of other commonly encountered dermatological terms.

Macule

A macule is a localized area of colour or textural change in the skin. Macules can be hypopigmented, as in vitiligo; pigmented, as in a freckle (Fig. 7-1a); erythematous, as in a capillary haemangioma (Fig. 7-1b).

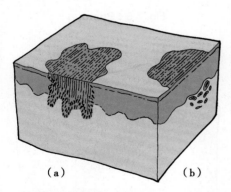

Fig. 7-1   **Macule. (a)** Pigmented macule in a freckle. **(b)** Erythematous macule in a capillary haemangioma.

Papule

A papule is a small solid elevation of the skin, generally defined as less than 10mm in diameter. Papules may be flat topped, as in lichen planus; dome shaped, as in xanthomas; or spicular if related to hair follicles (Fig. 7-2).

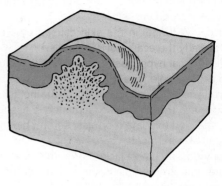

Fig. 7-2   **Papule.**

Nodule

Similar to a papule but larger (i.e. greater than 10mm in diameter), nodules can involve any layer of the skin and can be oedematous or solid. Examples include a dermatofibroma (Fig. 7-3) and secondary deposits.

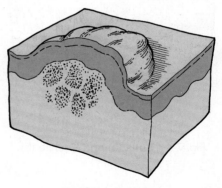

Fig. 7-3   **Nodule.**

Bulla

A bulla is similar to a vesicle but larger: greater than 10mm in diameter. The blisters of bullous pemphigoid (Fig. 7-4a) and pemphigus vulgaris are examples.

Vesicle

A vesicle is a small blister (less than 10mm in diameter) consisting of clear fluid accumulated within or

Glossary of other dermatological terms

- **Abscess:** A localized collection of pus formed by necrosis of tissue.
- **Alopecia:** Absence of hair from a normally hairy area.
- **Atrophy:** Loss of epidermis, dermis or both. Atrophic skin is thin, translucent and wrinkled with easily visible blood vessels.
- **Burrow:** A tunnel in the skin caused by a parasite, particularly the acarus of scabies.
- **Callus:** Local hyperplasia of the horny layer, often of the palm or sole, due to pressure.
- **Carbuncle:** A collection of boils (furuncles) causing necrosis in the skin and subcutaneous tissues.
- **Crust:** Dried exudate (normally serum, blood or pus) on the skin surface.
- **Ecchymosis:** A macular red or purple haemorrhage, more than 2mm in diameter, in the skin or mucous membrane.
- **Erosion:** A superficial break in the epidermis, not extending into the dermis, which heals without scarring.
- **Erythema:** Redness of the skin due to vascular dilatation.
- **Excoriation:** A superficial abrasion, often linear, which results from scratching.
- **Fissure:** A linear split in the epidermis, often just extending into the dermis.
- **Cellulitis:** A purulent inflammation of the skin and subcutaneous tissue.
- **Folliculitis:** An inflammation of the hair follicles.
- **Comedo:** A plug of sebum and keratin in the dilated orifice of a pilosebaceous gland.
- **Freckle:** A macular area in which there is increased pigment formation by melanocytes.

below the epidermis. Vesicles may be grouped as in dermatitis herpetiformis (subepidermal). Intraepidermal vesicles are shown in the figure (Fig. 7-4b).

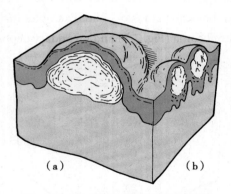

(a)   (b)

Fig. 7-4   **Bulla (a) and Vesicle (b).**

Fig. 7-5   **Pustule.**

Pustule

A pustule is a visible collection of free pus in a blister. Pustules may indicate infection (e.g. a furuncle), but not always, as pustules seen in psoriasis, for example, are not infected (Fig. 7-5).

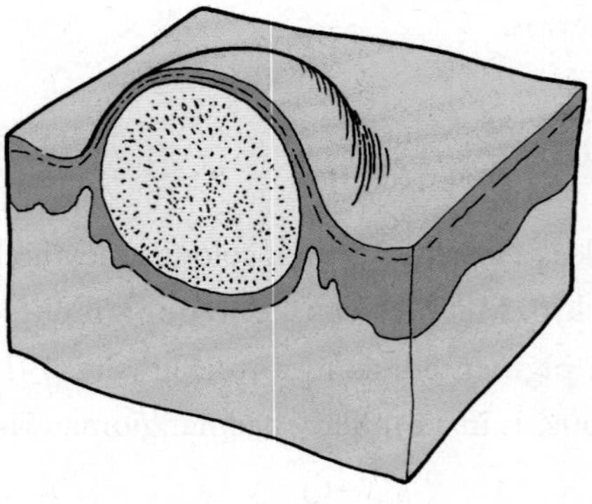

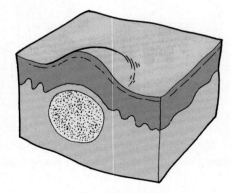

Fig. 7-6   **Cyst.**

Cyst

A cyst is a nodule consisting of an epithelial-lined cavity filled with fluid or semisolid material. An epidermal ('sebaceous') cyst is shown below (Fig. 7-6).

Wheal

A wheal is a transitory, compressible papule or plaque of dermal oedema, red or white in colour and usually signifying urticaria (Fig. 7-7).

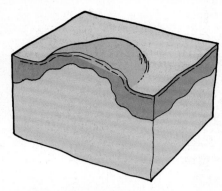

Fig. 7-7   **Wheal.**

Scale

A scale is an accumulation of thickened, horny layer keratin in the form of readily detached fragments. Scales usually indicate inflammatory change and thickening of the epidermis. They may be fine, as in 'pityriasis'; white and silvery, as in psoriasis (below); or large and fish-like, as seen in ichthyosis (Fig. 7-9).

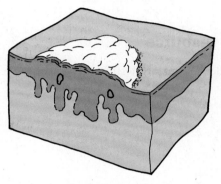

Fig. 7-9   **Scale.**

Plaque

A plaque is a palpable, plateau-like elevation of skin, usually more than 2cm in diameter. Plaques are rarely more than 5mm in height and can be considered as extended papules. Certain lesions of psoriasis (below) and mycosis fungoides are good examples (Fig. 7-8).

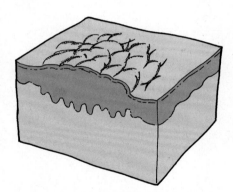

Fig. 7-8   **Plaque.**

Ulcer

An ulcer is a circumscribed area of skin loss extending through the epidermis into the dermis. Ulcers are usually the result of impairment of the vascular or nutrient supply to the skin, e.g. as a result of peripheral arterial disease (Fig. 7-10).

Glossary of other dermatological terms

- Furuncle: A pyogenic infection localized in a hair follicle.
- Hirsuties: Excessive male pattern hair growth.
- Hypertrichosis: Excessive hair growth in a non-androgenic pattern.
- Keloid: An elevated and progressive scar not showing regression.
- Keratosis: A horn-like thickening of the skin.
- Lichenification: Chronic thickening of the skin with increased skin markings, as a result of rubbing or scratching.
- Milium: A small white cyst containing keratin.
- Papilloma: A nipple-like projection from the skin surface.
- Petechia: A haemorrhagic punctuate spot measuring 1~2mm in diameter.
- Poikiloderma: A combination of hyperpigmentation, telangiectasia and atrophy seen together in a dermatosis.
- Purpura: Extravasation of blood resulting in red discoloration of the skin or mucous membranes.
- Scar: The replacement of normal tissue by fibrous connective tissue at the site of an injury.
- Stria: An atrophic linear band in the skin - white, pink or purple in colour. The result of connective tissue changes.
- Telangiectasia: Dilated dermal blood vessels giving rise to a visible lesion.

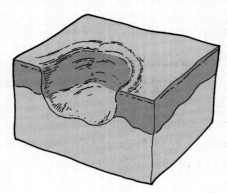

Fig. 7-10 **Ulcer.**

papule　丘疹
nodule　结节
bulla　大疱
vesicle　水疱
pustule　脓疱
cyst　囊肿
wheal　风团
plaque　斑块
scale　鳞屑
ulcer　溃疡
lichenification　苔藓样变

Web resource

http://dermnetnz.org/terminology.html

Key words

macule　斑疹

Review questions

1. What are the primary and secondary skin lesions?
2. What is the difference between erosion and ulcer?

(Hongzhong Jin)

Chapter 8   Taking a history

The truism that 'there is no substitute for a good history' is just as applicable in dermatology as in any other branch of medicine. The time needed to take a history depends on the complaint. For example, the history in a patient with hand warts can usually be completed quickly, but more time and detailed questioning are required for the patient with generalized itching.

History taking in dermatology can be divided into five basic investigations: the presenting complaint, past medical history, social and occupational history, family history, and drug history.

Presenting complaint

Chief complaint is the patient's reason for coming to the clinic including symptoms or signs and their duration. Before any diagnosis, it is essential to find out when, where and how the problem started, what the initial lesions looked like and how they evolved and extended. Symptoms, particularly itching, the prime dermatological complaint, must be recorded along with any aggravating or exacerbating factors, such as sunlight. It is useful to gauge the effect of the eruption on the patient's ability to perform everyday tasks. For chronic conditions, it is helpful to assess the effect on the patient's quality of life and mental wellbeing. Specific scoring systems can record these effects, e.g. the Dermatology Life Quality Index (DLQI). In brief, history of present illness should be well characterized with descriptions of: predisposing factors; the initial lesions and their development; timing including onset, duration and frequency; setting in which it occurs; factors that have aggravated or relieved the symptoms; associated manifestations such as fever; treatments attempted. To pay attention, presenting complaint should be written in chronological order.

> ### Case history 1
>
> An 18-year-old male bank clerk developed a scaly erythematous plaque on the left elbow (Fig. 8-1) 6 months before presentation. It spread to involve the other elbow and both knees, but was not itchy. He developed scaliness in the scalp and nail dystrophy. His mother once had a similar rash.
> Diagnosis: psoriasis.

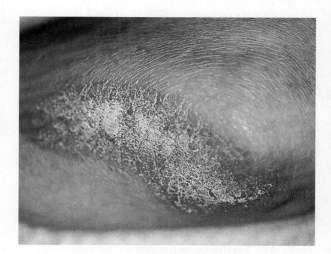

Fig. 8-1   **Psoriatic plaque on elbow.**

Past medical history

Patients must be asked about any previous skin disease or atopic symptoms, such as hay fever, asthma or childhood eczema. Internal medical disorders may be relevant; these can involve the skin directly or may be associated with certain skin diseases. For example, patients with generalized itching may have diabetes or malignant tumor. Prescribed or self-administered drugs may also cause an eruption. Medications should be noted, including name, dose, route and frequency of use. Ask patients about their allergies (food, drugs and environmental factors) including specific reactions to each identified. Dietary history is occasionally important, e.g. in some patients with atopic eczema, but diet is often erroneously blamed for skin disease.

Case history 2

A 29-year-old woman was referred from the depart-ment of respiratory medicine where she had recently been diagnosed as having pulmonary sarcoidosis. Three weeks previously, she had developed tender, warm erythematous nodules (Fig. 8-2) on the shins. She was on no medication. An incisional biopsy con-firmed the clinical impression.
  Diagnosis: erythema nodosum.

being considered), as well as other factors. Living or travelling in warm climates potentially exposes an individual to a wide range of tropical and subtropical infections, and to strong sunlight.

Case history 3

A 45-year-old male printer engineer gave a 6-month history of hand dermatitis (Fig. 8-3). A few months previously, he had started to use the solvent trichlo-roethylene in his job. Patch testing was negative. On substituting a different solvent, the eruption cleared.
  Diagnosis: irritant contact dermatitis.

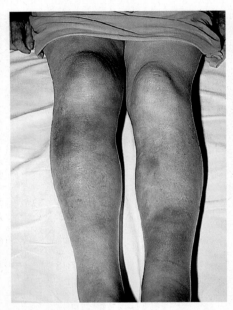

Fig. 8-2 **Erythema nodosum on the lower legs.**

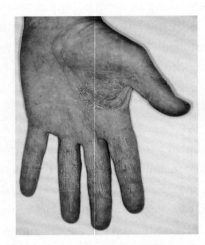

Fig. 8-3 **Irritant contact dermatitis on the palm of the hand.**

Social and occupational history

Many social factors can cause, influence or be influ-enced by a patient's skin complaint. Occupational factors can induce contact dermatitis or other skin changes, and it is often necessary to ask the patient to explain exactly his present and previous occupations. If the eruption improves when the patient is away from work, occupational factors should be suspected. Hobbies may also involve contact with objects or chemicals that could produce contact dermatitis.

Knowledge of the patient's living conditions and home background can be helpful in understanding a problem and deciding on treatment. For example, children with tinea capitis are sometimes keeping pets at home. Alcohol intake should be noted (espe-cially if the use of potentially hepatotoxic drugs is

Family history

A full family history is essential. Outlines age, health and cause of death of siblings, parents, and grand-parents and whether they have similar lesions, symp-toms or diseases. Some disorders with prominent skin signs are genetically inherited, e.g. tuberous sclerosis. Others, such as psoriasis or atopic eczema, have a strong hereditary component. In addition to genetic syndromes, a family history may reveal that other family members have had a recent onset of an eruption similar to that of the patient, suggesting an infection or infestation such as condyloma acu-minate or scabies. It is sometimes also necessary to enquire about sexual contacts.

Case history 4

An 18-year-old male student gave a 3-month history of an intensely itchy papular eruption affecting the hands, wrists and penis (Table 8-1). Several lesions were excoriated (Fig. 8-4). Treatment with a potent topical steroid was of little benefit. His girlfriend had also recently developed itchy lesions. Close examination showed burrows in the skin.

　Diagnosis: scabies.

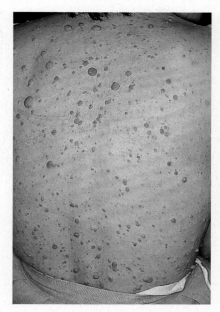

Fig. 8-5 **Multiple neurofibromas on the back.**

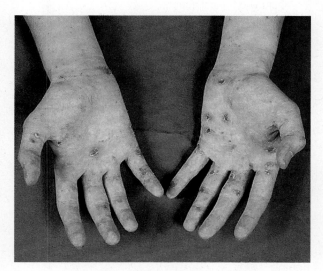

Fig. 8-4 **Excoriated lesions of scabies.**

Table 8-1	**Itchy eruption: diagnosis**
Symptom	**Intensely itchy eruption**
Possible diagnosis	Scabies
	Lichen planus
	Dermatitis herpetiformis
	Urticaria
	Eczema
	Insect bites

Case history 5

A 25-year-old female shop assistant complained of brownish macules over her back (Fig. 8-5) and chest, which had first appeared in childhood and had gradually increased in number and size. During her teens, she had developed several soft pinkish, painless nodules on the trunk, some of which had become pedunculated. Her father had developed a few similar nodules in later life, and one of her two brothers had brown patches on his skin.

　Diagnosis: von Recklinghausen's neurofibromatosis (NF-1).

Drug history

Both prescribed and self-administered medicaments can result in a 'drug eruption'. Almost all patients try an over-the-counter topical preparation (or a friend or relative's ointment) on rashes, and many have had a variety of treatments prescribed that may be inappropriate or may cause irritant or allergic reactions. It is important to quiz the patient about all medicament use in different delivery routes not just oral drugs, including the use of over-the-counter tablets or creams or eye drops that the patient may well not think relevant, home remedies and alternative medical practices, traditional Chinese medicines, vitamins, minerals, contraceptives. Cosmetics, cleansing wipes and moisturizing creams can cause dermatitis, and it is often necessary to ask specifically about their use.

Case history 6

A 68-year-old woman had a minor irritating eruption on her forehead. She applied an antihistamine-containing cream that she bought in a pharmacy. Within 24 hours of applying it, her face became severely swollen (Fig. 8-6). Patch testing carried out later showed an allergic reaction to the cream.

　Diagnosis: medicament dermatitis.

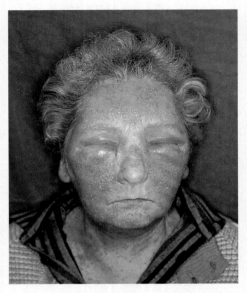

Fig. 8-6   **Acute allergic contact dermatitis to a topical antihistamine cream.**

Case history 7

An 18-year-old female secretary was given griseofulvin for a fungal infection. She went sunbathing and, 12 hours later, developed an eruption with a distribution in light-exposed areas (Fig. 8-7).
 Diagnosis: phototoxic drug eruption.

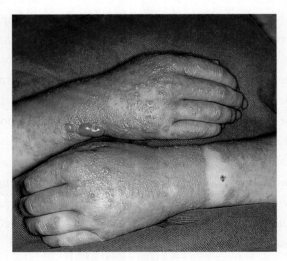

Fig. 8-7   **Acute phototoxic drug eruption.**

Taking a history
- Elicit the nature and temporal course of the eruption or lesion.
- Enquire about atopic symptoms, general medical conditions and foreign travel.
- Take a social, occupational and family history - it may be relevant. Ask about eczema or psoriasis in relatives.
- Identify any influence of the illness on day-to-day functions including work.
- Record the recent use of drugs and medications, including topical agents.
- Ask about the use of cosmetics and, in relevant cases, exposure to sun or ultraviolet radiation (e.g. sunbeds).

Key words

taking a history   病史采集
presenting complaint   现病史
chief complaint   主诉
past medical history   既往史
social and occupational history   社会和职业史
family history   家族史
drug history   用药史
Itching   瘙痒
pain   疼痛
numbness   麻木

Review questions

1. What elements should be characterized in descriptions of presenting history in dermatology?
2. Do you know some genetic disorders with prominent skin signs?
3. What is the importance of taking the patient's drug history?

(Jinhua Xu)

Chapter 9   Examining the skin

The skin needs to be examined in good, preferably natural, light. The whole of the skin should be examined, ideally; this is essential for atypical or widespread eruptions (Fig. 9-1). Looking at the whole skin often reveals diagnostic lesions that the patient is unaware of or may think unimportant. In the elderly, thorough skin examination often allows the early detection of unexpected but treatable skin cancers. Skin examination is difficult for the non-dermatologist, and the novice needs a pattern to follow. It is important to:

- note the distribution and colour of the lesions
- examine the morphology of individual lesions, their size, shape, border changes and spatial relationship; touch the skin - palpation reveals the consistency of a lesion
- assess the nails, hair and mucous membranes, sometimes in combination with a general examination (e.g. for lymphadenopathy)
- wear gloves when examining the mouth, genitals and perineum or if lesions may be infected
- use special techniques, e.g. dermoscopy, microscopy of scrapings to look for fungal elements, or the use of Wood's (ultraviolet A) light, where applicable.

Distribution of eruption or lesions

Stand back from the patient and observe the pattern of the eruption (Fig. 9-1). Determine whether it is localized (e.g. a tumour) or widespread (e.g. a rash). If the latter, determine whether the eruption is symmetrical and, if so, peripheral or central. Note whether it involves the flexures (e.g. atopic eczema) or the extensor aspects (e.g. psoriasis). Is it limited to sun-exposed areas? Is it linear?

Dermatomal patterns are also seen. Herpes zoster (shingles) is the commonest example of this, but some naevi also appear in this guise or follow Blasch-

ko's lines. Regional patterns (Fig. 9-1), e.g. involvement of the groin or axilla, will suggest certain diagnoses to the experienced physician. For example, guttate psoriasis and tinea versicolor tend to occur on the trunk, whereas lichen planus often occurs around the wrists, and contact dermatitis frequently affects the face, feet or hands. The factors resulting in these patterns are complex but include skin anatomy, e.g. blood vessels, nerves, appendages or embryonic lines, and environment, e.g. moist conditions in the axillae, chemical contacts and sun exposure.

Morphology of individual lesions

A hand lens or dermoscope is often helpful in looking at individual lesions. Palpation (often neglected by medical students) is also important to determine the consistency, depth and texture. Definitions of lesions are given in the chapter of "Terminology of skin lesions".

Lesions may be monomorphic (e.g. guttate psoriasis) or pleomorphic (e.g. chickenpox). There may also be secondary changes on top of primary lesions. The local configuration of lesions is often of diagnostic help (Table 9-1). Determine whether the lesions are grouped, linear or annular, or if they show the Koebner phenomenon, whereby lesions appear in an area of trauma which is often linear, e.g. a scratch.

Table 9-1	**Configuration of lesions**
Configuration	**Disease**
Linear	Psoriasis, lichen striatus, linear epidermal naevus, lichen planus, morphoea
Grouped	Dermatitis herpetiformis, insect bites, herpes simplex, molluscum contagiosum
Annular	Tinea corporis (ringworm), mycosis fungoides, urticaria, granuloma annulare, annular erythemas
Koebner phenomenon	Lichen planus, psoriasis, viral warts, molluscum contagiosum, sarcoidosis, vitiligo

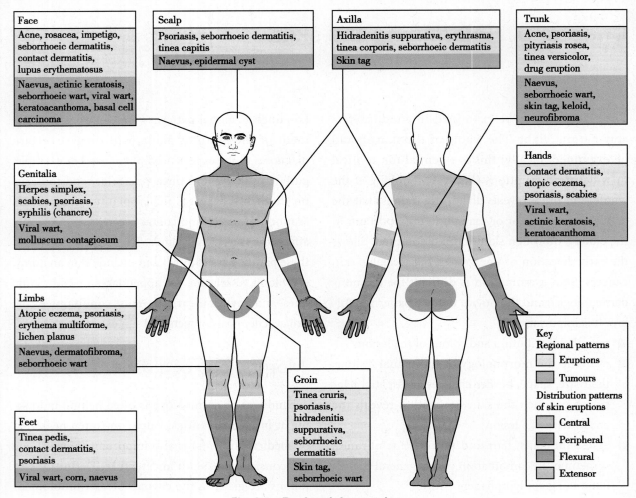

Face

Acne, rosacea, impetigo, seborrhoeic dermatitis, contact dermatitis, lupus erythematosus

Naevus, actinic keratosis, seborrhoeic wart, viral wart, keratoacanthoma, basal cell carcinoma

Scalp

Psoriasis, seborrhoeic dermatitis, tinea capitis

Naevus, epidermal cyst

Axilla

Hidradenitis suppurativa, erythrasma, tinea corporis, seborrhoeic dermatitis

Skin tag

Trunk

Acne, psoriasis, pityriasis rosea, tinea versicolor, drug eruption

Naevus, seborrhoeic wart, skin tag, keloid, neurofibroma

Genitalia

Herpes simplex, scabies, psoriasis, syphilis (chancre)

Viral wart, molluscum contagiosum

Hands

Contact dermatitis, atopic eczema, psoriasis, scabies

Viral wart, actinic keratosis, keratoacanthoma

Limbs

Atopic eczema, psoriasis, erythema multiforme, lichen planus

Naevus, dermatofibroma, seborrhoeic wart

Groin

Tinea cruris, psoriasis, hidradenitis suppurativa, seborrhoeic dermatitis

Skin tag, seborrhoeic wart

Feet

Tinea pedis, contact dermatitis, psoriasis

Viral wart, corn, naevus

Key
Regional patterns

☐ Eruptions

☐ Tumours

Distribution patterns of skin eruptions

☐ Central

☐ Peripheral

☐ Flexural

☐ Extensor

Fig. 9-1   **Regional dermatology.**

Nails, hair and mucous membranes

The nails, scalp and hair frequently show diagnostic and even pathognomonic signs. With any unusual or atypical eruption, the mucous membranes of the mouth and genitalia may show important changes, such as oral involvement by Wickham striae in lichen planus, oral lesions in Kaposi's sarcoma or vulval involvement with lichen sclerosus.

General examination

Palpation of lymph nodes is important in patients with skin malignancy. In patients with a skin lymphoma, a full examination is needed, looking particularly for lymphadenopathy and hepatospleno-megaly. Palpation of pedal pulses is vital in patients with leg ulcers.

Special techniques and assessment of disease morbidity

The diagnoses of many skin conditions can be helped by special techniques. Photography is often used to record the state of a patient's skin disease and allows comparisons at follow-up visits.

In the current management of skin diseases, it is sometimes necessary to make a quantitative evaluation of the disease and its impact on a patient's life. For example, the National Institute for Health and Clinical Excellence (NICE) states that a patient's psoriasis must be of a certain severity, according to the psoriasis area and severity index, before treatment with a biologic agent is recommended.

- Psoriasis Area and Severity Index (PASI). The PASI is a numerical score of the extent and activity of a patient's psoriasis. It is calculated by a reproducible formula based on the surface area and cutaneous features of the disease.
- Severity Scoring for Atopic Dermatitis (SCORAD). The SCORAD gives a numerical value to the severity of a patient's atopic eczema.
- Dermatology Life Quality Index (DLQI). The DLQI is a measure of the impact of a skin disease on a patient's social, work and personal activities over the preceding week.

Case history 1

An 8-year-old girl gave a 12-month history of an itchy eruption affecting the antecubital and popliteal fossae (Fig. 9-2). Her mother had had a similar rash as a child. The pattern and the morphology were characteristic.

   Diagnosis: atopic eczema.

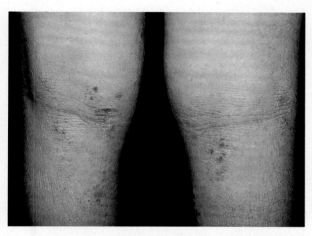

Fig. 9-2   **Atopic eczema affecting the popliteal fossae.**

Case history 2

Six weeks ago, a 25-year-old man developed a slightly itchy linear area running down the medial aspect of his left leg (Fig. 9-3). Dermatological conditions giving a linear eruption include lichen planus, morphoea, psoriasis and linear epidermal naevus.

   Diagnosis: lichen striatus, a self-limiting inflammatory dermatitis of unknown origin.

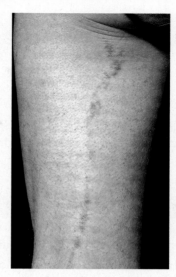

Fig. 9-3   **Lichen striatus affecting the left leg.**

Examining the skin

- Examine the entire skin surface.
- Use a hand lens and adequate illumination. Consider dermoscopy.
- Gently palpate lesions to assess texture.
- Look at the nails, hair and mucous membranes (oral and genital).
- Observe for distribution, individual lesion morphology and configuration.
- Always microscope scrapings if a fungal infection is a possibility.

Key words

dermatomal pattern   皮区模式

Psoriasis Area and Severity Index (PASI)   银屑病面积与严重程度指数

Dermatology Life Quality Index (DLQI)   皮肤病生活质量指数

Review questions

1.   What should be included when you do skin examination?
2.   Please describe four type of configuration of skin lesions.

(Hong Fang)

Chapter 10   Practical clinic procedures

Dermatologists make use of several diagnostic and therapeutic procedures in their everyday clinical practice.

Diagnostic procedures

The ability to diagnose a skin disease is improved by the use of better methods observing lesions and by appropriate use of samples for laboratory investigation. These diagnostic methods can be divided into non-invasive diagnostic method and histopathologic examination.

Non-invasive diagnostic method Dermoscopy

A hand lens helps when looking at small lesions such as nits on hair shafts (Fig. 10-1) or scabetic burrows, but dermoscopy gives added information, especially for pigmented lesions.

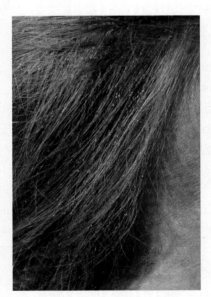

Fig. 10-1 **Head lice and nits are evident on a hair shaft, best visualized using a hand lens.**

Dermoscopy employs a ×10 magnification illuminated lens system, which can visualize a lesion after the application of a drop of oil or water between the skin and the applied lens. Detailed visualization of the epidermal structures is possible, particularly the pigment network (Fig. 10-2). Analysis takes account of:

- the symmetry of the lesion
- patterns of pigmentation
- blue-white structures in the pigment network.

Dermoscopy allows an opinion to be made about the nature and malignant potential of the lesion.

Microbiology samples

Swabs for bacterial and viral culture should be sampled from areas showing pus or exudation. Scrapings for fungal microscopy and culture are obtained by the following techniques:

- the active scaly edge of an eruption is sampled using a disposable scalpel blade held vertically to the skin.
- nail samples are taken from the distal portion or from debris beneath the nail using clippers or a scalpel.
- hair sampling requires plucking of hairs as the hair root is often infected (a scalp scraping is also worthwhile).

Samples are taken onto a small sheet of black paper or a microscope slide (Fig. 10-3). Direct microscopy of scrapings mounted in 20% potassium hydroxide solution will show hyphae (Fig. 10-4).

Demonstrating the acarus of scabies

Dermatologists sometimes need to demonstrate the mite to themselves or their patients. This can be achieved by:

- removing the acarus using a small needle (the end of the burrow with the mite in can be difficult to see) and mounting it on a microscope slide
- visualizing the acarus by dermo-scopy: it appears as a dark triangle
- taking a superficial scalpel scraping, which is examined by microscopy.

(i)

(ii)

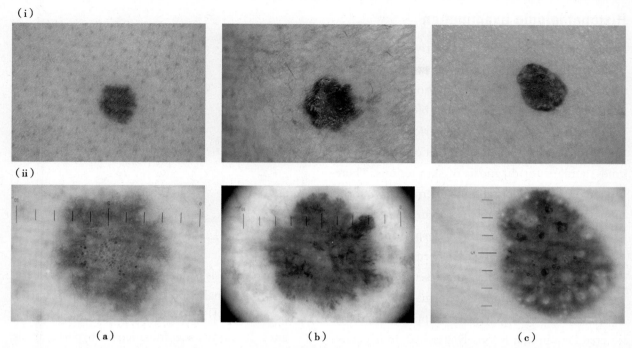

(a)   (b)   (c)

Fig. 10-2 **Use of the dermoscope in (a) a benign melanocytic naevus, (b) a malignant melanoma, (c) a seborrhoeic wart.** Comparison of the macroscopic (i) and dermoscopic (ii) appearances in each case.

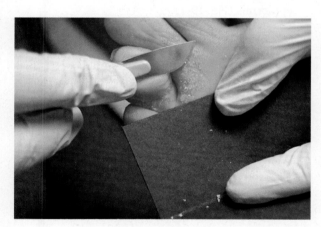

Fig. 10-3 **Take a scraping from the edge of an area of suspected fungal infection by using a disposable scalpel blade.**

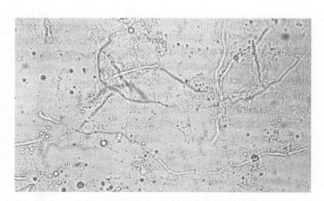

Fig. 10-4 **Microscopy of skin scrapings showing fungal hyphae.**

Wood's light examination

Wood's light is a hand-held ultraviolet A (UVA) source that can be shone on the skin in a darkened room to diagnose certain skin diseases that show particular patterns of fluorescence in UV radiation. It is used especially for:

- determining the extent of vitiligo
- showing hypopigmented macules in tuberous sclerosis
- diagnosing bacterial infections such as erythrasma
- diagnosing tinea capitis due to *Microspora* species.

Dermographism

Stroking the skin in patients with symptomatic dermographism will induce whealing. Cold-induced urticaria can be provoked by the application of an ice cube to the skin. Rubbing a lesion of urticaria pigmentosa will produce a localized wheal.

Doppler studies

The measurement of the ankle/brachial blood pressure index (ABPI) is essential in the management of patients with leg ulcers. The ABPI must be >0.8 for compression therapy.

Histopathologic examination

Sometimes, dermatologists can't arrive at a diagnosis based on the medical history, physical examination and non-invasive diagnostic methods. In order to achieve a reliable diagnosis, a skin biopsy and histopathologic examination will be performed. Most of the times, histopathologic examination is considered gold-standard for diagnosis of skin lesions. Therefore, in order to understand the interpretation of skin biopsies by dermatopathologists accurately, we should know some basic concepts of dermatopathology, especially these terminologies in dermatopathology:

■ Hyperkeratosis implies increased thickening of the stratum corneum. The normal appearance of this layer is the "basket weave" appearance, or layered keratin that is loosely attached. In hyperkeratosis the stratum corneum usually appears solid, in addition to thick (Fig. 10-5). Synonym: orthokeratosis. Clinically the hyperkeratotic processes are manifested by scales that peel-off with relative ease. In the case of keratodermas, the thickening of the stratum corneum may be extraordinary.

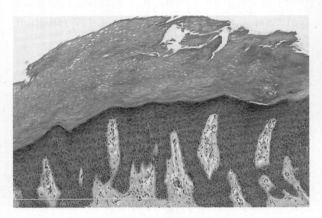

Fig. 10-5 **Hyperkeratosis**

■ Acanthosis implies hyperplasia or increased thickening of the stratum Malpighii. Usually the rete ridges are preserved, elongated and/or thickened. The suprapapillary portions of the epidermis may appear thinned (psoriasis), normal or thickened. Acanthosis is subdivided into regular, when the rete ridges end at about the same level and irregular (Fig. 10-6).

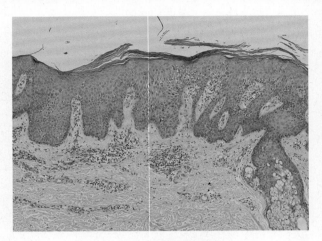

Fig. 10-6 **Acanthosis**

■ Papillomatosis results from the upward proliferation of dermal papillae causing the epidermis to be undulated. It results a "warty" clinical appearance. It is often accompanied by hyperkeratosis, parakeratosis and acanthosis, but the hallmark of papillomatosis is the upward projections of the epidermis (Fig. 10-7).

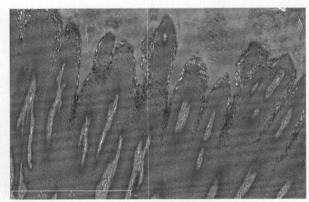

Fig. 10-7 **Papillomatosis**

■ Spongiosis is a process in which intercellular edema between the squamous cells of the epidermis causes an increase in the widths of the spaces between the cells (Fig. 10-8). There is also intracellular edema manifested by intracytoplasmic vacuoles. When the intracellular edema is very prominent, reticular degeneration, characterized by bursting of cell walls with formation of vesicles, ensues.

■ A blister is fluid filled space in the epidermis or immediately below the epidermis. Depending on the size, blisters are classified as vesicles when less than 1cm in diameter or bulla, larger than 1cm. In addition to fluid, blisters often contain inflammatory cells and/or epidermal cells.

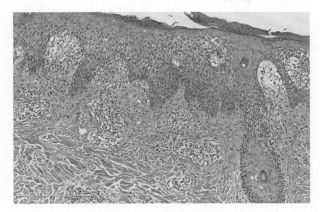

Fig. 10-8　**Spongiosis**

■ Vesicles and Bullae: The vesicular dermatoses are classified regarding the location of the vesicle in relation to the epidermis, as well as the mechanism of blister formation. The vesicular dermatoses are classified regarding the location of the vesicle in relation to the epidermis, as well as the mechanism of blister formation. Regarding location, vesicles and bulla are classified as subcorneal, intraepidermal (Fig. 10-9), or subepidermal.

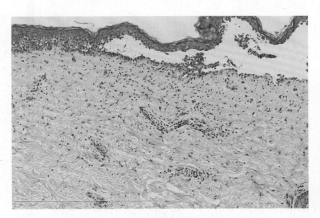

Fig. 10-9　**Acantholytic vesicle**

■ Interface dermatitis is characterized by the presence of inflammatory cells at the dermo-epidermal junction, associated with vacuolar degeneration of the cytoplasm of the basal cells, so-called hydropic degeneration. When this phenomenon is very prominent it may result in separation of the epidermis from the dermis. The inflammatory cells are usually lymphocytes and sprinkle

from the capillaries of the papillary dermis. Interface dermatitis should be distinguished from lichenoid dermatitis, in which there is a lichenoid infiltrate in addition to the interface changes.

■ Lichenoid infiltrate or lichenoid dermatitis is defined as a band-like infiltrate of lymphocytes running parallel to the epidermis and usually involving the dermoepidermal junction (Fig. 10-10). Lichenoid dermatitis is a type of interface dermatitis; however, many of the interface dermatitides lack a lichenoid infiltrate.

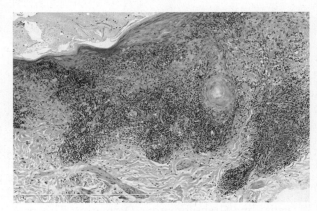

Fig. 10-10　**Lichenoid change**

■ Panniculitis means inflammation of the subcutaneous tissue. The subcutaneous fat is roughly organized in lobules separated by thin fibrous septa (Fig. 10-11).

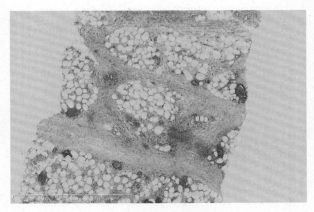

Fig. 10-11　**Panniculitis**

■ A cyst is an epithelial-lined space in the skin. The lining of the cyst may be derived from one of many different sources, including eccrine ducts, hair follicles, and sebaceous ducts. The contents of the cysts are variable depending on the tissue of origin, often being made by keratin.

- Perivascular Dermatitis: Entities in this category are characterized by the absence of significant epidermal change and the presence of an inflammatory infiltrate that is largely restricted to the superficial, or superficial and deep dermis around blood vessels (Fig. 10-12).

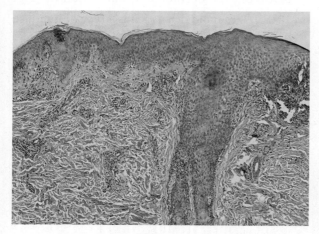

Fig. 10-12 **Perivascular dermatitis**

- Palisading Granulomatous Dermatitis: This pattern is characterized by an interstitial infiltrate of histiocytes admixed with other inflammatory cells, principally lymphocytes, and zones of altered collagen (Fig. 10-13). Classically, the inflammatory infiltrate surrounds the zones of altered collagen in a wall-like or fence-like fashion, hence the term "palisading." The classic entities in this differential diagnosis include granuloma annulare, necrobiosis lipoidica, and rheumatoid nodule.

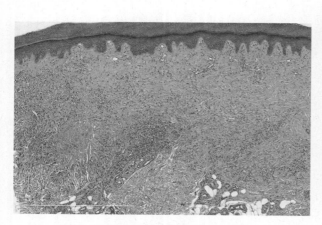

Fig. 10-13 **Palisading dermatitis**

- Nodular and Diffuse Dermatitis: There is a significant overlap with the nodular and diffuse pattern and the superficial and deep perivascular pattern. The primary difference in the nodular and diffuse patterns from the perivascular pattern is that the inflammation is not just centered on vessels. On scanning magnification, nodular dermatitis is characterized by discrete areas of inflammation, separated by uninvolved areas (Fig. 10-14). In contrast, the diffuse pattern demonstrates dense dermal inflammation without intervening areas of sparing. Distinction in individual cases is admittedly arbitrary and subject to individual interpretation. As with automobiles, your mileage may vary.

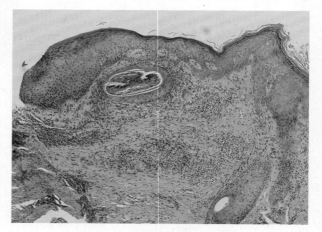

Fig. 10-14 **Nodular dermatitis**

- Sclerosing Dermatitis: The sclerosing dermatitis pattern is generally characterized by dermal sclerosis, usually with little inflammation (Fig. 10-15).

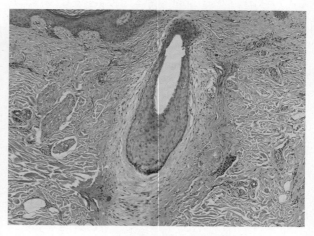

Fig. 10-15 **Fibrosing dermatitis**

Therapeutic procedures

Dermatologists use some non-surgical techniques in their clinical work. Surgical methods and cryotherapy are dealt with elsewhere.

Intralesional steroid injection

The injection of steroid into the skin is useful in the management of several diseases, including:

- alopecia areata
- keloid or hypertrophic scars
- acne cysts
- granuloma annulare
- hypertrophic lichen planus
- prurigo nodularis
- nail psoriasis

Triamcinolone acetonide (10mg/ml) is normally used in an insulin syringe, which has an integral needle. An injection of 0.1~1.0ml of the solution is given into the mid or deep dermis (Fig. 10-16). Compound betamethasone is also widely used for intralesional injection. The main side-effects are skin atrophy, hypopigmentation and telangiectasia. Occasionally, injection of other substances into the skin is used, e.g. bleomycin for viral warts.

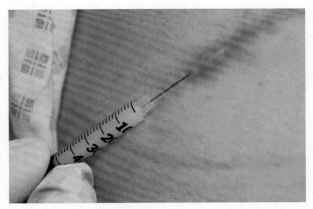

Fig. 10-16 **Intralesional injection of steroid into a hypertrophic scar.**

Paring of skin

The paring down of hyperkeratotic areas on the hands or feet using a disposable scalpel often helps in:

- diagnosis, as it can reveal the underlying lesion, e.g. the punctate thrombosed capillaries of a viral wart or a small haematoma within the epidermis (such as that produced by the friction of shoes on the heel)
- therapy, e.g. for callosities under the metatarsals, by reducing the pressure that results from the callus. For onychomycosis, thinning the nails helps the topical medicine penetration.

On the feet, callosities often develop as a result of the interaction of external forces and an abnormal anatomy of the foot. The advice of a chiropodist or podiatrist will usually be helpful.

Use of caustics

Xanthelasma around the eyes can be treated by the careful application of the caustic trichloroacetic acid (30%~50%) solution on an almost dry cotton applicator. Great care is needed to protect the eyes. Trichloroacetic acid (30%~60%) solution also can be used to treat condyloma acuminatum alone or in combination with other treatments. The treatment should be carried out only by those experienced in the procedure. The xanthelasma turns white with 'frosting' within seconds of application of the acid, and subsequently the treated skin peels off over a period of days.

> *Procedures in the skin clinic*
> - Dermoscopy is useful in deciding whether or not a pigmented lesion might be a malignant melanoma.
> - Skin scrapings for mycology should be taken from the edge of a suspect area using a disposable scalpel blade onto a piece of black paper.
> - Wood's light can show the extent of vitiligo or diagnose erythrasma or tinea capitis.
> - Intralesional triamcinolone is a useful treatment for alopecia areata, keloid, acne cysts and other diseases. Skin atrophy is a potential side-effect.
> - Paring of skin can reveal the underlying condition, e.g. a viral wart, or be a treatment for callosity.
> - Application of caustic: trichloroacetic acid is used with care in the treatment of xanthelasma.

Key words

dermoscopy   皮肤镜

Wood's light   伍德灯

dermographism   皮肤划痕症

paring of skin　皮肤刮削
caustics　腐蚀剂
dermatopathology　皮肤病理学

Review questions

1. How to acquire fungi samples from nails?

2. Which diseases are indicated when a localized wheal appear after rubbing the lesions?

3. What's the difference between interface dermatitis and lichenoid dermatitis?

(Xiuli Wang)

Chapter 11   Basics of medical therapy

The treatment of skin disease includes topical, systemic, intralesional, radiation and surgical modalities. Specific treatments are detailed below. First is an overview of dermatological therapies.

Topical therapy

Topical treatment has the advantage of direct delivery and reduced systemic toxicity. It consists of a *vehicle* or base, which often contains an active ingredient (Table 11-1).

Vehicles are defined as follows:

■ **Lotion.** A liquid vehicle, often aqueous based (also known as solution, which may contain a salt in solution.) or alcohol based (also known as tincture and spiritus). Tincture is typically an alcoholic extract of plant or animal material or alcoholic solution of nonvolatile substance. Spiritus is an alcoholic solution of volatile substance. A *shake lotion* contains an insoluble powder (e.g. calamine lotion).

■ **Cream.** A semisolid emulsion of oil-in-water; containing an emulsifier for stability and a preservative to prevent overgrowth of micro-organisms.

■ **Gel.** A transparent semisolid, non-greasy aqueous emulsion.

Table 11-1	**An overview of topical medicaments**	
Drug	**Indications**	**Pharmacology**
Corticosteroids	Eczemas, psoriasis, lichen planus, discoid lupus erythematosus, sunburn, pityriasis rosea, mycosis fungoides, photodermatoses, lichen sclerosus	Mode of action is through vasoconstrictive, anti-inflammatory and antiproliferative effects; medication is available in different strengths; side-effects need to be considered
Antiseptics	Skin sepsis, leg ulcers, infected eczema	Chlorhexidine, benzalkonium chloride, silver nitrate and potassium permanganate are used
Antibiotics	Acne, rosacea, folliculitis, impetigo, infected eczema	Chlortetracycline, neomycin, bacitracin, gramicidin, polymixin B, sodium fusidate and mupirocin; resistance and sensitization are problems Metronidazole is used for rosacea
Antifungals	Fungal infections of the skin, *Candida albicans* infections	Nystatin, clotrimazole, miconazole, econazole, terbinafine, ketoconazole, sulconazole and amorolfine
Antiviral agents	Herpes simplex, herpes zoster	Aciclovir, penciclovir
Parasiticidals	Scabies, lice	Benzyl benzoate, permethrin and malathion for scabies; malathion, permethrin and phenothrin for lice - applied as a lotion or shampoo
Coal tar	Psoriasis, eczema	Presumed anti-inflammatory and antiproliferative effects; available as creams, shampoos and in paste bandages
Dithranol	Psoriasis	Antiproliferative effects; available as creams, pastes and ointments
Vitamin D analogues	Psoriasis	Calcitriol, calcipotriol and tacalcitol inhibit keratinocyte proliferation and promote differentiation
Keratolytics	Acne, scaly eczemas	Salicylic acid, benzoyl peroxide and tretinoin
Retinoids	Acne, psoriasis	Isotretinoin (acne), tazarotene (psoriasis)
Topical immunomodulators (calcineurin inhibitors)	Atopic eczema (and off-licence use in other diseases)	Tacrolimus and pimecrolimus

- **Ointment.** A semisolid grease or oil, containing little or no water but sometimes with added powder. No preservative is usually needed. The active ingredient is suspended rather than dissolved.
- **Paste.** An ointment base with a high proportion of powder (starch or zinc oxide) producing a stiff consistency.
- **Powder.** Powder is composed of a large number of very fine dry particles.
- **Oil.** Active ingredients can be mixed or dissolved in vegetable or mineral oil.

Therapeutic properties of the vehicle

Lotions evaporate and cool the skin and are useful for inflamed or exudative conditions, e.g. for wet wraps. The high water content of a cream means that it mostly evaporates; it is also non-greasy and easy to apply or remove. Ointments are best for dry skin conditions such as eczema. They rehydrate and occlude, but being greasy are difficult to wash off and are less acceptable to patients than creams. Pastes are ideal for applying to well-defined surfaces, such as psoriatic plaques, but are also hard to remove.

Quantities required

One application to the whole body requires 15~20g of ointment. The adult face or neck requires 1g, trunk (each side) 3g, arm 0.5g, hand 0.5g, leg 3g and foot 1g. A useful guide for patients is the '*fingertip unit*' (FTU) - the amount of cream or ointment that can be applied to the terminal phalanx of the index finger (Fig. 11-1). One FTU equals 0.5g. The weekly amount required for the twice-daily use of an emollient in an adult is 250g. Doctors often underestimate the quantities needed.

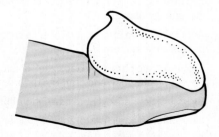

Fig. 11-1 **The fingertip unit (FTU) = 0.5g.**

The safe maximum amount varies with the strength of the steroid, the age of the patient and the length of treatment. For 1% hydrocortisone, adults can use 150~200 g/week, but children can use only 60g and babies as little as 20g. Creams/ointments are applied twice daily except for mometasone, fluticasone and tacalcitol, which are used once daily.

Pharmacokinetics

The ability of a drug to penetrate the epidermis depends on several factors. These include:
- the drug's molecular size and structure and its lipid/water solubility
- the vehicle used and whether application is occluded
- the site on the body - absorption is greatest through the eyelid and genitalia
- whether or not the skin is diseased.

Emollients

Emollients help dry skin conditions such as eczema and ichthyosis by re-establishing the surface lipid layer and enhancing rehydration of the epidermis. One of common emollients is emulsifying ointment. Sometimes emollients contain urea or antimicrobials. Oils added to bath water can also help.

Dressings and hospital admission

Many departments have treatment centres where daily dressings and ultraviolet (UV) treatments are given. If outpatient management is unsuccessful, hospital admission may be needed. Dressings, for either the outpatient or the inpatient, consist of stockinette gauze applied to the trunk or limbs after the ointments have been put on. These must be changed once or twice a day. Leg ulcer dressings may be changed less frequently, depending on the type of application used.

Bandages impregnated with tar are sometimes helpful for leg ulcers and eczema. Many types of paraffin gauze, hydrocolloid and alginate dressing are now available for leg ulcers.

Topical steroids

A summary of the indications for topical treatment with corticosteroids is given in Table 11-1. The relative potencies of the more commonly prescribed preparations are shown in Table 11-2.

Table 11-2	**Relative potencies of topical steroids**
Potency	**Example (generic name)**
Mild	Hydrocortisone 1% and 2.5%
Moderately potent	Clobetasone butyrate 0.05%
	Fludroxycortide 0.0125%
	Alclometasone dipropionate 0.05%
	Triamcinolone acetonide 0.025%~0.1%
Potent	Betamethasone valerate 0.1%
	Betamethasone dipropionate 0.05%
	Fluocinolone acetonide 0.025%
	Fluocinonide 0.05%
	Fluticasone propionate 0.05%
	Hydrocortisone butyrate 0.1%
	Mometasone furoate 0.1%
	Triamcinolone acetonide 0.1%
Very potent	Clobetasol propionate 0.05%
	Diflucortolone valerate 0.3%
	Halcinonide 0.1%

Side-effects of topical steroid therapy

The use of topical steroids carries the potential for harmful side-effects. These include:

■ atrophy of the skin - thinning, erythema, telangiectasia, purpura and striae

■ induction of acne or perioral dermatitis, and exacerbation of rosacea

■ atypical fungal infection (tinea incognito); bacterial or viral infections may be potentiated

■ allergic contact dermatitis, resulting from a component of the preparation or the steroid itself

■ systemic absorption - suppression of the pituitary-adrenal axis, Cushingoid appearance, growth retardation

■ tachyphylaxis - reduced responsiveness to the steroid after prolonged use.

Systemic therapy

Systemic treatments are used when topical treatment is ineffective, for serious skin diseases and for infections. Details are given in Table 11-3.

Other treatments

Corticosteroids are sometimes injected directly into lesions (e.g. to treat keloids). Certain disorders respond to phototherapy. Iontophoresis is a treatment for excess sweating of the palms in which a direct electric current is passed into skin in contact with tap water.

In the past, X-irradiation was used to treat psoriasis, acne, tinea capitis, tuberculosis of the skin and hand eczema. There are now very few indications for X-ray treatment of non-malignant disease, although irradiation is of great value in several types of skin tumour.

Cryotherapy, in which liquid nitrogen is applied to the skin, is extensively used in dermatology. It is mainly employed for the treatment of benign or pre-malignant skin tumours.

Basics of medical therapy

■ Correct diagnosis is essential to ensure appropriate treatment.

■ When using topical steroids:
  - use the lowest potency that is effective
  - look out for side-effects, especially atrophy of the skin
  - emollients can help reduce the amount of topical steroid required.

■ Explain the treatment to the patient and preferably give a written handout; this aids compliance. The fingertip unit is a convenient way to indicate the amount of cream the patient should apply.

■ Use the simplest treatment possible; patients easily get mixed up if they have several different topical preparations to apply to different parts of the body.

■ Prescribe adequate amounts. Patients are often given too small quantities of their creams, 'run out' and return to the clinic no better because the treatment has been inadequate.

Web resource

http://dermnetnz.org/treatments/topical-treatment.html

Table 11-3　**An overview of systemic therapy**

Group	Drug	Indications
Corticosteroids	Prednisolone usually	Bullous disorders, connective tissue disease, vasculitis
Cytotoxics	Methotrexate Hydroxycarbamide Azathioprine, mycophenolate mofetil	Psoriasis, sarcoidosis, eczema Psoriasis Bullous disorders, chronic actinic dermatitis, atopic eczema
Biologics	Etanercept, infliximab, adalimumab, ustekinumab	Psoriasis unresponsive to other systemic agents, off-licence use in other diseases
Immunosuppressants	Cyclosporin Gold	Psoriasis, atopic eczema, pyoderma gangrenosum Bullous disorders, lupus erythematosus
Retinoids	Acitretin Isotretinoin Alitretinoin	Psoriasis, other keratinization disorders Acne Hand dermatitis
Antifungals	Griseofulvin, terbinafine Ketoconazole Itraconazole, fluconazole	Fungal infection Fungal infection (*Candida aIbicans* too) Fungal infection, candidiasis
Antibiotics	Various	Skin sepsis, acne, rosacea
Antivirals	Acyclovir, valaciclovir Famciclovir	Herpes simplex, herpes zoster Herpes zoster, genital herpes simplex
Antihistamines	H1 blockers First-generation agents: chlorpheniramine; diphenhydramine; hydroxyzine; cyproheptadine. Second-generation agents: Astemizole; mizolastine; ebastine; epinastine; azelastine; olopatadine; fexofenadine; loratadine; desloratadine; cetirizine; levocetirizine; acrivastine; rupatadine	Urticaria, eczema
Antiandrogens	Cyproterone acetate	Acne (females only)
Antimalarials	Hydroxychloroquine	Lupus erythematosus, porphyria cutanea tarda
Antileprotic	Dapsone	Dermatitis herpetiformis, leprosy, vasculitis

Key words

lotion　洗剂

solution　溶液

tincture　酊剂

spiritus　醑剂

shake lotion　振荡剂

cream　乳膏或霜剂

gel　凝胶

ointment　软膏

paste　糊剂

powder　粉剂

oil　油剂

fingertip unit (FTU)　指尖单位（用于估算外用药物的剂量）

emollients　润肤剂

tachyphylaxis　快速耐受

corticosteroids　类固醇皮质激素

steroids　类固醇

cryotherapy　冷冻疗法

Review questions

1. Please give examples of common vehicles or bases in topical therapy.
2. What are the indications for topical treatment with corticosteroids?
3. What are side-effects of topical steroid therapy?

(Wei He)

Chapter 12   Epidemiology of skin disease

Skin disease is very common. About 10% of a general practitioner's workload and 6% of hospital outpatient referrals can be accounted for by skin problems. Skin disease is also economically significant; it is a major occupational cause of loss of time from work and the third most common industrial disease.

In any discussion of epidemiology, it is important first to define the terms used:

- *Prevalence* refers to the proportion of a defined population affected by a disease at any given time.
- *Incidence* is defined as the proportion of a population experiencing the disorder within a stated period of time (usually 1 year).

The type, prevalence and incidence of skin disease all depend on social, economic, geographical, racial, cultural and age-related factors.

Skin disease in the general population

Reliable population statistics are difficult to obtain, but it appears that, in Europe, the prevalence of skin disease needing some sort of medical care is about 20%. Eczema, acne and infective disorders (including warts) are the commonest complaints (Fig. 12-1). Only a minority seek medical advice.

Skin disease in community and specialized clinics

The precise proportion of skin disorders seen in a community setting (Fig.12-2) will vary with the age structure of the population served, the amount and type of industry in the area and socioeconomic factors. Demographic studies may reveal a trend; for example, for unknown reasons, atopic eczema has become more common over the last 30 years.

Patients seen in a specialist dermatology clinic are a selected population (Fig. 12-3). In some countries, e.g. the UK, a general practitioner will have referred them; in other places, self-referral may depend on the availability of medical insurance. Referral patterns

vary between different regions, depending on local facilities, interests and customs. In Europe, within a year, just over 1% of the population is referred for a dermatological opinion. In the early 2010s, a quarter of all new referrals required a surgical procedure.

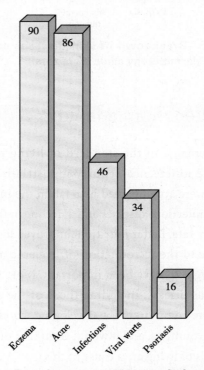

Fig. 12-1 **Prevalence per 1000 population for skin disease of any severity.**

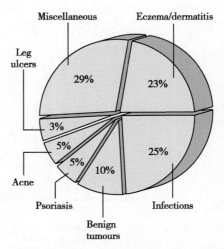

Fig. 12-2 **Breakdown of skin diseases seen in general practice (% of total).**

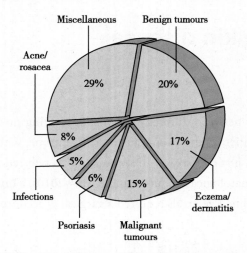

Fig. 12-3 **Breakdown of skin diseases seen in a hospital dermatology clinic (% of total).**

Socioeconomic factors

Improvements in the standard of living resulting from the nineteenth-century industrialization of Europe were accompanied by a fall in the incidences of most infectious diseases and a decline in the infant mortality rate. Better nutrition, improved living conditions and the introduction of hygienic measures are thought to have been important. Most forms of infectious disease, including those of the skin, are now more common in the developing world than in western countries, and it would seem that the poorer standards of living are a cause of this.

However, industrialization brings its own problems. Occupational dermatitis is quite common in industrialized countries, and mild cases are often not reported. Increased sophistication in western countries also means that patients now want something done about disorders or minor imperfections that would not have bothered past generations.

Changes in social fashion have also brought about changes in skin disease. For example, the habit of sunbathing, which became popular in the 1970s, seems to have resulted in an increase in the incidence of malignant melanoma from the 1980s to the present.

The media have also had an effect: the numerous articles and programmes on the potential problems associated with a change in pigmented naevi have produced a flood of referrals of worried patients seeking reassurance about their lesions! However, it is still true that many people with minor skin problems do not consult a doctor.

Geographical factors

Humid conditions found in hot countries predispose to fungal and bacterial infections, and to other conditions such as 'prickly heat' (miliaria: an itchy eruption due to blocked sweat ducts). Ultraviolet radiation in sunny climes will result in actinic damage and malignant change in the skin of non-pigmented migrants to the area.

Figure 12-4 shows a comparison between some common complaints in different geographical loca-

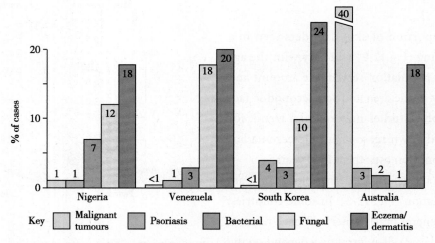

Fig. 12-4 **Geographical variations in hospital attendances (%) with some common dermatological disorders.**

tions. The rates for bacterial and fungal infections show variation, and skin cancers are more common in Australia. However, the figures for eczema/dermatitis are remarkably constant.

Racial and cultural factors

Quite apart from the obvious differences in pigmentation, the skin structure varies between the different races. For example, hair is often spiral in black Africans but straight in mongoloids. In caucasians, hair is more variable and may be straight, wavy or helical. Skin tumours and actinic damage are seen more in caucasians than in black Africans, with mongoloids showing an intermediate incidence. Keloids and hair problems, such as pseudofolliculitis, are more common in black Africans, whereas mongoloid skin has a tendency to become lichenified and acne may be less frequent. Vitiligo appears to have a similar incidence in all races, but is more conspicuous and may have a greater psychological impact in those with a dark skin.

Cultural factors may bring problems. For example, tight braiding of the hair, practised by some black Africans, may result in alopecia, whereas the use of certain traditional oils or cosmetics can produce dermatitis or a change in pigmentation.

Age and sex prevalence of dermatoses

Different disorders are associated with different times of life (Table 12-1). Some disorders occur throughout life but are more common at certain ages, whereas others are almost exclusively encountered in defined age groups. For example, atopic eczema is most common in infants, acne is mainly seen in adolescents and psoriasis has its peak onset in the second and third decades of life. Certain disorders tend to appear in middle age, e.g. pemphigus and malignant melanoma. In old age, degenerative and malignant skin conditions are often found. Thus, the age structure of the population will influence the type of dermatology practised.

Table 12-1	**Age-related onset of selected skin disorders**
Age	**Disorder**
Childhood	Port wine stain and strawberry naevi, ichthyosis, erythropoietic protoporphyria, epidermolysis bullosa, atopic eczema, infantile seborrhoeic dermatitis, urticaria pigmentosa, viral exanthems, viral warts, molluscum contagiosum, impetigo
Adolescence	Melanocytic naevi, acne, psoriasis (notably guttate), seborrhoeic dermatitis, vitiligo, pityriasis rosea
Early adulthood	Psoriasis, seborrhoeic dermatitis, lichen planus, dermatitis herpetiformis, lupus erythematosus, vitiligo, tinea versicolor
Middle age	Porphyria cutanea tarda, lichen planus, rosacea, pemphigus vulgaris, venous ulceration, malignant melanoma, basal cell carcinoma, mycosis fungoides
Old age	Asteatotic eczema, generalized pruritus, bullous pemphigoid, venous and arterial ulcers, seborrhoeic warts, solar keratosis, solar elastosis, Campbell-de-Morgan spots, basal cell carcinoma, squamous cell carcinoma, herpes zoster

Some conditions are more common to a specific gender (Table 12-2).

Table 12-2	**Skin disorders with a male or female preponderance**
Sex	Disorder
Female	Palmoplantar pustulosis, lichen sclerosus, lupus erythematosus, systemic sclerosis, morphoea, rosacea, dermatitis artefacta, venous ulceration, *in situ* squamous cell carcinoma, malignant melanoma
Male	Seborrhoeic dermatitis, dermatitis herpetiformis, porphyria cutanea tarda, polyarteritis nodosa, pruritus ani, tinea pedis and cruris, mycosis fungoides, squamous cell carcinoma, actinic keratosis

Epidemiology
- The commonest skin diseases in the general community are eczema, acne and infections, including viral warts.
- About 20% of the general population have some sort of skin disorder requiring medical attention.
- Skin disease accounts for more than 10% of all consultations in general practice.
- Better living conditions reduce skin infection, but excess sun on a white skin predisposes to skin cancer.

Web resource

http://www.who.int/child_adolescent_health/documents/fch_cah_05_12/en/index.html.

Key Words

epidemiology 流行病学

prevalence 患病率

incidence 发病率

dermatoses 皮肤病

hospital outpatient 医院门诊患者

clinic 诊所

community clinics 社区诊所

specialized clinics 专科诊所

Review questions

1. Please give five examples of skin disorders with female preponderance.
2. How many percent of general population have skin disorders requiring medical attention?

(Qing Sun)

Chapter 13   Body image, the psyche and the skin

The stress of having skin disease

The potentially harsh psychological effects of having chronic skin disease tend to be underestimated. Up to 30% of skin outpatients suffer 'psychological distress' from their condition. This is particularly understandable in the teenager with acne, or in someone who has extensive psoriasis or eczema. In both these situations, the individual's devalued body image may be out of proportion to the objective severity of his or her skin problem. Skin diseases can thus make patients into 'social lepers' who feel that their social lives are restricted because other people do not want to mix with them. These effects on 'quality of life' can be assessed by specific questionnaires, e.g. the Dermatology Life Quality Index (DLQI).

Patients sometimes feel that their disorder is either caused directly by, or exacerbated by, 'stress'. This is difficult to prove, as it is often impossible to differentiate reactive from aetiological states. Many dermatologists believe that psychological factors can, for example, make eczema and psoriasis worse, but most would also agree that these are stressful conditions in their own right. However, it is accepted that there are a small number of conditions that are of psychogenic origin. Management with a liaison psychiatrist can be helpful.

Skin disorders of psychogenic origin

Dermatitis artefacta

Dermatitis artefacta (Fig. 13-1) should be suspected from the presence of lesions with bizarre shapes (often linear or angular and in accessible sites) that do not conform to natural disease. The lesions are often ulcerated or crusted and do not heal as expected, although they do heal if occluded. Blisters or bruises are also sometimes found.

The condition tends to occur in young women. Confrontation is not recommended, as this may lead to an angry denial. Management is aimed at excluding genuine disease, establishing a rapport with the patient and gently trying to investigate the presence of psychological stresses, e.g. in the home or work environment or in social or sexual relationships.

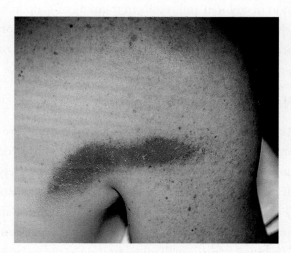

Fig. 13-1   **Dermatitis artefacta: a linear lesion.**

Delusions of body image

Patients may present with no objective skin disease but still complain of symptoms such as burning or redness of the face, or display a preoccupation with an imagined problem such as excessive facial hair. This condition, sometimes known as dysmorphophobia, is usually seen in women, although it does occur in men, who may complain of a burning scrotum. Most of these patients are depressed, although some may show signs of schizophrenia. Psychiatric referral is needed for those with true delusions.

Delusions of parasitosis

Patients with this condition are convinced that their skin is infested with parasites, and they often bring collections of keratin and debris to support their contention. Self-induced excoriation of the skin may be seen. It mainly occurs in women over the age of 40 years. Most patients do not have an organic psychosis, but they are often obsessional and do have a monosymptomatic hypochondriacal psychosis. Treatment is difficult. It is necessary to exclude a true parasitosis. The antipsychotic drugs pimozide, risperidone or olanzapine may be helpful but all have significant potential side-effects that require monitoring.

Trichotillomania

Rubbing, pulling and twisting the hair is not uncommon in children and results in thinning of scalp hair, which recovers spontaneously. When the condition occurs in adults, the hair may be cut using scissors or a razor, and the prognosis is not so good.

Neurogenic excoriations

Accessible areas of the skin, particularly the forearms and back of the neck, are commonly involved in this condition, with excoriated lesions in a variety of stages of evolution from ulcers to healed scars (Fig. 13-2). The damage is inflicted as a result of an uncontrollable itch, but there is no primary lesion. Effective occlusion will allow healing. *Acné excoriée* is a variant seen in young women who squeeze and pick their acne lesions, resulting in artefactual erosions.

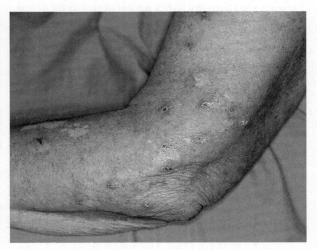

Fig. 13-2 **Neurogenic excoriations on the arm.** Some have healed to leave hypopigmented scars.

> *Body image, the psyche and the skin*
> - Psychological stress is commonly associated with skin disease, and the patient's psychological state should be routinely assessed. Quality of life questionnaires are available.
> - Some skin disorders (e.g. eczema and psoriasis) may get worse at times of stress in certain patients. It may be helpful for the patient to recognize this.
> - A small number of skin diseases are psychogenic in origin. A liaison psychiatrist may offer assistance.

Web resource

http://www.ncbi.nlm.nih.gov/pubmed/17883417

Key words

dermatitis artefacta　人工皮炎
dysmorphophobia　丑形恐怖 / 畸形恐惧
psychiatric referral　精神科会诊
trichotillomania　拔毛癖
psychological distress　心理压抑
neurogenic excoriations　神经官能病性表皮剥脱

Review questions

1. How can we assess the patient's psychological state?
2. Please give three examples of common skin disorders with psychogenic origins and describe them briefly.

(Qing sun)

Diseases

Chapter 14   Psoriasis - Epidemiology, pathophysiology and presentation

Definition

Psoriasis is a chronic, non-infectious, polygenic inflammatory dermatosis characterized by well-demarcated erythematous plaques topped by silvery scales (Fig. 14-1).Various environmental triggering factors, e.g. infections, trauma, or medications can elicit disease in predisposed individuals.

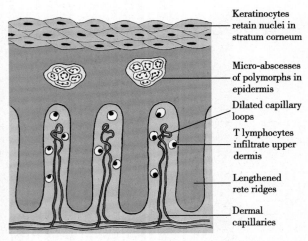

Keratinocytes retain nuclei in stratum corneum

Micro-abscesses of polymorphs in epidermis

Dilated capillary loops

T lymphocytes infiltrate upper dermis

Lengthened rete ridges

Dermal capillaries

Fig. 14-1   **Histopathology of psoriasis.**

Epidemiology

Psoriasis affects 1.5%~3% of the population in Europe and North America, but is less common in Africa, China and Japan. The sex incidence is equal. The condition may start at any age, even in the elderly. The two peaks of onset are the second to third and the sixth decades. It is unusual in children under 8 years old. The most frequent form of the disease in children is plaque psoriasis.

Aetiopathogenesis

Genetics

Inherited factors predispose to the development of psoriasis: genetic factors appear to be polygenic.

About 35% of patients show a family history, and identical twin studies show a concordance of 64%. There is a 14% probability that a child with one parent who has psoriasis will be affected, but this increases to 41% if both parents have psoriasis. There are strong correlations with the human leucocyte antigens (HLAs), e.g. HLA-Cw6. HLA-Cw6 is strongly linked to the age of onset. Most patients with early-onset psoriasis expressed HLA-Cw6.It has been identified at least nine psoriasis susceptibility regions (PSORS1-9) in different chromosomal locations. The most important genetic region is PSORS1 on chromosome locus 6p, which is estimated to account for up to 50% of psoriasis risk. Environmental factors are thought to trigger the disease in susceptible individuals.

Epidermal kinetics and metabolism

Psoriatic lesions result from abnormal reactivity of skin T cells with alteration of the epidermal barrier and of inflammatory signalling. The number of cycling epidermal cells is increased seven-fold because of an increase in the basal and suprabasal proliferating cell compartment. The cell cycle time is not reduced. Growth factors, especially transforming growth factor-α, mediate these events. The upper dermal capillary plexus is expanded.

Precipitating factors

A number of precipitating factors are associated with the disorder:

- *Koebner phenomenon.* Trauma to the epidermis and dermis, such as a scratch or surgical scar, can precipitate psoriasis in the damaged skin (Fig. 14-2).
- *Infection.* Typically, a streptococcal sore throat may precipitate guttate psoriasis.
- *Drugs.* Beta-blockers, IFNs, lithium and antimalarials can make psoriasis worse or precipi-

tate it. Rapid taper of systemic corticosteroids can induce pustular psoriasis as well as flares of plaque psoriasis.

■ *Sunlight.* Exposure to sunlight can aggravate psoriasis (in about 6%), although it has a beneficial effect in the majority.

■ *Psychological stress.* Stress can cause and exacerbate psoriasis.

■ *Cigarettes and alcohol.* These seem to make psoriasis worse.

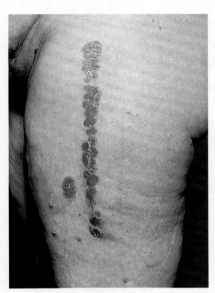

Fig. 14-2   **The Koebner phenomenon.** Psoriasis has developed in a surgical scar.

Pathology

The epidermis is thickened, with keratinocytes retaining their nuclei (Fig. 14-1). There is no granular layer, and keratin builds up loosely at the horny layer. The rete ridges are elongated, and polymorphs infiltrate up into the stratum corneum where they form micro-abscesses. Capillaries are dilated in the papillary dermis. T lymphocytes infiltrate the earliest psoriatic lesions.

Clinical presentation

Psoriasis varies in severity from the trivial to the life-threatening. Its appearance and behaviour also range widely from the readily recognizable chronic plaques on the elbows to the acute generalized pustular form.

Psoriasis can be confused with other conditions (Table 14-1).

Table 14-1	**Differetial diagnosis of psoriasis**
Variant of psoriasis	**Differential diagnosis**
Plaque psoriasis	Psoriasiform drug eruption (due to beta-blockers) Hypertrophic lichen planus
Palmoplantar psoriasis	Hyperkeratotic eczema Reiter's disease
Scalp psoriasis	Seborrhoeic dermatitis
Guttate psoriasis	Pityriasis rosea
Flexural psoriasis	Candidiasis of the flexures
Nail psoriasis	Fungal infection of the nails

Presentation patterns of psoriasis include:

■ plaque

■ guttate

■ flexural

■ localized forms

■ generalized pustular

■ nail involvement

■ erythroderma

Plaque

Well-defined, raised disc-shaped plaques (Fig. 14-3) involving the elbows, knees, scalp, hair margin or sacrum are the classic presentation. The plaques are usually red and covered by waxy white scales which, if detached, may leave bleeding points. Plaques vary in diameter from 2cm or less to several centimetres, and are sometimes pruritic.

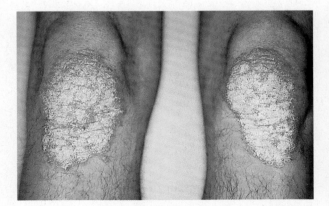

Fig. 14-3   **Typical scaly plaques of psoriasis on the knees**.

Guttate

Guttate psoriasis is an acute symmetrical eruption (a 'flurry') of 'drop-like' lesions with little scale in the early stage, usually on the trunk and limbs. This form mostly occurs in adolescents or young adults (Fig. 14-4).

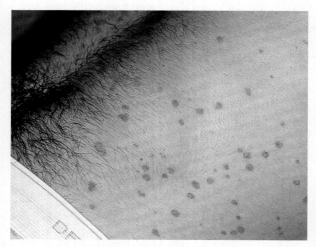

Fig. 14-4 **The drop-like lesions of guttate psoriasis.**

Flexural

This variant of psoriasis affects the axillae, submammary areas, groin and natal cleft (Fig. 14-5). Plaques are smooth and often glazed. It is mostly found in the elderly.

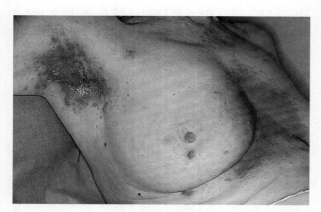

Fig. 14-5 **Smooth, non-keratotic involvement in flexural.**

Localized forms

Psoriasis can also present in a number of localized forms:

■ *Palmoplantar pustulosis* is characterized by yel-low- to brown-coloured sterile pustules on the palms or soles (Fig. 14-6). A minority of subjects have classic plaque psoriasis elsewhere. It is most common in middle-aged women who are ciga-rette smokers, and it follows a protracted course.

■ *Acrodermatitis of Hallopeau* is an uncommon indolent form of pustular psoriasis affecting the digits and nails (Fig. 14-10).

■ *Scalp psoriasis* may be the sole manifestation of the disease (Fig. 14-9). It can be confused with dandruff but is generally better demarcated and more thickly scaled.

■ *Napkin psoriasis* is a well-defined psoriasiform eruption in the nappy area of infants, few of whom later develop true psoriasis.

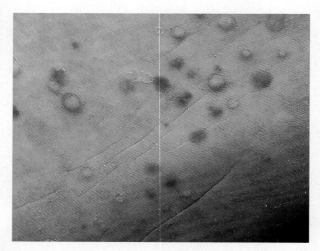

Fig. 14-6 **Palmoplantar pustulosis: a localized vari-ant of psoriasis on the sole of the foot.**

Generalized pustular

Generalized pustular is a rare but serious and even life-threatening form of psoriasis. Sheets of small, sterile yellowish pustules develop on an erythema-tous background and may spread rapidly (Fig. 14-7). The onset is often acute. The patient is unwell, with fever and malaise, and requires hospital admission.

Nail involvement

Psoriasis affects the matrix or nail bed in 25%~50% of cases (Fig. 14-8). Thimble pitting is the common-est change, followed by *onycholysis* (separation of the distal edge of the nail from the nail bed). An oily

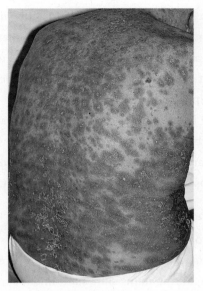

Fig. 14-7 **Generalized pustular psoriasis in an elderly patient.**

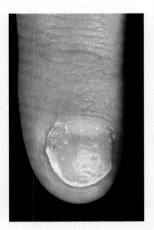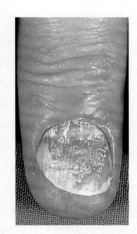

Fig. 14-8 **Nail involvement in psoriasis: pitting (left) and subungual hyperkeratosis with onycholysis (right).**

Psoriasis
- Psoriasis affects 1.5%~3% of western populations.
- Inheritance is polygenic: 35% have a family history.
- Geneticists have identified loci for possible psoriasis genes, e.g. *PSOR1* on chromosome locus 6p.
- Peaks of onset are in the second to third and the sixth decades.
- The number of proliferating keratinocytes is increased seven-fold, but the epidermal cell cycle time is not shortened.
- Presentation is variable: the chronic plague form affecting the elbows, knees and scalp is the commonest.
- Precipitating factors include streptococcal infection, drugs, sunlight, alcohol, smoking and psychological stress.
- Nail involvement is found in 25%~50% of cases and is difficult to treat.

or salmon pink discoloration of the nail bed is seen, often adjacent to onycholysis. Subungual hyperkeratosis, with a build-up of keratin beneath the distal nail edge, mostly affects the toenails. Nail changes are frequently associated with psoriatic arthropathy. Treatment is often difficult.

Web resource

http://www.psoriasis-association.org.uk/

Psoriasis - Management and complications

Management

The non-infectious nature of psoriasis, its relapsing nature and the likely need for long-term therapy should be explained. A sympathetic approach is helpful, and patients often obtain support from the self-help group (The Psoriasis Association). Treatment is tailored to the patient's particular requirements, taking into account the type and extent of the disease, and the age and social background (Table 14-2).

Table 14-2 **A guide to psoriasis therapy**	
Type of psoriasis	**Treatment options**
Stable plaque	Vitamin D analogue with topical steroid Dithranol (short contact), coal tar, tazarotene Narrow-band ultraviolet B
Extensive plaque	Narrow-band ultraviolet B (plus topicals) Methotrexate, cyclosporin, PUVA or Re-PUVA Biologics
Guttate	Topical steroids (mild/moderate), coal tar Narrow-band ultraviolet B
Facial/flexural	Topical steroids (mild/moderate); tacalcitol
Palmoplantar	Topical steroids (potent) Acitretin, PUVA or Re-PUVA
Generalized pustular; erythrodermic	Acitretin, methotrexate, cyclosporin Biologics

Topical therapy

It is usual to prescribe topical agents as the first-line treatment.

Vitamin D analogues

Calcipotriol (Dovonex), *tacalcitol* (Curatoderm) and *calcitriol* (Silkis) are topical synthetic vitamin D analogues for use in mild and moderate chronic plaque psoriasis. They inhibit cell proliferation and stimulate keratinocyte differentiation, correcting some of the epidermal cell proliferation changes in psoriasis. Patient acceptability is good as the preparations do not smell or stain, are easy to apply and do not have the risk of skin atrophy seen with topical steroids. Skin irritation may be a problem. Efficacy is commensurate with dithranol or topical steroids.

Hypercalcaemia is possible if the maximum dose is exceeded. Calcipotriol cream can be used up to 100g/week (40% of the body surface on a twice-daily basis), and tacalcitol ointment up to 35g/week (20% of body surface as a once-daily dose). Tacalcitol is tolerated on the scalp and face, where calcipotriol tends to irritate. Calcipotriol is available as a scalp preparation. Vitamin D analogues are often used in alternation with a topical steroid, and in combination with ultraviolet B or psoralen plus ultraviolet A (PUVA) therapy.

Topical corticosteroids

Topical steroids have the advantage of being clean, non-irritant and easy to use. However, against this must be balanced the risk of side-effects and of precipitating an unstable form of psoriasis, especially on their withdrawal. Topical steroids are the treatment of choice for face, genitalia and flexures, and are useful for stubborn plaques on hands, feet and scalp. Potent steroids should not be applied to the face, although they may be used judiciously on palms and soles. Elsewhere, moderately potent steroids normally suffice. Their use must be monitored carefully. Creams are often preferred to ointments. Lotions and gels are available for the scalp.

Coal tar preparations

Coal tar distillates have been used for decades to treat psoriasis. They are safe and seem to act by inhibiting DNA synthesis. The main disadvantages of tar are that it smells and is messy. Despite this, it can be useful for inpatient care, e.g. combined with ultraviolet B - the Goeckermann regimen. Refined tar (1%~10%) is available in a cream or lotion base for outpatient use (e.g. Carbo-Dome, Exorex, Psoriderm). These preparations are suitable for chronic plaque psoriasis or guttate psoriasis once the acute phase is past.

Dithranol (anthralin)

Dithranol has an antimitotic effect and is irritant to normal skin. It cannot be used on the face or genitalia, and it stains skin, hair, linen, clothes and bathtubs a purple-brown colour. For inpatient use, the usual base is Lassar's paste (zinc and salicylic acid paste BP). It is applied to the plaques of psoriasis initially in the 0.1% strength, increasing up to 2% if necessary. The surrounding skin is protected with a bland preparation such as white soft paraffin, and the treated area is covered with tube gauze. The combination of this with a daily tar bath and ultraviolet B is called the Ingram regimen. Psoriasis clears within 3 weeks in most patients on this treatment.

The 'short contact regimen', in which dithranol is applied for 30min each day, is suitable for outpatients with stable plaque psoriasis. The dithranol is best washed off in a shower. Dithrocream is a suitable preparation and comes in concentrations from 0.1% to 2%.

Retinoids

A topical retinoid, tazarotene (0.05% and 0.1%; Zorac gel), is effective for chronic plaque psoriasis. It may irritate and is often used alternating with a topical steroid.

Keratolytics and scalp preparations

Hyperkeratotic psoriasis of the palms and soles can be treated with 5% salicylic acid ointment. Scalp psoriasis (Fig. 14-9) responds to 3% salicylic acid in a cream base (sometimes with 3% precipitated sulphur) applied daily or every 2 or 3 days, and is used in combination with a tar-containing shampoo (e.g.

Alphosyl 2 in 1, Capasal, Polytar, T/Gel). Coconut oil compound (e.g. Cocois, with tar, salicylic acid and sulphur) also helps scaly scalps.

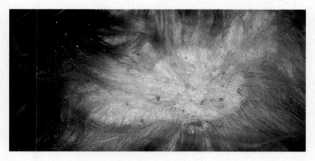

Fig. 14-9 **Scaly plaques of psoriasis in the scalp, with localized hair loss.**

Systemic therapy

Psoriasis that is life-threatening, unresponsive to adequate topical treatment or restricting the ability to work (Fig. 14-10) may require systemic therapy. Benefits must be weighed against side-effects. The use of potentially toxic drugs is justified by their ability to transform a patient's life from severely restricted to nearly normal.

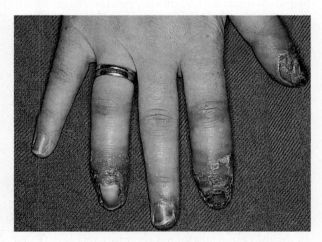

Fig. 14-10 **Acrodermatitis continua variant of psoriasis.** Sterile pustular changes with dactylitis are present on three fingers.

Methotrexate

The folate antagonist methotrexate is well established as for severe psoriasis and may have anti-inflammatory as well as immune modulatory effects. It is given once a week orally as a single dose (usually 7.5~15mg), although it can be given subcutaneously or intramuscularly. Normal liver, kidney and bone marrow function must be established before starting methotrexate, and these functions must be monitored during treatment. Liver disease, alcoholism and acute infection are contraindications to methotrexate, and drug interaction (e.g. with aspirin, non-steroidal anti-inflammatory drugs or co-trimoxazole) must be avoided. Improvement is seen within 2~4 weeks. Minor side-effects (e.g. nausea) are common, but liver fibrosis or cirrhosis is a risk long term. Liver damage can be monitored using the serum procollagen III aminopropeptide. Most authorities now regard the morbidity and cost of routine liver biopsy to be unjustified. Methotrexate is also a teratogen.

Retinoids

The vitamin A derivative acitretin (Neotigason) is particularly effective in treating pustular psoriasis and in thinning hyperkeratotic plaques. Acitretin may be used with topical therapies or with UVB or PUVA ('Re-PUVA'), when it allows a more rapid clearance at a lower total dose of UV. Most patients develop minor side-effects, such as dry mucous membranes, itching and peeling skin. More serious complications include hyperostosis, abnormal liver function, hyperlipidaemia and teratogenicity. The last virtually precludes the use of acitretin in women of child-bearing age. Although acitretin has a half-life of 50 days, in some patients it is metabolized to etretinate, a retinoid that takes 2 years to be excreted.

Cyclosporin

Cyclosporin, an immunosuppressant widely used to prevent rejection of organ transplants, is effective in severe psoriasis. It acts by inhibiting T lymphocyte activation and interleukin-2 production. Dose-dependent reversible nephrotoxicity is a side-effect. Blood pressure and kidney function are monitored during treatment. There may be a risk of skin cancer or lymphoma, and concomitant UV treatment is avoided.

Biologic agents and other systemic treatments

Other immunosuppressive drugs can control psoriasis, but they are not as potent as methotrexate.

Hydroxycarbamide has the advantage of not affecting the liver, but it can suppress the bone marrow. Fumaric acid esters are effective in some cases. Biologic agents are very effective but expensive.

Complications

Psoriasis may be complicated by arthropathy, erythroderma and the Koebner phenomenon (Fig. 14-2). It is associated with the metabolic syndrome and an increased risk of cardiovascular disease.

Psoriatic arthropathy

Psoriatic joint disease occurs in 20%~30% of patients with psoriasis and is associated with more severe skin disease. It shows an equal sex ratio and takes three forms:

1. *Asymmetrical arthritis.* A small number of joints are usually involved, with few erosions and good preservation of function.
2. *Symmetrical polyarthritis.* This form is associated with erosions, deformity and loss of function (Fig. 14-11). It is distinguished from rheumatoid arthritis by predominantly affecting distal interphalangeal joints and by the rheumatoid factor test being negative.
3. *Predominant spondylitis.* This type is similar to ankylosing spondylitis and may be accompanied by a peripheral arthritis, although it behaves independently of it.

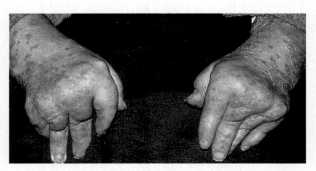

Fig. 14-11 **Severe mutilating symmetrical arthritis with widespread psoriasis.**

Erythrodermic psoriasis

Inpatient treatment is needed for this condition, often with systemic drugs.

Treatment of psoriasis

Side-effects are often the limiting factor in psoriasis treatment.

Topical treatment is usually the first approach:
- ■ *Steroids*: popular and effective but beware of side-effects.
- ■ *Vitamin D analogues*: clean and effective but may irritate.
- ■ *Coal tar*: safe but messy and not very popular with patients.
- ■ *Dithranol*: effective, irritant, rather impractical for home use.
- ■ *Keratolytics*: useful for scalp disease combined with tar or sulphur.

Systemic treatment is used for serious or severe psoriasis:
- ■ *PUVA*: popular but long-term risk of skin cancer.
- ■ *Retinoids*: good for pustular psoriasis and as Re-PUVA; teratogenic.
- ■ *Methotrexate*: a well-established systemic drug; hepatotoxic.
- ■ *Cyclosporin*: effective but potentially nephrotoxic.
- ■ *Biologics*: offer potential for targeted therapy. Expensive.

Web resource

http://www.nhs.uk/Conditions/Psoriasis/Pages/Treatment.aspx

Psoriasis - Biologics

The biological response modifiers are breakthrough treatments for moderate-to-severe psoriasis and for other diseases such as rheumatoid arthritis and Crohn's disease. Biologics are based on recombinant cytokines, fusion proteins or monoclonal antibodies (mouse or human) that bind to tumour necrosis factor-α (TNF-α), cytokine receptors or block T cell receptors to have their effect (Fig. 14-12).

Scientific background

Research has confirmed psoriasis to be an immune-mediated inflammatory disease and has identified associated genes that are involved in immune regulation. These discoveries allow the pharmaceutical industry to design drugs that should work in psoriasis and in other diseases where the pathomechanisms are well understood (Fig. 14-13). The 'biologics'

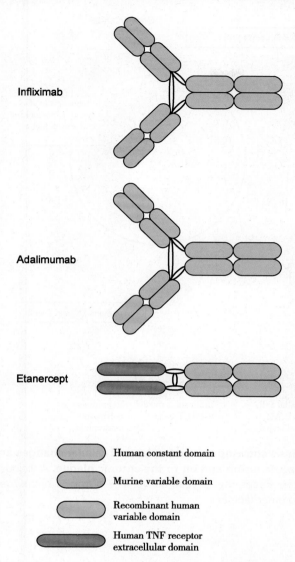

Infliximab

Adalimumab

Etanercept

Human constant domain

Murine variable domain

Recombinant human variable domain

Human TNF receptor extracellular domain

Fig. 14-12   **Diagram of the structure of the biologics.** Infliximab and adalimumab are similar to normal human immunoglobulins. Etanercept contains the extracellular TNF receptor domain fused to parts of the human immunoglobulin heavy chain.

work by having a blocking effect on TNF-α, other cytokines (e.g. interleukin (IL)-12 and -23), dendritic cells and T lymphocytes involved in causing the disease. TNF-α is derived from Th1 cells and mediates inflammation by initiating a cascade of cytokines. IL-12 (derived from dendritic cells) and IL-23 are central to defining T helper cell types and T cell differentiation.

Effects of activated chronic inflammatory cytokines

The chronic inflammatory cytokines that are active

in severe psoriasis may be one reason why patients with the disease have higher rates of cardiovascular morbidity. In addition, some genes associated with psoriasis may predispose to cardiovascular disease and diabetes.

Associated joint disease

Psoriasis is associated with an arthropathy in 20%~30% of cases. Some but not all biologics will improve psoriatic arthritis in addition to the skin disease.

Types of biologic available

The most commonly used biologics for psoriasis are the anti-TNF-α agents *infliximab*, *etanercept* and *adalimumab*, and the anti-IL-12/IL-23 drug *ustekinumab*. The biologics are very effective drugs, producing better responses than agents such as methotrexate. They are given by intravenous infusion or subcutaneous injection, at intervals that vary from twice weekly to once every 3 months. The most commonly used biologics will be discussed individually.

- *Etanercept*: a fusion protein that acts by binding to soluble and receptor-bound TNF-α. It was the first biologic to be approved by the National Institute for Health and Clinical Excellence (NICE) for use in patients whose psoriasis is moderate to severe and has failed to respond to other systemic drugs such as cyclosporin and methotrexate, or photochemotherapy (PUVA). In psoriasis, the severity of skin involvement is measured by the Psoriasis Area and Severity Index (PASI) and the impact on a patient's life by the Dermatology Life Quality Index (DLQI). High scores on both of these parameters are required for the use and funding of this and other biologic drugs within the National Health Service in England, according to NICE. Etanercept is given by subcutaneous injection once or twice weekly (in a dose of 25mg or 50mg).

- *Adalimumab*: a human recombinant IgG1 monoclonal antibody directed against TNF-α approved by NICE and administered by subcutaneous injection (40mg every 2 weeks).

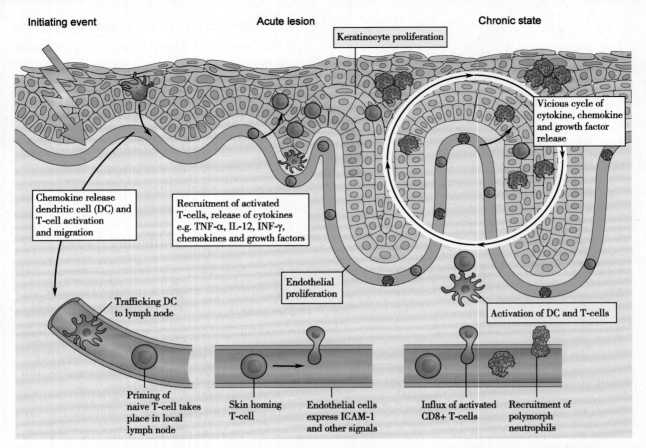

Initiating event Acute lesion Chronic state

Keratinocyte proliferation

Vicious cycle of cytokine, chemokine and growth factor release

Chemokine release dendritic cell (DC) and T-cell activation and migration

Recruitment of activated T-cells, release of cytokines e.g. TNF-α, IL-12, INF-γ, chemokines and growth factors

Endothelial proliferation

Trafficking DC to lymph node

Activation of DC and T-cells

Priming of naive T-cell takes place in local lymph node

Skin homing T-cell

Endothelial cells express ICAM-1 and other signals

Influx of activated CD8+ T-cells

Recruitment of polymorph neutrophils

Fig. 14-13 **A model of the immunopathogenesis of psoriasis showing the molecular and cellular changes as they progress from the intitiating event through to the acute lesion and on to the chronic plaque.** A vicious cycle of release of cytokines, chemokines and growth factors keeps the disease active. The biologics break the cycle by negating the inflammatory action of TNF-α, IL-12 and other factors.

- *Infliximab*: a combined murine and human monoclonal antibody against TNF-α given by intravenous infusion at a dose of 5mg/kg every 8 weeks. It is approved by NICE for severe psoriasis.

- *Ustekinumab*: this human monoclonal biologic blocks the p40 subunit common to IL-12 and IL-23. IL-12 has a critical role in the development of Th1 cells and NK cell activation, whereas IL-23 is necessary for the generation of Th17 cells. Ustekinumab is approved by NICE and is given by subcutaneous injection (45mg or 90mg for patients weighing >100kg) every 12 weeks after a loading regimen.

Pretreatment screening

Prior to initiating treatment, patients are counselled about potential side-effects of biologics (as shown below) and screened for other risk factors, as follows:

- Detailed history to exclude past or present cardiovascular or demyelinating disease and serious infections.

- Note the presence of coexisting joint disease that may influence the selection of biologic.

- Screen for infections including viral hepatitis, HIV and tuberculosis (the latter by chest X-ray and interferon-gamma release assay).

- In females of childbearing age, exclude pregnancy.

Effectiveness of biologics

The biologics show varying degrees of effectiveness in treating psoriasis. Response to treatment can be compared by looking at the proportion of patients treated who achieve a 75% improvement in their PASI score (the 'PASI 75') after 10~12 weeks of bio-

Table 14-3	**Use of biologics in other skin diseases**	
Biologic	**Type**	**Disease treated**
Rituximab	IgG chimeric antibody directed against CD20 that potently depletes B cell numbers. Given as an intravenous infusion	Used successfully in B cell malignancies and in autoimmune diseases including systemic lupus erythematosus, dermatomyositis, systemic sclerosis and pemphigus
Infliximab	Combined murine and human monoclonal antibody against TNF-α	Beneficial off-licence use in hidradenitis suppurativa, pyoderma gangrenosum, sarcoidosis, Behçet's disease and certain types of vasculitis
Omalizumab	Humanized monoclonal antibody that binds to IgE and thus inhibits the binding of IgE to high-affinity receptors on mast cells and basophils	Use is being considered in chronic urticaria and atopic dermatitis. Preliminary results are said to be mixed

logic therapy. If there has been no response after 12~16 weeks, the drug is withdrawn. Etanercept, adalimumab and infliximab are also effective in psoriatic arthritis.

Therapeutic algorithm

Biologics are approved by NICE (in the UK) for use in patients with severe psoriasis who have a PASI >10 and a DLQI >10, and who have failed on (or are intolerant of) standard systemic treatments such as cyclosporin, methotrexate or PUVA. Etanercept, adalimumab and ustekinumab are all approved for use in this situation. If the psoriasis is very severe, inflixumab may be most appropriate as it seems to have a more rapid onset of action. Occasionally methotrexate is used in combination with etanercept or infliximab. Patients who have failed on one biologic may be tried on an alternative. Ustekinumab may be an appropriate alternative to etanercept or adalimumab due to its different mode of action.

Side-effects of biologics

The main problems with biologics are related to injection site reactions, serious infections (e.g. reactivation of latent tuberculosis), cancers, demyelination and cardiovascular events. Occasionally biologics actually cause a worsening of psoriasis. They are expensive in comparison to other treatments. Generally the biologics are well tolerated by patients.

Use of biologic agents in other skin diseases

These are detailed in Table 14-3.

Biologics

- **Exciting new class of immunologically active drugs:** biologics are selectively directed against the molecular pathways known to be involved in the pathogenesis of psoriasis.
- **Properly controlled clinical trials:** have demonstrated the efficacy of these agents in reducing the severity and extent of psoriasis and in improving quality of life.
- **NICE approval:** in the UK, etanercept, adalimumab and ustekinumab can be used in patients with moderate-to-severe psoriasis who have appropriate PASI and DLQI scores.
- **Infliximab infusion:** is approved for use in more severe cases of resistant psoriasis.
- **Administration:** biologics are given by subcutaneous injection or intravenous infusion. The frequency of dosing is very variable, ranging from twice weekly to once every 3 months.
- **Infliximab in other diseases:** off-licence reports indicate infliximab to be beneficial in severe cases of pyoderma gangrenosum, hidradenitis suppurativa and sarcoidosis.
- **Rituximab:** a biologic that depletes B cells. It can be beneficial in pemphigus and some autoimmune diseases (off-licence use).

Key words

Koebner phenomenon   Koebner 现象

generalized pustular psoriasis   泛发性脓疱型银屑病

guttate psoriasis   点滴状银屑病

erythrodermic psoriasis   红皮病型银屑病

psoriatic arthritis   银屑病关节炎

Review questions

1. What is the etiology and pathogenesis of psoriasis?
2. What are the clinical manifestation and classification of psoriatic arthropathy?
3. What is the topical and systemic treatment of psoriasis?

(Hongzhong Jin)

Chapter 15   Eczema - Basic Principles

Definition

Eczema is a non-infective inflammatory skin condition that shows itching, redness and scaling. Eczema represents a reaction pattern to a variety of stimuli, some of which are recognized but many of which are unknown. Eczema and dermatitis mean the same thing and may be used interchangeably. 'Atopy' defines those with an inherited tendency to develop asthma, allergic rhinitis, conjunctivitis or atopic eczema and is present in 15%~25% of the population. Atopics produce high levels of circulating immunoglobulin (Ig) E antibodies, commonly to inhalant allergens (e.g. house dust mite).

Classification

The current classification of eczema is unsatisfactory in that it is inconsistent. However, it is difficult to provide a suitable alternative as the aetiology of most eczema is not known. Different types of eczema may be recognized by morphology, site or cause. A division into endogenous (due to internal or constitutional factors) and exogenous (due to external contact agents) is convenient (Table 15-1). However, in clinical practice, these distinctions are often blurred and, not infrequently, the eczema cannot be classified. A further division into acute (Fig. 15-1) and chronic (Fig. 15-2) eczema can be made in many cases according to the morphology of the eruption.

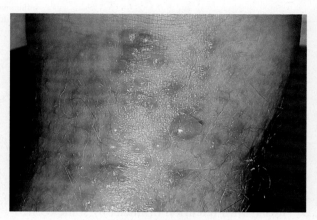

Fig. 15-1   **Acute dermatitis (eczema).** Erythema and oedema are seen with papules, vesicles and sometimes large blisters. Exudation and crust formation follow. The eruption is painful and pruritic. This case resulted from a contact allergy to a locally applied cream.

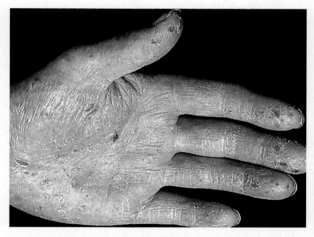

Fig. 15-2   **Chronic dermatitis (eczema).** Lichenification, scaling and fissuring of the hands due to repeated exposure to irritants. Allergic contact dermatitis cannot be excluded on the appearance alone.

Table 15-1 **A classification of eczema**	
Type	**Variety**
Exogenous (contact)	Allergic, irritant Photoreaction
Endogenous	Atopic Seborrhoeic Discoid (nummular) Venous (stasis, gravitational) Pompholyx
Unclassified	Asteatotic (eczéma craquelé) Lichen simplex (neurodermatitis) Juvenile plantar dermatosis

Acute eczema

In acute eczema, epidermal oedema (spongiosis), with separation of keratinocytes, leads to the formation of epidermal vesicles (Fig. 15-3a). Dermal vessels are dilated, and inflammatory cells invade the dermis and epidermis.

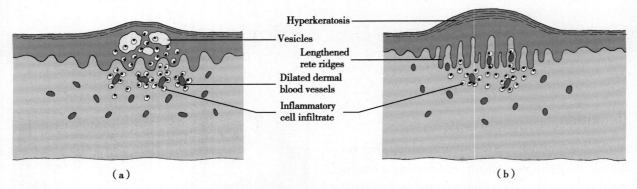

Fig. 15-3 **The histology of (a) acute and (b) chronic dermatitis.**

Chronic eczema

In chronic eczema, there is thickening of the prickle cell layer (acanthosis) and stratum corneum (hyperkeratosis) with retention of nuclei by some corneocytes (parakeratosis) (Fig. 15-3b). The rete ridges are lengthened, dermal vessels dilated and inflammatory mononuclear cells infiltrate the skin.

Contact dermatitis

Definition

Dermatitis precipitated by an exogenous agent, often a chemical, is known as contact dermatitis. It is particularly common in the home, among women with young children and in industry, where it is a major cause of loss of time from work.

Aetiopathogenesis

Irritants cause more cases of contact dermatitis than allergens, although the clinical appearances are often similar. Often, there is an inherited susceptibility to react to irritants. Allergic contact dermatitis is an example of type IV hypersensitivity.

Irritants cause dermatitis in a number of different ways, but usually by a direct noxious effect on the skin's barrier function. The most important irritants are:

- water and other fluids
- abrasives, i.e. frictional irritancy
- chemicals, e.g. acids and alkalis
- solvents, soaps and detergents.

A strong irritant causing necrosis of epidermal cells will produce a reaction within hours but, in most cases, the effect is more chronic. Repetitive and cumulative exposure over several months or years to water, abrasives and chemicals can induce dermatitis, commonly on the hands. Individuals with a history of atopic eczema are more susceptible to irritants.

Clinical presentation

Contact dermatitis may affect any part of the body, although the hands and face are common sites. The appearance of a dermatitis at a particular site (Fig. 15-4) suggests contact with certain objects. For example, an eczema on the wrist of a woman with a history of reacting to cheap earrings suggests a nickel allergic response to a watchstrap buckle (Fig. 15-5). Diagnosis is often not easy as a history of irritant or allergen exposure is not always forthcoming. Knowing the patient's occupation, hobbies, past history and use of cosmetics or medicaments helps in listing possible causes.

Nickel sensitivity is the commonest contact allergy, affecting 10% of women and 1% of men. Usually, it causes only an inconvenient eczema at jewellery or metal contact sites, but an industrial dermatitis can result, e.g. in nickel platers or metal machinists.

Environmental sources of common allergens are shown in Table 15-2. Medicaments and cosmetics can also induce allergic or irritant reactions. Allergic contact dermatitis occasionally becomes generalized by secondary 'autosensitization' spread. Activation by ultraviolet (UV) radiation of a topical agent, e.g. UV

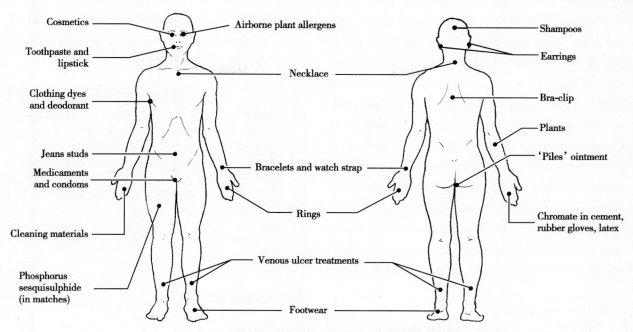

Fig. 15-4 **Distribution clues for contact dermatitis.**

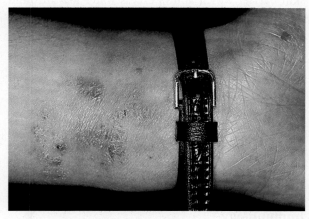

Fig. 15-5 **Allergic contact dermatitis to nickel in a watchstrap buckle.**

Table 15-2	**The sources of common allergens**
Allergen	**Source**
Chromate	Cement, tanned leather, primer paint, anticorrosives
Cobalt	Pigment, paint, ink, metal alloys
Colophonium	Glue, plasticizer, adhesive tape, varnish, polish
Epoxy resins	Adhesive plastics, mouldings
Fragrances	Cosmetics, creams, soaps, deodorants, aromatherapy
Nickel	Jewellery, zips, fasteners, scissors, instruments
Paraphenylenediamine	Dye (clothing, hair), shoes, colour developer
Plants	*Primula obconica*, chrysanthemums, garlic, poison ivy/oak (USA)
Preservatives	Cosmetics, creams and oils
Rubber chemicals	Gloves, clothing, shoes, masks, tyres, condoms

sunscreen filters or previously some perfumes, produces a photocontact reaction in sun-exposed sites.

Differential diagnosis

Contact dermatitis of the hands needs to be differentiated from endogenous eczema, latex contact urticaria, psoriasis and fungal infection. Acute contact dermatitis of the face may resemble angioedema or erysipelas.

Management

The management of contact dermatitis is not always easy because of the many and often overlapping factors that can be involved in any one case. The *identification* of any offending allergen or irritant is the overriding objective. *Patch testing* helps to identify any allergens involved and is particularly useful in dermatitis of the face, hands and feet. The exclusion of an offending allergen from the environment is desirable and, if this can be achieved, the dermatitis may clear.

However, it is difficult to eliminate fully all contact with ubiquitous allergens such as fragrance or colophonium. Similarly, irritants are often impossible to exclude. Some contact with irritants may be inevitable owing to the nature of certain jobs, but occupational hygiene can often be improved. Unnecessary contact with irritants should be limited, protective clothing worn (notably nitrile gloves) and adequate washing and drying facilities provided. *Barrier creams* are seldom the answer, although they do encourage personal skin care. *Topical steroids* (moderately potent or potent) help in contact dermatitis, but avoidance measures should predominate.

Contact dermatitis

- **Irritant factors of various types** cause more contact dermatitis than allergens.
- **Irritant contact dermatitis**, in many cases, can be difficult to distinguish from allergic or endogenous eczema on morphological grounds alone.
- **Atopics and those with 'a sensitive skin'** are more susceptible to the effects of irritants.
- **Patch testing** is helpful to confirm allergic contact dermatitis, particularly of the face, hands and feet. Specific immunoglobulin (Ig) E tests or prick tests may also be needed, e.g. for latex.
- **Common allergens:** nickel, rubber chemicals, fragrances, chromate, cobalt, colophonium, preservatives, plant allergens and paraphenylenediamine.
- **Common irritants:** water, frictional abrasives, chemicals (especially alkalis), solvents, oils, detergents, soaps, low humidity and temperature extremes.
- **Elimination and avoidance** of allergens and irritants are useful, although prevention is the ideal.

Web resource

http://www.eczema.org/

Eczema - Atopic eczema

Definition

Atopic eczema is predominantly a disease of childhood that gives rise to poorly demarcated chronic pruritic papular inflammation of the skin. Uncontrollable scratching is prominent. Most cases improve with age, although approximately 50% of children retain evidence of the condition into adult life. For diagnostic criteria, see Table 15-3.

Table 15-3　**Diagnostic criteria for atopic dermatitis**
Evidence of itchy skin, or parental report of scratching or rubbing plus three or more of the following:
■ History of involvement of the skin creases.
■ History of asthma or hay fever (or first-degree relative if under 4 years).
■ History of generally dry skin in the past year.
■ Onset under 2 years old (not used if child is under 4 years).
■ Visible rash on the flexures (including face if under 4 years).

Aetiopathogenesis

Skin barrier

Individuals with atopic eczema have an impaired skin barrier which allows excess water loss through the skin (drying effect) and an increased potential for exogenous irritants and allergens to penetrate (inducing inflammation). Discovery of a strong association between loss-of-function mutations in the gene encoding filaggrin, which is a skin barrier protein expressed in the outer layers of the epidermis, and individuals with atopic eczema has shown how critical epidermal function is to development of atopic eczema.

Immunology

Individuals with atopic eczema make aberrant immune responses to environmental allergens which become skewed towards Th2 responses, inducing allergen-specific IgE production. The basic cause of these immune defects is still unclear. However, the serum IgE is normal in 20% of atopic eczema subjects.

Incidence

About 20%~30% of UK infants are affected. The condition usually starts within the first 6 months of life and, by 1 year, 60% of those likely to develop atopic eczema will have done so. Two-thirds have a family history of atopy. Remission occurs within 10~20 years in 40%~60%, although some relapse later.

Clinical presentation

The appearance of atopic eczema differs depending on the age of the patient.

Infancy

Babies develop an itchy vesicular exudative eczema on the face (Fig. 15-6), head and hands, often with secondary infection. About half continue to have eczema beyond 18 months.

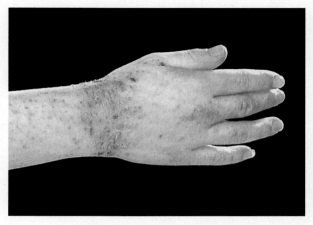

Fig. 15-7   **Atopic eczema in a child, showing excoriations and lichenification at the wrist.**

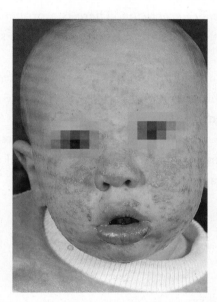

Fig. 15-6   **Atopic eczema in an infant.** Secondary bacterial infection was present.

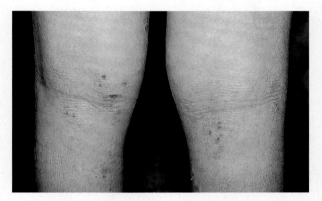

Fig. 15-8   **Atopic eczema involving the popliteal fossa in a child.**

Childhood

After 18 months, the pattern often changes to the familiar involvement of the flexures (antecubital and popliteal fossae, neck, wrists and ankles) (Figs 15-7 and 15-8). The face often shows erythema and infra-orbital folds. Lichenification, excoriations and dry skin (Fig. 15-9) are common, and palmar markings may be increased. Postinflammatory hyperpigmentation occurs in those with dark skin. Scratching and rubbing cause most of the clinical signs and are a particular problem at night when they can interfere with sleep. Behavioural difficulties can occur, and a child's eczema can disrupt family life. Occasionally, a 'reverse pattern' of eczema is seen, with involvement of the extensor aspects of the knees and elbows.

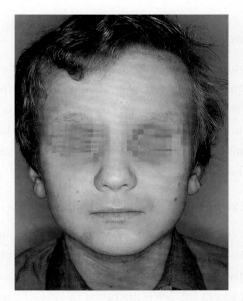

Fig. 15-9   **A 'dry' pruritic type of atopic eczema.** Note the loss of eyebrows due to constant rubbing of the face.

Adulthood

The commonest manifestation in adult life is hand dermatitis, exacerbated by irritants, in someone with a past history of atopic eczema. However, a small number of adults have a chronic severe form of generalized and lichenified atopic eczema (Fig. 15-10), which may interfere with their employment and social activities. Stressful situations, such as examinations or marital problems, often coincide with exacerbations.

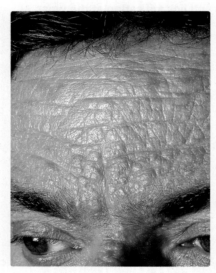

Fig. 15-10 **Grossly lichenified and nodular atopic eczema on the face of an adult.**

Differential diagnosis

Infantile seborrhoeic eczema may sometimes develop into the atopic variety and, occasionally, the distinction from scabies is necessary. Rarely, infants with immune deficiency syndromes (e.g. Wiskott-Aldrich) or with Langerhans cell histiocytosis have an eczematous eruption.

Investigations

Prick tests or the allergen-specific IgE tests to inhalant and (sometimes) food allergens are frequently positive, although the relevance is often unclear. Total serum IgE levels are raised in 80% of patients. Swabs for bacterial and viral culture may be helpful during an exacerbation.

Complications

Atopic eczema is subject to several complications - some common and some rare:

- ■ *Bacterial infection.* Most individuals with atopic eczema are colonized with *Staphylococcus aureus* and invasive infection is a common cause of disease exacerbations.
- ■ *Viral infection.* Patients have an increased susceptibility to infection with molluscum contagiosum and possibly with viral warts.
- ■ *Eczema herpeticum.* There is a propensity to develop widespread lesions with herpes simplex (Fig. 15-11).
- ■ *Cataracts.* A specific form of cataract infrequently develops in young adults with severe atopic eczema.
- ■ *Growth retardation.* Children with severe atopic eczema may have short stature. Topical steroid therapy is unlikely to be causal.

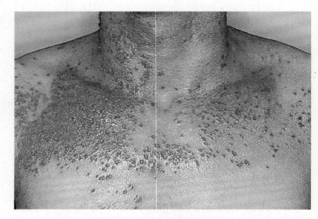

Fig. 15-11 **Eczema herpeticum.** Herpes simplex infection complicating atopic eczema.

Management

General measures include explaining the disorder and its treatment to the patient and the parents, stressing the normally good prognosis. Nails should be kept short. The exclusion of house dust mite from the home environment is difficult. Careers advice to avoid wet work jobs (e.g. nursing, hairdressing, cleaning) and those with exposure to irritant oils is important. Some sufferers obtain support from groups such as the National Eczema Society.

Specific treatments for atopic eczema are summarized in Table 15-4.

Table 15-4	Treatment of atopic eczema
Treatment	**Indication**
Emollients	Most eczema; ichthyosis
Topical steroids	Most types of eczema
Topical tacrolimus	Steroid-resistant eczema
Tar bandage	Lichenified/excoriated eczema
Oral antihistamine	Pruritus
Oral antibiotic	Bacterial superinfection
Exclusion diet	Food allergy/resistant eczema
UVB, ciclosporin and azathioprine	Resistant and severe eczema unresponsive to topical therapy

Topical therapy

Washing and emollient therapy

Soap and 'bubbly' products should be completely avoided. Emollients should be used regularly on the skin and to wash with. They moisturize the dry skin, diminishing the desire to scratch and reducing the need for topical steroids. The greasy emollients (ointments) are more effective at repairing the skin barrier and therefore are usually more effective. Creams containing antiseptics such as chlorhexidine and bath oils may also help.

Topical steroids and calcineurin inhibitors

In children, 1% hydrocortisone ointment applied twice a day is usually adequate (ointments are generally preferred to creams for eczema). Moderate potency steroid may be used for a short time in children with resistant eczema, and for more prolonged periods in adults. Steroids in conjunction with topical antibiotics may be of help in infected eczema. Tacrolimus ointment (0.03% children, 0.1% adults) or pimecrolimus are alternatives to steroids, especially in facial and hand eczema.

Therapeutic bandaging/clothing

Coal tar or ichthammol paste bandages normally left on overnight are useful for lichenified or excoriated eczema. Wet wraps or dry wraps are often required for a short time on an exudative eczema. Elasticated or silk impregnated clothing are often well tolerated and useful in children. Wool clothing irritates and should be avoided.

Systemic therapy

Sedative antihistamines, given at night, are helpful principally through the sedative effect. Infected exacerbations frequently require the intermittent use of an oral antistaphylococcal antibiotic. Eczema herpeticum should be assessed urgently and treated with acyclovir. Patients with severe and resistant forms of atopic eczema may be treated with narrow-band UVB, azathioprine or ciclosporin.

Dietary manipulation

Symptoms such as urticaria or angioedema following ingestion of food should be investigated by a specialist with an interest in allergy but routine testing for specific IgE does not reliably predict those foods that may exacerbate eczema. Eczema around the mouth or perianal region, gastrointestinal symptoms and failure to thrive are suggestive of food allergy relevant to eczema. Dietician-supervised exclusion diets are reserved for a minority who have not improved with standard therapy.

> **Atopic eczema**
> - Affects 20%~30% of UK infants: onset at less than 1 year in 60% of cases.
> - Loss of skin barrier function including filaggrin mutations is central to the disease pathogenesis.
> - Classically affects the face in infants, later knee and elbow flexures.
> - Itch-scratch cycle induces lichenification.
> - Exacerbations are often due to infection, particularly staphylococcal.
> - Treatment involves emollients, topical steroids, tacrolimus, clothing, systemic antihistamines and antibiotics.

Web resource

http://guidance.nice.org.uk/CG57

Eczema - Other Forms

The other main types of eczema are seborrhoeic, discoid, venous, asteatotic and hand dermatitis.

Seborrhoeic dermatitis

Seborrhoeic dermatitis is a chronic, red, scaly, inflammatory eruption usually affecting the scalp and face (Table 15-5).

Table 15-5 Differential diagnosis of seborrhoeic dermatitis	
Site of seborrhoeic dermatitis	Differential diagnosis
Face	Psoriasis, contact dermatitis, rosacea
Scalp	Psoriasis, fungal infection
Trunk	Psoriasis, pityriasis versicolor, fungal infection

Aetiopathogenesis

Sebum production is normal, but the eruption often occurs in the sebaceous gland areas of the scalp, face and chest. Endogenous and genetic factors, and an overgrowth of the commensal yeast *Malassezia* (previously *Pityrosporum ovale*) are involved. The condition is severe in some patients with HIV infection.

Clinical presentation

There are four common patterns:

1. *Scalp and facial involvement.* Excessive dandruff, with an itchy scaly erythematous eruption affecting the sides of the nose, scalp margin, eyebrows and ears (Fig. 15-12). Blepharitis may occur. Most common in young adult males.

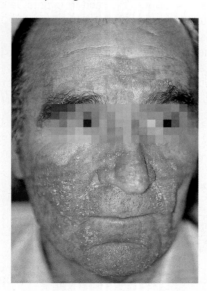

Fig. 15-12 **Seborrhoeic dermatitis affecting the face.**

2. *Petaloid.* A dry, scaly patch of eczema over the presternal area.
3. *Pityrosporum folliculitis.* An erythematous follicular eruption with papules or pustules over the back (Fig. 15-13).
4. *Flexural.* Involvement of the axillae, groin and submammary areas by a moist intertrigo, often secondarily colonized by *Candida albicans*. Seen in the elderly (do not confuse with the similarly named infantile eruption).

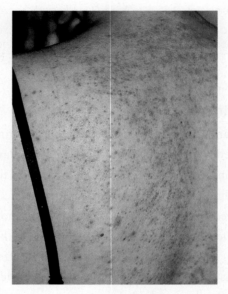

Fig. 15-13 **Seborrhoeic dermatitis of the *Pityrosporum* folliculitis type affecting the back.**

Management

The scalp lesions require the use of a medicated shampoo (e.g. containing coal tar, selenium sulphide or ketoconazole), either alone or following the application of 2% sulphur and 2% salicylic acid cream left on for several hours. Facial, truncal and flexural involvement responds to an imidazole or antimicrobial, often combined with 1% hydrocortisone, in a cream or ointment base. Oral itraconazole is also effective. Recurrence is common and repeated treatment often necessary.

Discoid (nummular) eczema

Discoid eczema is an eczema of unknown aetiology characterized by coin-shaped lesions on the limbs; it typically affects middle-aged or elderly men (Fig.

15-14). Younger subjects, especially in dark skin types, may have atopic eczema.

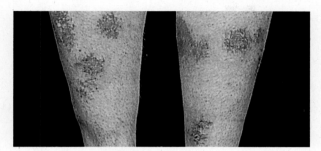

Fig. 15-14　**Discoid eczema of the lower leg.**

Clinical presentation

The coin-shaped eczema lesions are often symmetrical and can be intensely itchy. The eczema may be vesicular or chronic and lichenified. It may clear after a few weeks, but tends to recur. Secondary bacterial infection is common.

Management

The condition can often be confused with tinea corporis and contact dermatitis. A potent or very potent topical steroid, often combined with an antimicrobial or antibiotic, is helpful.

Venous (stasis) eczema

Venous eczema affects the lower legs (Fig. 15-15) and is associated with underlying venous disease. Incompetence of the deep perforating veins increases hydrostatic pressure in dermal capillaries. Pericapillary fibrin deposition impedes oxygen diffusion and leads to clinical changes.

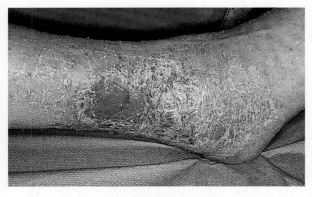

Fig. 15-15　**Venous eczema.**

Clinical presentation

Most patients are middle-aged or elderly women. Leashes of venules and haemosiderin pigmentation around the ankles are early signs. Eczema develops, sometimes with fibrosis of the dermis and subcutaneous tissue (lipodermatosclerosis) and ulceration. Contact allergy to an applied medicament can complicate the picture.

Management

An emollient, alone or with a mild or moderately potent steroid ointment, is needed. Tar-impregnated bandages applied once or twice a week are useful, especially when ulceration coexists. Venous disease or ulceration is treated on its own merit.

Hand dermatitis

Hand dermatitis is a common, often recurrent condition that varies from being acute and vesicular to chronic, hyperkeratotic and fissured. The condition results from a variety of causes, and several factors are often involved. In children, hand dermatitis is mostly due to atopic eczema. An atopic predisposition often underlies adult hand dermatitis, especially if caused by repeated exposure to irritants.

Allergic causes need excluding, and most adults with hand dermatitis require patch testing. Fungal infection is ruled out by microscopy and culture, especially in unilateral hand dermatitis, and the feet are examined because tinea pedis can provoke a hand dermatitis as an 'id' phenomenon. A core of patients are left who have an endogenous recurrent hand dermatitis often characterized by sago-like vesicles on the sides of the fingers, on the palms and sometimes on the soles.

Clinical presentation

Hand dermatitis often presents as a chronic eczema, but may appear as a vesicular eruption known as *pompholyx*. Vesicles may be seen with atopic eczema or contact dermatitis but, in pompholyx, there is usually no associated disorder. The onset is in young adults, particularly in warm weather, and it is often recurrent. Involvement can be confined to a few microvesicles on the fingers, or it can be extensive with bullae affecting the whole hand (Fig. 15-16). Some of these patients are nickel sensitive.

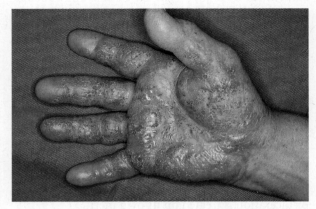

Fig. 15-16 **Acute pompholyx involving the entire palmar surface of the hand in a nickel-sensitive woman.**

Management

Acute pompholyx requires drainage of large blisters and the application (once or twice a day) of wet dressings (e.g. immersed in 0.01% aqueous potassium permanganate or Burow's solution of 0.65% aqueous aluminium acetate). Oral antibiotics are given if bacterial infection is present. Some dermatologists prescribe systemic steroids, but these are usually not necessary. Once the acute stage settles, potent or highly potent steroid lotions or creams are used with cotton gloves. For chronic or subacute cases, a steroid ointment and emollients are helpful. Advice for patients with hand dermatitis is given in Table 15-6. Alitretinoin has recently been licensed for severe chronic hand eczema refractory to potent topical corticosteroids.

Asteatotic eczema (eczéma craquelé)

Asteatotic eczema is a dry eczema with fissuring and cracking of the skin, often affecting the limbs in the elderly (Fig. 15-17).

Overwashing of patients in institutions, a dry winter climate, hypothyroidism and the use of diuretics can contribute to eczema in the atrophic skin of old people. The skin of the limbs and trunk is erythema-

Table 15-6 **Hints on hand care for patients with hand dermatitis**
Hand washing Use warm water and unscented soap; avoid paper towels and hot air dryers; instead use a dry cotton towel.
Protection Avoid wet work if possible, or otherwise wear cotton gloves under vinyl or nitrile gloves; wear gloves in cold weather and for dusty work.
Medicaments Use emollients regularly throughout the day; apply steroid ointments twice a day.
Avoid handling Shampoos, hair preparations, detergents, solvents, polishes, certain vegetables (e.g. tomatoes, potatoes), peeling fruits (e.g. oranges) and cutting raw meat.

tous, dry and itchy and shows a fine crazy-paving pattern of fissuring. Emollients applied to the skin and used in the bath often suffice to clear up the condition, but sometimes a mild steroid is necessary.

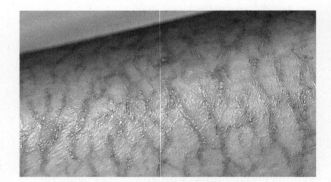

Fig. 15-17 **Asteatotic eczema.**

Other eczemas

Other types of eczema are occasionally encountered. They include: lichen simplex chronicus, lichen striatus, juvenile plantar dermatosis and napkin (diaper) eruption.

Lichen simplex chronicus (neurodermatitis)

Neurodermatitis is an area of lichenified eczema due to repeated rubbing or scratching, as a habit or due to 'stress'. It usually occurs as a single plaque on the lower leg, back of the neck or in the perineum (*pruritus vulvae/ani*). The skin markings are exaggerated, and pigmentation may occur. Asian and Chinese people are particularly susceptible. Sometimes a nodular lichenification known as *prurigo nodularis* develops on the shins and forearms. Emollients, topical steroids, weak tar paste and tar-impregnated bandages are the mainstay of treatment.

Lichen striatus

Lichen striatus is a rare self-limiting linear eczema affecting a limb and occurring in adolescents.

Eczema

- **Seborrhoeic dermatitis** commonly affects the scalp and face. It responds to combined antimicrobial/hydrocortisone creams.
- **Discoid eczema** often presents as coin-shaped lesions on limbs of the middle-aged or elderly. It improves with moderate potency topical steroids.
- **Venous eczema** is associated with venous disease. It responds to emollients and low or moderate potency topical steroids.
- **Hand dermatitis:** multiple and mixed aetiology; determine causes by exclusion.
- **Asteatotic eczema:** the eczéma craquelé of elderly skin. Treat with emollients or low potency topical steroids.
- **Lichen simplex chronicus:** an area of lichenified eczema induced by persistent scratching, often found on the posterior neck or lower leg.
- **Lichen striatus:** a rare linear eczema.

Web resource

http://www.merckmanuals.com/professional/sec11.html

Key words

eczema   湿疹
contact dermatitis   接触性皮炎
irritant contact dermatitis   刺激性接触性皮炎
allergic contact dermatitis   变应性接触性皮炎
patch test   斑贴试验
endogenous eczema   内源性湿疹
exogenous eczema   外源性湿疹
pompholyx   汗疱疹
atopic eczema   特应性湿疹
pruritus   瘙痒
filaggrin gene   丝聚蛋白基因
skin barrier   皮肤屏障
allergen-specific IgE   变应原特异性 IgE
prick test   点刺试验
food allergy   食物过敏
eczema herpeticum   疱疹性湿疹
staphylococcus aureus colonization   金黄色葡萄球菌定植
seborrhoeic dermatitis   脂溢性皮炎
discoid eczema   盘状湿疹
lichen simplex chronicus   慢性单纯性苔藓
asteatotic eczema   乏脂性湿疹
lichen striatus   线状苔藓
prurigo nodularis   结节性痒疹

Review questions

1. What's the main clinical presentation of contact dermatitis?
2. Please describe the main characteristic manifestation of atopic dermatitis in different stages.
3. What are the main treatment strategies for atopic dermatitis?
4. What are the diagnostic criteria for atopic dermatitis?
5. What is the differential diagnosis for seborrhoeic dermatitis?

(Qing Sun)

Chapter 16 Lichenoid eruptions

Lichen planus and other disorders with a lichenoid appearance of shiny flat-topped papules are presented here.

Lichen planus

Lichen planus is a relatively common pruritic papular dermatosis involving the flexor surfaces, mucous membrane and genitalia. Two-thirds of cases occur in the 30~60-year-old age group. It is uncommon at the extremes of age, and the sex incidence is equal.

The cause is unknown, but an immune pathogenesis for lichen planus is suspected as T cells infiltrate the skin, immunoglobulin M is found at the dermo-epidermal junction, a lichenoid eruption is part of graft-versus-host diseaseand there is an association with some autoimmune diseases.

Pathology

In lichen planus, the granular layer is thickened, basal cells show liquefaction degeneration and lymphocytes infiltrate the upper dermis in a band-like fashion (Fig. 16-1).

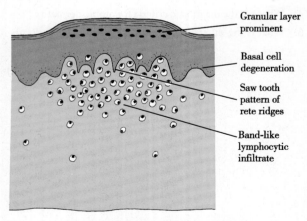

Granular layer prominent

Basal cell degeneration

Saw tooth pattern of rete ridges

Band-like lymphocytic infiltrate

Fig. 16-1 **Histopathology of lichen planus.**

Clinical presentation

Lichen planus tends to start on the limbs. It may spread rapidly to become generalized within 4 weeks, but the commoner localized forms progress more slowly. Typical lesions are very itchy flat-topped polygonal papules, a few millimetres in diameter, which may show a surface network of delicate white lines (Wickham striae). Initially, the papules are red, but they become violaceous (Fig. 16-2).

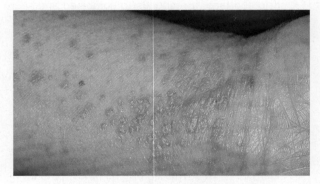

Fig. 16-2 **Typical violaceous papules of lichen planus at the wrist.**

The eruption is symmetrical and affects:
- the forearms and wrists
- the lower legs and thighs
- the genitalia, mucous membranes
- the palms and soles.

Mucous membrane involvement, especially of the buccal mucosa, occurs in up to two-thirds of cases, and may be present without skin lesions (Fig. 16-3). Large lacy white network on buccal mucosa, less often on tongue, lips or labial mucosa. Painful erosions also present, often on hard palate. Similar reticulate pattern with erosions can be seen on genital mucosa. Lichen planus also shows the Koebner phenomenon which may explain some linear lesions. Follicular and other variants are found (see below). In most cases, papules flatten after a few months to leave pigmentation, but some become hypertrophic. Half of all patients are clear within 9 months, but 15% have continuing symptoms even after 18 months. Up to 20% have a further attack. Lichen planus may be confused with other conditions, as shown in Table 16-1.

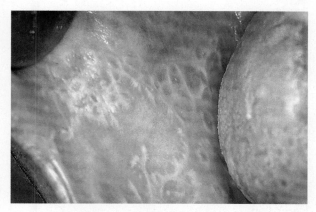

Fig. 16-3 **White lace-like Wickham striae on the buccal mucosa.**

Table 16-1	**Differential diagnosis: lichen planus**
Type of lichen planus	**Differential diagnosis**
Generalized	Lichenoid drug eruption, Guttate psoriasis, Atypical pityriasis rosea
Genital	Psoriasis, scabies, Lichen sclerosus
Hypertrophic	Lichen simplex

Complications

Lichen planus may be complicated by the following:

■ *Nail involvement.* Found in 10% of patients. Longitudinal grooving and pitting are reversible, but dystrophic/atrophic lesions can produce scarring or permanent nail loss.

■ *Scalp lesions.* May be follicular, but pseudopelade-like permanent scarring alopecia is more common.

■ *Malignant change.* Very infrequent.

Management

Lichen planus disease is self-limiting in most patients. There is no specific therapy for lichen planus. Moderate to high potency topical steroids usually produce symptomatic improvement. Oral lesions are helped by a steroid-containing paste (e.g. Adcortyl in Orabase) or topical tacrolimus. Hypertrophic lichen planus may require highly potent topical steroids, sometimes under occlusion, or intralesional steroid injection. Extensive involvement, ulcerative mucous membrane lesions or a potentially scarring nail dystrophy warrant a trial of oral prednisolone (in a dose of 10~20mg/day) for 1~3 months. Long-term systemic steroids are not justified. Acitretin or psoralen with ultraviolet A (PUVA) may help resistant cases.

Lichen sclerosus

Lichen sclerosus is an uncommon disorder typified by white lichenoid atrophic lesions on the genitalia. Although associated with autoimmune disease, the cause is unknown.

Pathology

The upper dermis is oedematous with few cells; collagen is hyalinized. Lymphocytes infiltrate the lower dermis.

Clinical presentation

Lichen sclerosus occurs 10 times more frequently in women. It is commonest in middle age, although it may develop in childhood (with a better prognosis). Genital lesions are almost invariable, but involvement of the trunk or arms is seen. Individual lesions are a few millimetres in diameter, porcelain white and slightly atrophic, and may aggregate into wrinkled plaques (Fig. 16-4). Hyperkeratosis, telangiectasia, purpura and even blistering occur. Vulval and perianal lesions cause itching and soreness. Involvement in the male results in urethral stricture and phimosis

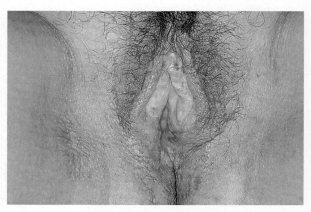

Fig. 16-4 **Lichen sclerosus of the vulva.**

(balanitis xerotica obliterans). Occasionally, lesions are found in the mouth. Lichen sclerosus is chronic and usually permanent in adults. Spontaneous resolution is most likely at puberty in childhood cases.

Differential diagnosis

Female genital involvement may resemble lichen simplex chronicus, Bowen's disease and extramammary Paget's disease. Male genital lesions mimic lichen planus, psoriasis and some rare inflammatory and premalignant forms of balanitis.

Complications

Shrinkage of the vulva occurs, and dyspareunia is a problem in females. Males may experience recurrent balanitis and ulceration of the glans. Squamous cell carcinoma develops infrequently in the longstanding lesions of both sexes.

Management

Non-genital lesions require no treatment. In female genital involvement, a moderate or potent strength steroid cream will reduce the itch and prevent scarring. Vulvectomy is contraindicated in uncomplicated cases.

Treatment is similar for the male genital lesions, although circumcision is performed if phimosis develops. Both sexes need long-term follow-up and biopsy of any suspicious areas.

Lichen planus-like drug eruption

An eruption resembling lichen planus can follow the ingestion of several drugs.

Clinical presentation

A lichen planus-like rash has been recognized with gold and mepacrine therapy for many years. The eruption, which can be severe, is often more 'psoriasiform' and hyperpigmented than true lichen planus (Fig.16-5) and, on histology, shows a greater number of eosinophils. Resolution after withdrawal of the drug is often slow. Table 16-2 lists some of the drugs responsible.

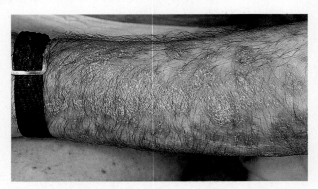

Fig. 16-5   **A lichenoid drug eruption with psoriasiform features, here due to quinine.**

Table 16-2   **Drugs causing a lichen planus-like eruption**

Type of agent	Drug
Antiarthritic	Gold, penicillamine, non-steroidal anti-inflammatory drugs
Antibiotic	Streptomycin, tetracyclines
Antimalarial	Chloroquine, mepacrine, quinine
Antituberculous	Isoniazid, ethambutol
Diuretic	Thiazides, furosemide
Antihypertensive	Captopril, enalapril, beta-blockers, amlodipine
Antidiabetic	Tolbutamide, chlorpropamide
Antipsychotic	Phenothiazines, lithium
Statin	Simvastatin, pravastatin

Lichenoid eruptions

■ **Lichen planus** is a relatively common pruritic papular eruption, which resolves in most cases within 18 months.
■ **Lichen planus-like drug eruption** resembles lichen planus but is more persistent; it is seen, for example, with gold, chloroquine and thiazides.
■ **Lichen sclerosus** is most common in women, and frequently affects the genitalia. Vulval shrinkage may occur. Topical steroids are helpful. There is a risk of malignant change.

Web resource

http://emedicine.medscape.com/article/1123213-overview

Key words

lichen planus   扁平苔藓
Wickham striae   威克姆纹
hypertrophic lichen planus   肥厚性扁平苔藓

Review qusetions

1. The typical manifestation of what kind of disease is Wickham striae?

2. Why the incidence of lichen sclerosis of the female is more than male?

3. What is the most effective treatment for lichen planus?

Chapter 17   Papulosquamous eruptions

Papulosquamous eruptions are raised, scaly and marginated, and include psoriasis, lichen planus and other conditions listed in Table 17-1. Eczema is not included as it does not usually have a sharp edge. These eruptions are not related aetiologically. Several are characterized by fine scaling and have the prefix 'pityriasis', which means 'bran-like scale'.

Table 17-1   **Papulosquamous eruptions**
Chronic superficial dermatitis
Drug eruption
Lichen planus
Pityriasis rubra pilaris
Pityriasis versicolor
Pityriasis alba
Pityriasis lichenoides
Pityriasis rosea
Psoriasis
Reiter's disease
Secondary syphilis
Tinea infection

Pityriasis rosea

Pityriasis rosea is an acute, self-limiting disorder probably infective in origin, characterized by scaly oval papules and plaques that occur mainly on the trunk.

Clinical presentation

The generalized eruption is preceded in most patients by the appearance of a single lesion, 2~5cm in diameter, known as a 'herald patch' (Fig. 17-1). Some days later, many smaller plaques appear, mainly on the trunk but also on the upper arms and thighs. Individual plaques are oval, pink and have a delicate peripheral 'collarette' of scale. They are distributed parallel to the lines of the ribs, radiating away from the spine. Itching is mild or moderate. The eruption fades spontaneously in 4~8 weeks. It tends to affect teenagers and young adults. The cause is unknown, but epidemiological evidence of 'clustering' suggests an infective aetiology.

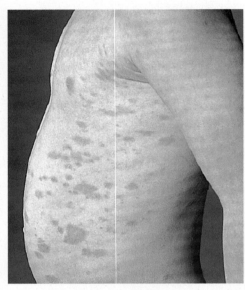

Fig. 17-1   **Pityriasis rosea, showing a herald patch on the lower abdomen and associated oval scaly plaques.**

Differential diagnosis and management

Guttate psoriasis, pityriasis versicolor and secondary syphilis may cause confusion. A serological test for syphilis is needed in doubtful cases. The condition is self-limiting, and treatment does not hasten clearance, although a moderate potency topical steroid can help to relieve pruritus.

Pityriasis (tinea) versicolor

Pityriasis versicolor is a chronic, often asymptomatic, fungal infection characterized by pigmentary changes and involving the trunk.

Clinical presentation

The condition is caused by overgrowth of the mycelial form of the commensal yeast *Malassezia* (previously *Pityrosporum ovale*) and is particularly common in humid or tropical conditions. In Europe, it mainly affects young adults, appearing on the trunk and proximal parts of the limbs (Fig. 17-2). In untanned, white caucasians, brown or pinkish oval or round superficially scaly patches are seen, but, in tanned or racially pigmented skin, hypopigmentation is found as a result of the release by the organism of dicarboxylic acids that inhibit melanogenesis.

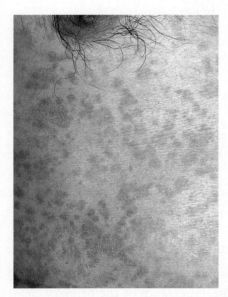

Fig. 17-2 **Pityriasis versicolor on the chest: brown scaly patches are evident.**

Differential diagnosis

Differentiation from vitiligo is important: usually pityriasis versicolor has a fine scale, and scrapings readily show the 'grapes and bananas' appearance of the spores and short hyphae on microscopy. Pityriasis rosea and tinea corporis may occasionally appear similar.

Management

Treatment involves either the topical application of one of the imidazole antifungals (e.g. Canesten or Daktarin cream) or the use of 2.5% selenium sulphide (Selsun) shampoo applied for 30min (or ketoconazole (Nizoral) shampoo applied for 30 min) and showered off (use three times a week for 2 weeks). Itraconazole, 200mg by mouth daily for 7 days, is effective for resistant cases. Recurrences are common, and patients are advised that re-treatment may be required.

Reiter's disease

Reiter's disease is a syndrome of polyarthropathy, urethritis, iritis and a psoriasiform eruption.

Clinical presentation and management

Reiter's disease almost invariably affects males who have the HLA-B27 genotype and commonly follows a genitourinary or bowel infection. The joint and eye changes are often severe. Skin involvement includes a balanitis and red, scaly, pustular, psoriasiform plaques on the feet (keratoderma blenorrhagicum).

Severe skin changes are unresponsive to topical therapy, and methotrexate or acitretin by mouth is often needed.

Chronic superficial dermatitis

Previously known as parapsoriasis, a term best avoided, this is an uncommon chronic dermatitis of small scaly pink-brown oval or round-shaped plaques, mainly on the trunk. The variant with larger plaques may proceed to mycosis fungoides (cutaneous T cell lymphoma) or be this from the onset.

Clinical presentation

In chronic superficial dermatitis, scaly patches develop, usually on the abdomen, buttocks or thighs (Fig. 17-3). The onset is in young to mid-adult life, and the plaques are indolent. It may be difficult to

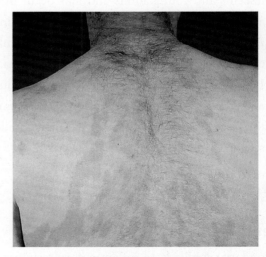

Fig. 17-3 **Plaques of chronic superficial dermatitis on the back of a middle-aged man.**

predict which cases will progress to mycosis fungoides, especially as the evolution may take place over many years, but the 'benign' lesions tend to be small and finger-like in shape, whereas the 'premalignant' plaques are larger, asymmetrical, atrophic and can show associated poikiloderma (reticulate pigmentation, telangiectasia and atrophy). Biopsy is necessary to look for the changes of mycosis fungoides, and further biopsy of any changed area is required. The disease is often indolent and may persist over a period of several years.

Differential diagnosis and management

Psoriasis, discoid eczema and tinea corporis may need to be considered in the diagnosis, but the plaques of chronic superficial dermatitis are distinguished by being fixed.

The first-line treatment with moderately potent topical steroids is sometimes helpful. Ultraviolet B (UVB) or psoralen with UVA (PUVA) will often be needed for the large plaque variant. Long-term follow-up is recommended.

Other pityriases

Other varieties of pityriasis include the following:
- *Pityriasis lichenoides.* A rare chronic eruption in which small papules topped by a fine single scale appear on the limbs and trunk. It is seen in adolescents and young adults and may occur in an acute form (Fig. 17-4), which heals with scarring.
- *Pityriasis rubra pilaris.* A rare, scaly follicular eruption, which may progress to erythroderma.
- *Pityriasis alba.* Occurs in children or young adults and is characterized by fine scaly white patches on the face or arms. It is a type of eczema and often seen in atopic patients.

Secondary syphilis

Definition

Secondary syphilis is an inflammatory response in the skin and mucous membranes to the disseminated

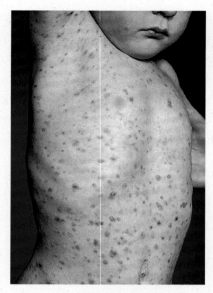

Fig. 17-4 **Pityriasis lichenoides (acute type) in a child.**

Treponema pallidum spirochaete. There has been a resurgence of syphilis in recent years.

Clinical presentation

The secondary phase of syphilis starts 4~12 weeks after the appearance of the primary chancre and consists of an eruption, lymphadenopathy and variable malaise. Pink or copper-coloured macules, which later develop into papules, appear in a symmetrical distribution on the trunk and limbs and are non-itchy (Fig. 17-5). Annular patterns are not

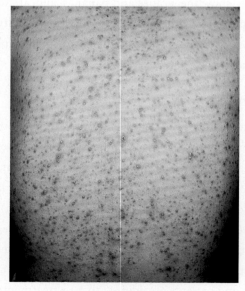

Fig. 17-5 **Secondary syphilis.** Coppery red-coloured macules and papules are evident on the trunk.

uncommon, and involvement of the palms and soles is distinctive. Other signs are moist warty lesions (condyloma lata) in the anogenital area, buccal erosions that may be arcuate (snail-track ulcers) and a diffuse patchy alopecia. Mucosal lesions are infectious. Without treatment, the lesions of secondary syphilis resolve spontaneously in 1~3 months.

Differential diagnosis and management

Pityriasis rosea, psoriasis, drug eruption, infectious mononucleosis, rubella and measles may need to be considered. Treponemal serology is positive in all patients with secondary syphilis. Treatment is with intramuscular benzathine benzylpenicillin. Patients with syphilis are best managed by physicians familiar with the treatment of genitourinary infections.

Papulosquamous eruptions

- **Pityriasis rosea** is a fairly common self-limiting eruption that involves the trunk of young adults. Scaly oval plaques follow a herald patch. It may be infective in origin.
- **Pityriasis versicolor** is a common truncal eruption of young adults and is due to *Malassezia*, a commensal yeast. It is often revealed in the summer as pale areas adjacent to tanned skin.
- **Reiter's syndrome** typically affects young males and follows a genitourinary or bowel infection. Keratotic skin lesions are seen with eye and joint changes.
- **Chronic superficial dermatitis** is an uncommon truncal eruption seen in young or middle-aged adults. The large plaque variant may represent early cutaneous T cell lymphoma.
- **Pityriasis lichenoides** is a rare chronic eruption of scaly-topped papules on the trunk and limbs. An acute form may scar.
- **Secondary syphilis** is a symmetrical, non-itchy truncal eruption with mucosal and palmar or plantar lesions, due to infection with *Treponema pallidum*.

Web resource

http://emedicine.medscape.com/article/762725-overview

Key words

papulosquamous eruptions　鳞屑性皮损
pityriasis rosea　玫瑰糠疹
pityriasis versicolor　花斑癣
pityriasis lichenoides　苔藓样糠疹
secondary syphilis　二期梅毒

Review questions

1. Describe the clinical presentation of pityriasis rosea.
2. What kind of complications may occur in patients with Reiter's disease?
3. Describe the main points of differential diagnosis of secondary syphilis.

(XiaoYong Man)

Chapter 18   Erythroderma

Definition

Erythroderma or generalized exfoliative dermatitis defines any inflammatory dermatosis with hot, red, oedematous, dry and exfoliating skin that involves all or nearly all the skin surface (sometimes stated as more than 90%). It is a secondary process and represents the generalized spread of a dermatosis or systemic disease throughout the skin.

Clinical presentation

Erythroderma is an uncommon but important dermatological emergency, as the systemic effects are potentially fatal.

General symptoms and signs

Some features are common to all patients with erythroderma, no matter what the cause. It is twice as common in men and mainly affects the middle-aged and elderly. The condition often develops suddenly, particularly when associated with leukaemia or an eczema. A patchy erythema may rapidly spread to be universal within 12~48h and be accompanied by pyrexia, malaise and shivering. Scaling appears 2~6 days later and, at this stage, the skin is hot, red, dry and obviously thickened. The patient experiences irritation and tightness of the skin and feels cold. The exfoliation of scales may be copious and continuous. Scalp and body hair is lost when erythroderma has been present for some weeks. The nails become thickened and may be shed. Pigmentary changes occur and, in those with a dark skin, hypopigmentation is seen. The picture is influenced by the patient's general condition and the underlying cause. The commonest causes of erythroderma are eczema, psoriasis and lymphoma (Table 18-1). Other dermatoses, including drug eruptions and pityriasis rubra pilaris, may also be implicated. Multiple skin biopsies may help in diagnosis.

Table 18-1 Causes of erythroderma and their relative frequencies	
Cause	**Frequency (%)**
Eczema (contact/atopic/seborrhoeic/unclassified)	40
Psoriasis	25
Lymphoma/leukaemia/Sézary syndrome	15
Drug eruption	10
Pityriasis rubra pilaris/ichthyosiform erythroderma	1
Other skin disease	1
Unknown	8

Eczema

Eczema or atopic dermatitis may become erythrodermic at any age. Erythroderma from eczema is most common in the elderly. Itch is often intense.

Psoriasis

At first, the eruption resembles conventional psoriasis but, when the exfoliative stage is reached, these specific features are lost (Fig. 18-1). The withdrawal of potent topical steroids or of systemic steroids, or an intercurrent drug eruption, can precipitate erythrodermic psoriasis.

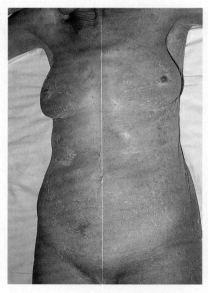

Fig. 18-1   **Erythrodermic psoriasis.**

Lymphoma/Sézary syndrome

Early biopsies may not be specific, and this may delay diagnosis, although universal erythroderma, infiltration of the skin and severe pruritus are helpful pointers. Lymphadenopathy is often prominent, but the nodes are not always involved by lymphoma. Sézary syndrome (Fig. 18-2) typically occurs in elderly males and is characterized by the presence of abnormal T lymphocytes with large convoluted nuclei (Sézary cells) in the blood and skin. Patients may be stable for a number of years, then deteriorate rapidly.

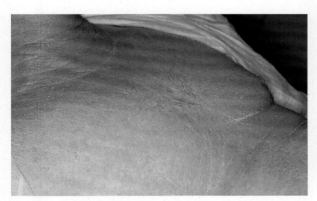

Fig. 18-2 **Erythroderma and infiltration of the skin due to Sézary syndrome.**

Drug eruption

An acute drug eruption, often of the drug hypersensitivity syndrome type, may become erythrodermic (Fig. 18-3). Carbamazepine, phenytoin, diltiazem, cimetidine, gold, allopurinol and sulphonamides are the commonest culprits.

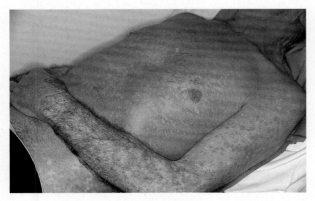

Fig. 18-3 **An erythrodermic reaction to an anti-inflammatory drug.**

Pityriasis rubra pilaris

Pityriasis rubra pilaris is a disorder of unknown aetiology that begins in adults with redness and scaling of the scalp and progresses to cover the limbs and trunk (Fig. 18-4). It is a follicle-based eruption and characteristically shows islands of sparing and a yellow keratotic thickening of the palms (Fig. 18-5). Treatment with acitretin may be considered. Clearance occurs spontaneously in 1~3 years. A relapsing childhood type is reported.

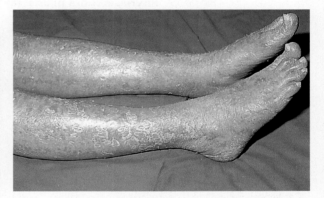

Fig. 18-4 **Pityriasis rubra pilaris affecting the legs.**

Other dermatoses

Ichthyosiform erythroderma is a type of inherited ichthyosis that is present from birth or early infancy. Acute graft-versus-host disease and, very occasionally, severe scabies or extensive pemphigus can cause erythroderma.

In about 10% of cases of erythroderma, no cause is found. The possibility of a latent lymphoma must be considered.

Complications

Erythroderma is associated with profound physiological and metabolic changes (Table 18-2). Cardiac failure and hypothermia are risks, especially in the elderly, and cutaneous or respiratory infection may also occur. Oedema is almost invariable and cannot be regarded as a sign of heart failure. The pulse rate is always increased. Cardiac failure and infection are difficult to diagnose. Blood cultures are easily contaminated with skin microflora. Lymphadenopathy is

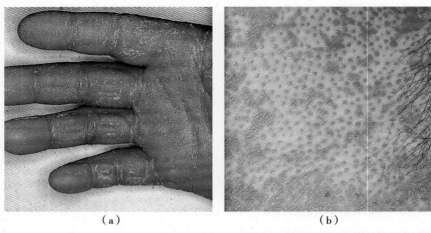

Fig. 18-5 **Pityriasis rubra pilaris. (a)** Yellowish hyperkeratosis of the palms.
(b) Typical follicular lesions.

common and does not necessarily signify lymphoma. In the pre-steroid era, erythroderma was fatal in one-third of cases, largely due to cardiac failure or infection.

Table 18-2	**Pathophysiology of erythroderma**
Clinical complication	**Pathophysiology**
Cardiac failure	Increased skin blood flow Increased plasma volume
Cutaneous oedema	Increased capillary permeability Increased plasma volume Hypoalbuminaemia
Hypoalbuminaemia	Increased plasma volume Reduced albumin synthesis, increased metabolism Protein loss in scaling
Dehydration	Increased transepidermal water loss Increased capillary permeability
Impaired temperature regulation	Excess heat loss Failure to sweat
Dermatopathic lymphadenopathy	Cutaneous inflammation and infection

Management

Inpatient treatment and skilled nursing care are mandatory. The patient is nursed in a comfortably warm room at a steady temperature (preferably 30~32℃), and the pulse, blood pressure, temperature and fluid balance are regularly monitored. A pressure-relieving mattress is sometimes used. Soothing emollient creams and mild to moderate topical steroids are a mainstay of local treatment and are often adequate. Systemic steroids are life-saving in severe cases. The maintenance of normal haemodynamics, attention to electrolyte equilibrium and adequate nutritional support (particularly with regard to minimizing protein losses) are vital for severely ill patients. Cardiac failure and intercurrent infections are treated as necessary.

> *Erythroderma*
> - A rare but potentially fatal eruption, often of sudden onset, showing near-universal skin involvement.
> - Commonest causes: eczema, psoriasis, lymphoma and drug eruption.
> - Characterized by hot, red, oedematous, dry and exfoliating skin.
> - Complications include cardiac failure, hypothermia, infection and lymphadenopathy.
> - Inpatient management and close supervision are required.
> - Treatment consists initially of bland emollients and topical steroids. Systemic steroids and full supportive therapy may be needed in life-threatening cases.

Web resource

http://emedicine.medscape.com/article/1106906-overview

Key words

erythroderma　红皮病

exfoliative dermatitis　剥脱性皮炎

eczema 湿疹

psoriasis 银屑病

drug eruptions 药疹

lymphoma 淋巴瘤

Sézary syndrome Sézary 综合征

pityriasis rubra pilaris 毛发红糠疹

Review questions

1. What are the causes of erythroderma?
2. What kind of complications may occur in patients with erythroderma?

(Wei He)

Chapter 19 Photodermatology

Photodermatoses - idiopathic

Polymorphic light eruption

Polymorphic light eruption is the most common form of photosensitivity and is an immunologically mediated photodermatosis, characterized by pruritic skin lesions of papules, plaques and sometimes vesicles that last for days in light-exposed areas.

Clinical presentation

This is the most common photodermatosis, and women are affected twice as frequently as men. Pruritic urticated papules, plaques and vesicles develop on light-exposed skin usually about 24h after sun or artificial ultraviolet (UV) exposure (Fig. 19-1). It starts in the spring and may persist throughout the summer. The degree of severity is variable.

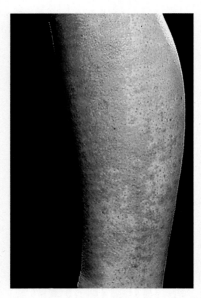

Fig. 19-1 **Polymorphic light eruption affecting the lower legs.**

Differential diagnosis and management

Photoallergic contact dermatitis, drug-induced photosensitivity and lupus erythematosus may need to be considered in the diagnosis of polymorphic light eruption.

The first-line treatment is to use sunscreens and protective measures. A short course of UV therapy (UVB or PUVA) in spring before the first intense sun exposure can 'harden' the skin so that the patient is able to have a disease-free summer.

Chronic actinic dermatitis (actinic reticuloid)

Chronic actinic dermatitis, characterized by pruritic eczematous eruption on sun-exposed skin, is a rare UV-induced disease with unknown pathogenesis usually affecting middle-aged or elderly male.

Histologically, the skin shows spongiotic dermatitis with lymphohistiocytic infiltrate and variable acanthosis.

Clinical presentation

There is often a long history of a chronic dermatitis that evolves into a photodermatitis, or a photoallergic contact dermatitis may have been present from the outset. Lichenified plaques of chronic dermatitis form on light-exposed sites and beyond, and are worse in the summer, although the eruption tends to become perennial (Fig. 19-2). The patients are sensitive to the UVA and UVB wavelengths and often to visible light as well. They may also have a contact or photocontact sensitivity to plant sesquiterpene lactones (airborne allergens) or to cosmetic ingredients, although the contribution remains unclear.

Differential diagnosis and management

Airborne contact dermatitis or drug-induced photosensitivity may need to be considered, but there is normally little doubt about the diagnosis with careful history taking, examination and phototesting.

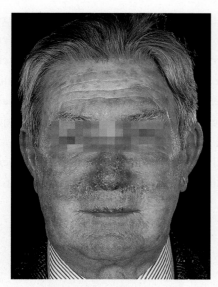

Fig. 19-2   Chronic actinic dermatitis involving the light-exposed areas of the face.

Strict photoprotection is essential in the management of chronic actinic dermatitis. Light avoidance, sunscreens and topical steroids are used at first. Subsequently, azathioprine, ciclosporin, mycophenolate or systemic steroids may be necessary.

Solar urticaria and actinic prurigo

Solar urticaria and actinic prurigo are rare conditions. In solar urticaria, wheals appear within minutes of exposure to sunlight. Differentiation is required from erythropoietic protoporphyria, especially in childhood. Actinic prurigo starts in childhood and is characterized by papules and excoriations, mainly on sun-exposed sites. Actinic prurigo is strongly associated with HLA-DRB1*0401 or 07. Its pathophysiology also includes an abnormal immunologic response with increase of lymphocytes infiltration.

Photodermatoses - other causes

Genetic disorders

Certain rare genetic disorders show photosensitivity. They may have chromosome instability (e.g. Bloom syndrome) or defective DNA repair (e.g. xeroderma pigmentosum).

Metabolic disorders

Porphyrias

Porphyrins are important in the formation of haemoglobin, myoglobin and cytochromes. The porphyrias are rare, mostly inherited, metabolic disorders in which deficiencies of enzymes in the porphyrin biosynthetic pathway lead to accumulations of intermediate metabolites. The metabolites are detectable in the urine, faeces and blood, causing toxic reaction of the nervous system and photosensitivity in the skin.

The main cutaneous porphyrias are the following:

- *Erythropoietic protoporphyria.* Autosomal dominant and usually beginning in infancy or childhood, this is a painful red blistering eruption with tingling, pain, and itching. Pitted linear scars are left on the nose and hands, and lunulae of the nails are lost. The treatment consists of protection from sunlight, beta carotene, cystein, etc.
- *Porphyria cutanea tarda.* This is the most common porphyria, often associated with liver disease and frequently alcohol related. Sun-induced subepidermal blisters on the face and hands (Fig. 19-3) leave fragile, scarred and hairy skin. Alcohol and aggravating drugs (e.g. oestrogens) are avoided. Venesection or low-dose chloroquine therapy may be used.
- *Variegate porphyria.* Autosomal dominant and common in South Africa. The most common manifestation of Variegate porphyria is adult-onset cutaneous blistering lesions of sun-exposed skin, especially the hands and face. The skin signs are like porphyria cutanea tarda. However, acute attacks with abdominal pain and neuropsychiatric symptoms resemble *acute intermittent porphyria*, which has no skin features. Other symptoms including constipation; dorsalgia, pectoralgia and pain in extremities; anxiety; seizures; and a primarily motor neuropathy-causing muscle weakness that may progress to quadriparesis and respiratory paralysis.

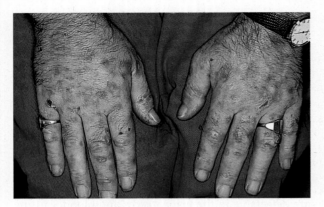

Fig. 19-3 **Porphyria cutanea tarda.** Changes can be seen on the dorsal aspects of the hands.

Pellagra

Dietary deficiency of vitamin B3 (nicotinic acid) may give a photosensitive dermatitis in association with diarrhoea and dementia.

Due to drugs or chemicals

Drug induced

Several drugs may produce an eruption in light-exposed areas by either toxic or allergic mechanisms. The morphology may be eczematous, blistering, pigmented or an exaggerated sunburn reaction. Rarely, photoonycholysis can occur (e.g. with tetracycline). Common photosensitizing drugs are shown in Box 19-1.

Box 19-1   Drugs causing photosensitivity
Amiodarone
Angiotensin-converting enzyme inhibitors
Ciprofloxacin
Furosemide
Nalidixic acid
Non-steroidal anti-inflammatory drugs
Nifedipine
Phenothiazines
Tetracyclines
Thiazides

Topically applied chemicals

The commonest topical photosensitizers (i.e. allergens) are sunscreen agents (e.g. benzophenones), non-steroidal anti-inflammatory drugs (NSAIDs), coal tar derivatives and fragrances. Topical phototoxicity (with an irritant mechanism) is usually due to plant-derived psoralens, as found, for example, in carrot, celery, fennel, parsnip, common rue and giant hogweed. Phytophotodermatitis describes a photocontact dermatitis that results from the local photosensitization of the skin through contact with psoralens from a plant (Fig. 19-4). In Berloque dermatitis, streaky pigmentation, often on the sides of the neck, results from the application of perfumes containing psoralens, usually oil of Bergamot.

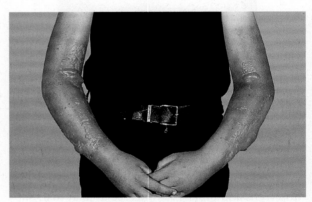

Fig. 19-4 **Phytophotodermatitis to common rue.** The patient had been gathering the plant in the bright sunlight and developed an extreme bullous reaction. The mechanism is toxic, i.e. irritant, rather than allergic.

Dermatoses improved or worsened by sunlight

UV improves certain conditions (Table 19-1) and is used as a treatment as natural sunlight, UVB or PUVA. However, benefit is not observed in every case, and UV can, for example, make a patient's psoriasis or atopic eczema worse. The sun may even precipitate psoriasis. The sun can aggravate several other conditions, listed in Table 19-1.

Table 19-1 Dermatoses improved or aggravated by sunlight	
Improved	**Worsened or provoked**
Vitiligo	Darier's disease
Atopic eczema	Herpes simplex
Mycosis fungoides	Lupus erythematosus
Pityriasis rosea	Porphyrias
Psoriasis	Rosacea
Uraemic pruritus	Acne

Photodermatology

- In normal skin, sunlight can cause tanning, sunburn, photoageing and photocarcinogenesis.
- The important idiopathic photodermatoses are polymorphic light eruption, chronic actinic dermatitis (actinic reticuloid) and solar urticaria. Photoprotective measures are essential in management.
- Other causes of photodermatoses include genetic, metabolic disorder and certain drugs or chemicals.
- Dermatoses worsened by sunlight include Darier's disease, herpes simplex, lupus erythematosus, cutaneous porphyrias, rosacea.
- Dermatoses improved by sunlight include acne, atopic eczema, mycosis fungoides, pityriasis rosea, psoriasis and the pruritus of renal failure.
- Drugs that are not infrequent causes of photosensitivity include tetracyclines, phenothiazines, angiotensin-converting enzyme (ACE) inhibitors, non-steroidal anti-inflammatory drugs (NSAIDs), furosemide and thiazides.

Web resource

http://www.photonet.scot.nhs.uk/

Key words

photodermatosis　光线性皮肤病

polymorphic light eruption　多形性日光疹

chronic actinic dermatitis　慢性光化性皮炎

solar urticaria　日光性荨麻疹

actinic prurigo　光化性痒疹

porphyria　卟啉症

pellagra　糙皮病（烟酸缺乏症）

Review questions

1. Please list at least three diseases that belong to idiopathic photodermatoses.

2. What is the cause of porphyrias and pellagra respectively?

3. Please list at least three drugs that cause photosensitivity.

(Xian Jiang)

Chapter 20 Bacterial infection - Staphylococcal and streptococcal

The skin is a barrier to infection but, if its defences are penetrated or broken down, numerous micro-organisms can cause disease (Table 20-1).

Table 20-1	**Bacterial diseases of the skin**
Organism	**Infection**
Commensals	Erythrasma, pitted keratolysis, tricho-mycosis axillaris
Staphylococci	Impetigo, ecthyma, folliculitis, second-ary infection
Streptococci	Erysipelas, cellulitis, impetigo, ecthyma, necrotizing fasciitis
Gram-negative	Secondary infection, folliculitis, cel-lulitis
Mycobacterial	TB (lupus vulgaris, warty tuberculosis, scrofuloderma), fish tank granuloma, Buruli ulcer, leprosy
Spirochaetes	Syphilis (e.g. primary, secondary), Lyme disease (erythema chronicum migrans)
Neisseria	Gonorrhoea (pustules), meningococ-caemia (purpura)
Others	Anthrax (pustule), erysipeloid (pustule)

The normal skin microflora

Normal skin has a resident flora of usually harmless micro-organisms, including bacteria, yeasts and mites. The bacteria are mostly staphylococci (e.g. *Staphylcoccus epidermidis*), micrococci, corynebacteria (diphtheroids) and propionibacteria. They cluster in the stratum corneum or hair follicles, and their number varies between individuals and between different sites on the body. Micrococci, for example, number 0.5 million/cm^2 in the axilla but only 60/cm^2 on the forearm. Some individuals are high carriers.

Staphylococcal infections

A third of people intermittently carry *Staphylococcus aureus* in the nose or, less often, the axilla or perineum. Staphylococci can infect the skin directly or secondarily, as in eczema or psoriasis.

Impetigo

Impetigo is a contagious superficial skin infection caused by either staphylococci or streptococci, or both. In China, impetigo is primarily caused by *Staphylococcus aureus*. Four clinical types are recognized: impetigo vulgaris, impetigo bullosa, impetigo neonatorum and ecthyma.

Clinical presentation

Impetigo is now relatively uncommon in the UK, mainly because of improved social conditions, but it is endemic in developing countries. It generally occurs in children and presents as thin-walled, easily ruptured vesicles, often on the face, which leave areas of yellow-crusted exudate (Fig. 20-1). Lesions spread rapidly and are contagious. A bullous form, with blisters 1~2cm in diameter, is often seen in all ages and affects the face or extremities. Impetigo neonatorum mostly occurs in babies at 4~10 days after birth, with the characteristics of acute onset and high contagiousness. Clinical symptoms of impetigo neonatorum are widespread distributed multiple large pustules with blush surrounded, and red erosion surfaces could form after rupture of pustules. Systemic symptoms such as fever may be associated, and sepsis, pneumonia and meningitis may be concomitant,

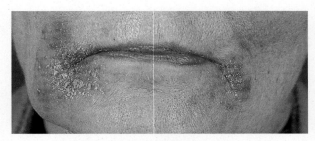

Fig. 20-1 **Impetigo of the face due to** *Staphylococcus aureus*.

which leads to a life-threatening condition. Atopic eczema, scabies, herpes simplex and lice infestation may all become impetiginized. Impetigo can be confused with herpes simplex or a fungal infection.

Management

Most mild and localized cases respond to the application of a topical antibiotic (e.g. mupirocin ointment, fusidic acid or neomycin/bacitracin). Systemic flucloxacillin or erythromycin is given for widespread infection. Impetigo caused by *Streptococcus pyogenes* may result in glomerulonephritis, a serious complication. Methicillin-resistant *Staph. aureus* (MRSA) carriage (and infection) has increased with the widespread use of antibiotics.

Ecthyma

Ecthyma is characterized by circumscribed, ulcerated and crusted infected lesions that heal with scarring. An insect bite or neglected minor injury may become infected with staphylococci or streptococci (or both). Ecthyma mostly occurs on the legs (Fig. 20-2) and buttocks and may be seen in drug addicts or debilitated patients. Treatment is with systemic and topical antibiotics.

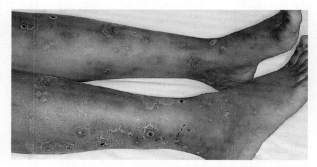

Fig.20-2 **Ecthyma, due to a streptococcus, affecting the lower legs.**

Folliculitis and related conditions

Infection can affect hair follicles. *Folliculitis* is an acute pustular infection of multiple hair follicles; a *furuncle* is an acute abscess formation in adjacent hair follicles; and a *carbuncle* is a deep abscess formed in a group of follicles giving a painful suppurating mass.

Clinical presentation

Follicular pustules are seen in hair-bearing areas, e.g. the legs, scalp or face. Physical of chemical injury to the skin may be associated with folliculitis. In men, folliculitis may affect the beard area (sycosis barbae). In women, it may occur on the legs after hair removal by shaving or waxing. *Staph. aureus* is usually, but not invariably, responsible. A Gram-negative folliculitis (e.g. with *Pseudomonas*) may occur with prolonged antibiotic treatment for acne. *Pityrosporum folliculitis* is a separate condition due to a commensal yeast.

Furuncles (boils) present as tender red pustules that suppurate and heal with scarring. They often occur on the face, neck, scalp, axillae and perineum. Some patients have recurrent staphylococcal boils of the axillae or perineum. Large suppurating carbuncles (Fig. 20-3) due to *Staph. aureus* may cause systemic upset.

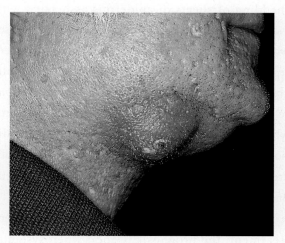

Fig. 20-3 **A carbuncle.** This required surgical drainage. The patient had had previous staphylococcal infection.

Carbuncle is a deep infection of a group of contiguous follicles accompanied by intense inflammatory changes in the surrounding and underlying connective tissues, including the subcutaneous fat. Most lesions are on the back of the neck, the shoulders or the hips and thighs.

Management

Swabs for bacterial culture are taken from the lesion and from carrier sites, e.g. the nose, axilla and groin.

Obesity, diabetes mellitus and occlusion from clothing are predisposing factors. Acute staphylococcal infections are treated with antibiotics, both systemic (e.g. flucloxacillin or erythromycin) and topical (e.g. fusidic acid, mupirocin or neomycin/bacitracin). Chronic and recurrent cases are more difficult. Carrier sites, e.g. the nose, need treatment with a topical antibiotic (e.g. mupirocin). General measures such as improved hygiene, regular bathing or showering, the use of antiseptics in the bath and on the skin (e.g. chlorhexidine) can help, but courses of oral antibiotics may be needed. Carbuncles often need prompt surgical drainage. An infrequent complication is thrombosis in the cavernous sinus, associated with facial infection.

Staphylococcal scalded skin syndrome

Staphylococcal scalded skin syndrome is an acute toxic illness, usually of infants, in which there is shedding of sheets of epidermis associated with localized staphylococcal infection in the skin or elsewhere. Large sheets of superficial epidermis are shed, resembling a scald, leaving denuded erythematous areas. Phage group Ⅱ type 71 *Staphylococci aureus* release into the bloodstream epidermolytic toxins, which cause the epidermis to split. Related conditions in adults with the same level of epidermal split are toxic epidermal necrolysis, pemphigus foliaceus or erythrodermia.

Although a serious condition requiring inpatient treatment, the prognosis is good when systemic flucloxacillin or erythromycin is prescribed. Anti-staphylococcal antibiotics, temperature regulation, maintaining fluid and electrolyte balance, nutritional management and skin care form the basics of treatment.

Streptococcal infections

Strep. pyogenes, the principal human skin pathogen, is occasionally found in the throat and may persist after an infection. It is sometimes carried in the nose and can contaminate and colonize damaged skin.

Erysipelas

Erysipelas is an acute infection of the dermis by *Strep. pyogenes*. It shows well-demarcated raised erythema, oedema and skin tenderness.

Clinical presentation

The skin lesions may be preceded by fever, malaise and 'flu-like' symptoms. Erysipelas usually affects the face (where it may be bilateral) or the lower leg, and appears as a painful hot red swelling (Fig. 20-4). The lesion has a well-defined edge and may blister. Cellulitis may coexist. According to the different clinical manifestations, erysipelas has some special types. When pustules occurs on the lesions, it is called pustular erysipelas. When Inflammation infiltrates to the subcutaneous tissue and caused gangrene, it is called gangrenous erysipelas. When lesions continued to expand and island-like spread, it is called migratory erysipelas. The streptococci usually gain entry to the skin via a fissure, e.g. behind the ear, or associated with tinea pedis between the toes.

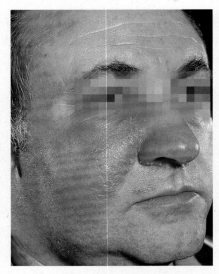

Fig. 20-4 **Erysipelas of the right cheek due to a streptococcal infection.**

Differential diagnosis and complications

On the face, erysipelas may be confused with angio-edema or allergic contact dermatitis, but the condition is usually distinguishable as it causes tenderness and systemic upset. Recurrent attacks in the same place can result in lymphoedema due to lymphatic damage. A fatal streptococcal septicaemia can occur in debilitated patients. Guttate psoriasis and acute glomerulonephritis may follow a streptococcal infection.

Management

A good response is usually seen with prompt treatment. Topical therapy is inappropriate, and penicillin should be prescribed. *Strep. pyogenes* is nearly always sensitive. Intravenous treatment is needed at first for a severe infection, usually with benzylpenicillin for about 2 days. Oral penicillin V can then be given for 7~14 days. In less severe cases, penicillin V is adequate. Erythromycin is used if there is penicillin allergy. Recurrent erysipelas, i.e. more than two episodes at one site, requires prophylactic long-term penicillin V (250mg once or twice a day), with attention to hygiene at potential portals of entry.

Necrotizing fasciitis

Necrotizing fasciitis is an acute and serious infection. It usually occurs in otherwise healthy subjects after minor trauma. An ill-defined erythema, often on the head or limbs and associated with a high fever, rapidly becomes necrotic. Early surgical debridement and systemic antibiotics are essential.

Staphylococcal and streptococcal infections
- **Normal skin microflora** includes staphylococci, micrococci, corynebacteria and propionibacteria, and may number 0.5 million/cm². Some individuals are higher carriers than others.
- **Staphylococcal infection** of the skin may be primary, e.g. impetigo, ecthyma or folliculitis, or secondary, e.g. superinfection of eczema, psoriasis or leg ulcers.
- **Streptococcal infections** may also be primary, e.g. erysipelas or cellulitis, or secondary, e.g. infection of dermatoses or leg ulcers.

Web resources

http://www.textbookofbacteriology.net/streptococcus.html

Key words

staphylococcus　葡萄球菌
streptococcus　链球菌
impetigo　脓疱病
ecthyma　臁疮
folliculitis　毛囊炎
furuncle　疖
carbuncle　痈
staphylococcal scalded skin syndrome　葡萄球菌烫伤样皮肤综合征
epidermolytic toxin　表皮溶解毒素
erysipelas　丹毒
necrotizing fasciitis　坏死性筋膜炎

Review questions

1. Please describe the clinical presentation, diagnosis and treatment of impetigo, folliculitis, furuncle and erysipelas.
2. What are the differences of folliculitis, furuncle and carbuncle?
3. What is the cause of staphylococcal scalded skin syndrome?
4. Which skin diseases are primarily caused by Staphylococcal infection?
5. Which skin diseases are primarily caused by Streptococcal infections?

(Meng Pan)

Chapter 21 Other bacterial infections

Diseases due to commensal overgrowth

Sometimes, 'normal' commensals can result in disease. Among the most common are the following:

■ *Pitted keratolysis.* Overgrowth of resident micro-organisms, that digest keratin; occurs with occluding footwear and sweaty feet (Fig. 21-1). Malodorous pitted erosions and punched out, discoloured areas result. Better hygiene, topical neomycin or soaks with 0.01% aqueous potassium permanganate or 3% aqueous formaldehyde usually help.

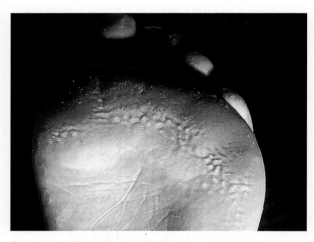

Fig. 21-1 **Pitted keratolysis, due to overgrowth of resident micro-organisms.**

■ *Erythrasma.* A dry, reddish-brown, slightly scaly and usually asymptomatic eruption that affects the body folds (Fig. 21-2). It fluoresces coral pink with Wood's light, owing to the production of porphyrins by the corynebacteria. Imidazole creams, topical fusidic acid or oral erythromycin are effective.

■ *Trichomycosis axillaris.* Overgrowths of corynebacteria form yellow concretions on axillary hair. Topical antimicrobials usually effect a cure.

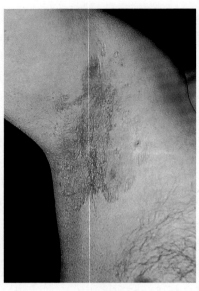

Fig. 21-2 **Erythrasma affecting the axilla.** This was caused by overgrowth of corynebacteria.

Mycobacterial infections

Mycobacterium tuberculosis and *M. leprae* are the most important mycobacteria in human disease, although other species can cause infections. Although tuberculosis is rare in the world, the incidence of TB in the world has resurgence, especially in developing countries. In western countries, tuberculosis (TB) has recently shown resurgence, related to immigration and co-infection with HIV. In the developing world, 50% of HIV-infected individuals also have TB. TB can produce a number of cutaneous manifestations (Table 21-1).

Table 21-1 **Skin manifestations of tuberculosis**
■ **Lupus vulgaris:** reddish-brown plaques, e.g. on the neck.
■ **Tuberculides:** cutaneous hypersensitivity reactions.
■ **Scrofuloderma:** skin involved from underlying node.
■ **Warty tuberculosis:** warty plaques, e.g. on buttock.

Lupus vulgaris

Reddish-brown plaques, often on the head or neck,

characterize lupus vulgaris. It is the commonest M. tuberculosis skin infection.

Clinical presentation

Lupus vulgaris follows primary inoculation and develops in individuals with some immunity. It begins as painless reddish-brown nodules that slowly enlarge to form a plaque (Fig. 21-3), leaving scarring and sometimes destruction of deeper tissues such as cartilage. Presentation in the elderly is often due to reactivation of inadequately treated pre-existing disease.

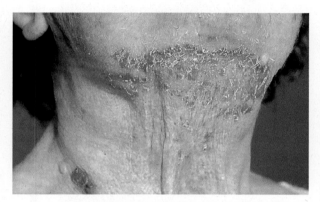

Fig. 21-3 **Lupus vulgaris, due to M. tuberculosis.**

Differential diagnosis and complications

Papules of lupus vulgaris typically show an 'apple-jelly' colour when compressed with a glass slide (diascopy). A biopsy will reveal tuberculoid granulomata with a few bacilli. The Mantoux test is positive. Sometimes it is necessary to consider:

- morphoeic basal cell carcinoma
- sarcoidosis or leprosy
- discoid lupus erythematosus.

Squamous cell carcinoma may develop in long-standing scarred lesions. The presence of M. tuberculosis somewhere in the body can induce cutaneous reactions called 'tuberculides'. Erythema nodosum is the best known example. Another is erythema induratum, which occurs as painful ulcerating nodules on the lower legs of women and is thought to be a hypersensitivity response to TB.

Management

Four drugs, normally rifampicin, isoniazid, pyra-zinamide and ethambutol, are given for the initial 8 weeks. After this, isoniazid and rifampicin are continued to complete a 6-month course. Directly observed therapy, in which ingestion of drugs is witnessed, improves cure rates if compliance could be a problem. Adverse reactions to TB drugs are common, including liver damage, alimentary symptom, peripheral neuritis and so on.

Scrofuloderma

A tuberculous lymph node or joint can directly involve the overlying skin, often on the neck and in children. Fistulae and scarring result.

Warty tuberculosis

A warty reddish or brown plaque, frequently on the hands, knees or buttock, results from inoculation of TB bacilli into the skin of someone with immunity from previous infection. It is rare in western countries, but is a common form of cutaneous TB in the developing world.

Other cutaneous mycobacterial infections

Fish tank granuloma

Typically, this is a reddish, slightly scaly plaque on the hand or arm of someone who keeps tropical fish. It is due to Mycobacterium marinum, which infects fish and is also found in swimming pools, sea water and fresh water.

Buruli ulcer

In tropical zones, Mycobacterium ulcerans-acquired from vegetation or water after trauma-produces a painless erythematous nodule usually on the leg or forearm. The nodule becomes necrotic and ulceration results.

Disseminated infection with Mycobacterium avium complex is seen in patients with HIV infection.

Spirochaetal infections

Spirochaetes are thin, spiral and motile organisms. Syphilis, due to Treponema pallidum, is the best known spirochaetal disease, but other spirochaetes, e.g. *Borrelia burgdorferi*, can be pathogenic.

Non-venereal treponemal infections

Non-venereal treponemal infections are endemic in tropical and subtropical areas where people live in conditions of extreme poverty. They are caused by spirochaetes that are very similar to *T. pallidum*. Serological tests for syphilis are positive. All three of the following diseases respond to long-acting penicillins.

- *Yaws* occurs in central Africa, central America and southeast Asia. In children, the treponeme enters the skin through an abrasion and, after a few weeks, results in an ulcerated papilloma that heals with scarring. Secondary lesions follow and, in the late stage, bone deformities develop.
- *Bejel* (endemic syphilis), found in rural Middle Eastern tribes living in unhygienic conditions, is similar to yaws but starts around the mouth. It is transmitted by skin contact.
- *Pinta* is confined to central and south America. It results in hyperkeratoses over extensor aspects of joints with both hypo- and hyperpigmentation.

Lyme disease

Lyme disease is a cutaneous and systemic infection caused by the spirochaete *Borrelia burgdorferi* and spread by tick bite. Most cases have been reported in the USA and Europe. At the site of the tick bite, usually a limb, a slowly expanding erythematous ring (erythema chronicum migrans) develops (Fig. 21-4). Arthritis and neurological and cardiac disease may follow. A response to high-dose amoxicillin or doxycycline is usual.

Further bacterial infections

Anthrax

A haemorrhagic bulla, associated with oedema and fever, forms at the site of inoculation of the skin with *Bacillus anthracis*, usually from contaminated animal products. It is now rare. Ciprofloxacin or amoxicillin is curative.

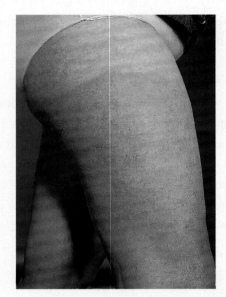

Fig. 21-4 **Erythema chronicum migrans of Lyme disease.**

Gram-negative infections

Bacilli such as *Pseudomonas aeruginosa* can infect skin wounds, notably leg ulcers. They may also cause folliculitis and cellulitis.

Cellulitis

Cellulitis is an infection of the subcutaneous tissues. It is often due to streptococci, but is deeper and more extensive than erysipelas. The cardinal features are swelling, redness and local pain with systemic upset and fever. The leg is often affected (Fig. 21-5). If the fingers and toes are involved, they are called panaritium with obvious local throbbing pain and tenderness. The organism may gain entry through fissures between the toes or via a leg ulcer. Lymphan-

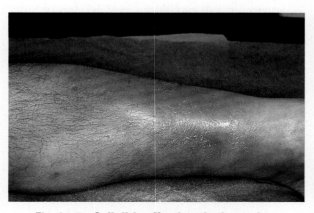

Fig. 21-5 **Cellulitis affecting the lower leg.**

gitis is common, and lymphatic damage may result. Hospital admission is usually indicated, particularly if the leg is involved. Antistreptococcal antibiotics are given for straightforward cases. However, a broad-spectrum antibiotic is prescribed for cellulitis complicating a leg ulcer, because a selection of organisms may be responsible. Blood cultures and ulcer swabs may give some guidance.

Other bacterial infections
- Overgrowth of commensal organisms can result in minor skin 'disease'.
- Cutaneous mycobacterial infection is mainly due to *M. tuberculosis*, but occasionally 'atypical' mycobacteria such as *M. marinum* cause disease.
- Syphilis is a chronic infectious disease due to *Treponema pallidum*. Penicillin is curative.
- Non-venereal treponematoses, e.g. yaws, are still important diseases of rural people living in poor conditions in the developing world.
- Lyme disease is a tick-transmitted infection with *Borrelia burgdorferi*; the skin signs are often associated with arthritis or neurological disease.
- Cellulitis often affects the leg and is frequently caused by streptococci, although other organisms may be involved.

Web resource

http://www.tballiance.org/
http://www.who.int/topics/tuberculosis/en/

Key words

lupus vulgaris　寻常狼疮
scrofuloderma　瘰疬性皮肤结核
warty tuberculosis　疣状皮肤结核
fish tank granuloma　水族馆肉芽肿
syphilis　梅毒
chancre　硬下疳
anthrax　炭疽
cellulitis　蜂窝织炎

Review questions

1. What are the clinical manifestations of lupus vulgaris?
2. What are the clinical features of cellulitis?

(Nan Yu)

Chapter 22   Viral infections - Warts and other viral infections

Unlike bacteria and yeasts, viruses are not thought to exist on the skin surface as commensals. However, studies in patients with viral warts have shown viral DNA in epidermal cells of seemingly normal skin next to warty areas.

Viral warts

Warts (verrucae) are common and benign cutaneous tumours due to infection of epidermal cells with human papillomavirus (HPV).

Aetiopathogenesis and pathology

Over a hundred subtypes of DNA HPV have been identified. The virus infects by direct inoculation and is caught by touch, sexual contact or at the swimming baths. Certain HPV subtypes are associated with specific clinical lesions, e.g. types 2, 27 and 57 with common hand warts, types 1, 2, 4, 27 and 57 with plantar warts, types 3 and 10 with plane warts, types 6 and 11 with genital warts. Certain genital HPV subtypes cause cytological dysplasia of the cervix, which may be precancerous. Immunosuppressed individuals, such as those with organ transplants, are particularly susceptible to viral warts. The epidermis is thickened and hyperkeratotic. Keratinocytes in the granular layer are often vacuolated.

Clinical presentation

Certain clinical patterns are well recognized:

- *Common warts.* These present as dome-shaped papules or nodules with a papilliferous surface. They are usually multiple, and are commonest on the hands (Fig. 22-1) or feet in children but also affect the face and genitalia. Their surface interrupts skin lines. Some facial warts are 'filiform' with fine digit-like projections.

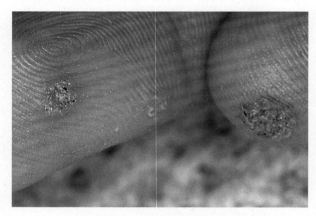

Fig. 22-1   **Common viral warts on the hand.**

- *Plane warts.* These are smooth flat-topped papules, often slightly brown in colour, and commonest on the face (Fig. 22-2) and dorsal aspects of the hands. They are usually multiple and resist treatment, but eventually resolve spontaneously, often after becoming inflamed. They can show the Koebner phenomenon.

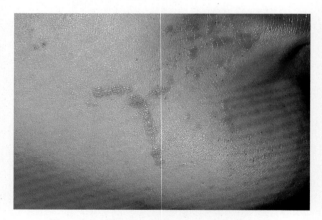

Fig. 22-2   **Plane viral warts on the face.**

- *Plantar warts.* These are seen in children and adolescents on the soles of the feet; pressure causes them to grow into the dermis. They are painful and covered by callus, which, when pared, reveals dark punctate spots (thrombosed capillaries). Mosaic warts are plaques on the soles that comprise multiple individual warts.

■ *Genital warts.* In males, these affect the penis and, in homosexuals, the perianal area. In females, the vulva, vagina and perianal area maybe involved (Fig. 22-3). The warts may be small or may coalesce into large cauliflower-like 'condylomata acuminata'. Proctoscopy (if perianal warts are present) and colposcopy (for female genital warts) are needed to identify and treat any rectal or cervical warts. Sexual partners need to be examined.

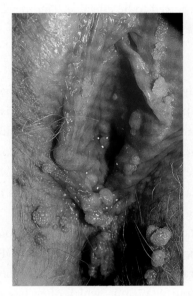

Fig. 22-3　**Viral warts on the vulva.**

Differential diagnosis and complications

The diagnosis of viral warts is usually obvious. Occasionally, corns on the sole or hand, or molluscum contagiosum elsewhere, are confused. With viral warts under the fingernails and toenails, it is important to consider amelanotic malignant melanoma, periungual fibroma (of tuberous sclerosis) and bony subungual exostosis. Genital warts may resemble the condyloma lata of secondary syphilis. HPV types 16 and 18 in genital warts carry a risk of malignant change. HPV infections in organ transplant patients have been linked with skin cancers.

Management

In children, 30%~50% of plantar warts disappear spontaneously within 6 months. Hand and foot warts should be pared by a scalpel or using an emery board. This gets rid of keratotic skin and allows easier treatment. Table 22-1 shows the available treatments. Immunosuppressed patients, especially those with organ transplants, are prone to wart infections. They need special management and should be inspected and treated for warts before being given their grafts.

Table 22-1	**Treatments for viral warts**		
Modality	**Details**	**Indication**	**Contraindications/side-effects**
Topical	Salicylic and lactic acids (e.g. Duo-film, Occlusal, Salactol, Salatac)	Hand and foot warts	Facial/anogenital warts, atopic eczema, contact allergy to colophoniurn in collodion preparations
	Glutaraldehyde (e.g. Glutarol)	Hand and foot warts	Facial/anogenital warts, atopic eczema
	Formaldehyde (e.g. Veracur)	Foot warts	Facial/anogenital warts, atopic eczema
	Podophyllotoxin (0.15%) cream	Anogenital warts	Pregnancy (teratogenic)
	Imiquimod cream	Anogenital warts	Pregnancy; local reaction
Cryotherapy	Applied every 3~4 weeks	Hand and foot, genital warts	Painful; may cause blistering
Curettage and cautery	Local anaesthetic (or general anaesthetic if large)	Solitary filiform warts, especially on face Large anogenital warts	Not recommended for hand or foot warts as scars may result; warts may recur
Other	Intralesional bleomycin	Resistant hand/foot warts	Procedure can be painful
	Laser surgery	Any type of wart	Postoperative pain; can scar
	Interferon-β or -γ	Resistant (genital) warts	Systemic side-effects
	Photodynamic therapy	Genital warts	Procedure takes time and can be painful
	Mild local hyperthermia at 44℃	Any type of warts	Burning; occasional blistering

Other viral infections

Other viral infections include molluscum contagiosum, orf, HIV and those in Table 22-2.

Molluscum contagiosum

Molluscum contagiosum are discrete pearly-pink umbilicated papules that are caused by a DNA pox virus. Mollusca mainly affect children or young adults. Spread is by contact, including sexual transmission or on towels. The dome-shaped papule, a few millimetres in diameter, has a punctum and, if squeezed, releases a cheesy material. The lesions are usually multiple and grouped, sometimes with a localized eczema. They are commonest on the face,

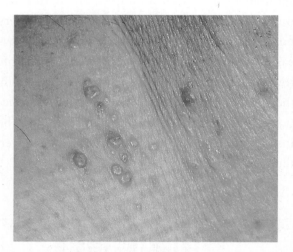

Fig. 22-4   **Molluscum contagiosum on the neck.**

neck and trunk (Fig. 22-4). Isolated ones may go unrecognized. Untreated, they may persist for several months.

If natural resolution is slow, imiquimod cream can be helpful. In the adult or older child, curettage under local anaesthesia or cryotherapy is appropriate. These measures are poorly tolerated in young children, and one approach is to instruct the parents to express the 'ripe' lesions gently after the child has been in the bath. Local hyperthermia at 44 °C for 30 mins is reported to be effective. The treatment procedure is tolerable to children.

Orf

Orf usually occurs as a solitary, rapidly growing papule, often on the hand. The orf pox virus is endemic in sheep and causes a pustular eruption around the muzzle area. Human infection is well recognized in country regions and occurs in shepherds, veterinary surgeons and, typically, a person who has been bottle-feeding a lamb.

A solitary red papule appears, usually on a finger, after an incubation period of about 6 days (Fig. 22-5). It grows rapidly to 1cm or so in size, evolving into a painful purple pustule, which often has a necrotic umbilicated centre. Erythema multiforme and lymphangitis are complications. Spontaneous resolution takes 2~4 weeks. Secondary infection requires a topical or systemic antibiotic.

Table 22-2 **Other viral infections**			
Disorder	**Cause**	**Clinical presentation**	**Course and management**
Fifth disease (erythema infectiosum)	Erythrovirus (Parvovirus) B19	Slapped cheek sign, lace-like erythema over hands, feet or trunk, sometimes arthralgia	Small outbreaks typically affect children aged 2~10 years; fades in 11 days; treatment unnecessary
Gianotti-Crosti syndrome	Hepatitis B and other viruses	Small red lichenoid papules on face, buttocks and extremities	Affects young children (peak 1~12 years); clears in 2~8 weeks
Hand, foot and mouth disease	Coxsackie A16 and others	Oral blisters/ulcers, red-edged vesicles on hands/feet, mild fever	Epidemics in young children; fades in 1 week; no treatment needed
Kawasaki disease	Unknown microorganism:? response to superantigens	Generalized erythema, peeling of hands/feet, strawberry tongue, fever, myocarditis, lymphadenopathy, coronary artery aneurysms	Affects young children; usually resolves in 2 weeks; investigate for cardiac involvement; treat with intravenous immunoglobulin and aspirin
Measles	RNA morbillivirus	Koplik's spots on buccal mucosa, morbilliform rash	Incubation period 10 days, prodrome; rash fades after 6~10 days

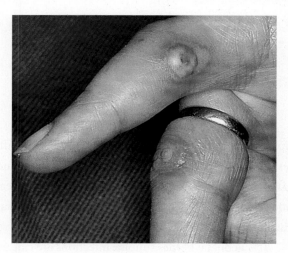

Fig. 22-5   **Orf on the fingers of a farmer's wife.**

Web resource

http://dermnetnz.org/viral/

Key words

virus   病毒

human papilloma virus   人乳头瘤病毒

wart   疣

molluscum contagiosum   传染性软疣

orf   羊痘

Review questions

1. To name a couple of warts caused by HPV.
2. What are the possible routes of infection by HPV?
3. Which cellular component is the host for HPV?
4. Who are most vulnerable population to orf?
5. What population by age is more often afflicted with molluscum contagiosum?

(Xinghua Gao)

Warts and other viral conditions

Viral warts

■ Hand and foot warts are common: overall, 65% clear spontaneously within 2 years.

■ Try wart paints for hand and foot warts before proceeding to other therapy.

■ Patients with anogenital warts need screening for other genital infections.

Molluscum contagiosum

■ Caused by a pox virus. Treated by imiquimod cream, curettage, cryotherapy or local hyperthermia.

■ Untreated, the lesions will remit spontaneously, although this may take several months.

Orf

■ Found in rural areas, affecting farmers and vets. The condition is endemic in sheep.

■ Diagnosis is usually obvious, but treat secondary infection and watch for erythema multiforme.

Chapter 23　Viral infections - Herpes simplex and herpes zoster

Herpes simplex

Herpes simplex is a very common, acute, self-limiting vesicular eruption due to infection with *Herpesvirus hominis*.

Aetiopathogenesis and pathology

Herpes simplex virus is highly contagious and is spread by direct contact with infected individuals. The virus penetrates the epidermis or mucous membrane epithelium and replicates within the epithelial cells. After the primary infection, the latent non-replicating virus resides mainly within the dorsal root ganglion, from where it can reactivate, invade the skin and cause recrudescent lesions. There are two types of herpes simplex virus. The HSV-1 is usually infected with facial or non-genital, and the HSV-2 with genital, although this distinction is not absolute. The pathological changes of epidermal cell destruction by the herpes virus result in intraepidermal vesicles and multinucleate giant cells. Infected cells may show intranuclear inclusions.

Clinical presentation

HSV infections have a wide range of clinical presentations, and asymptomatic infection is very common, it can be classified as either first episode or recurrent. Compared to recurrent type, primary infections have more subjective symptoms and longer latent period, which typically occur within 2 to 12 days after exposure.

First episode type

The majority of primary orolabial infections are asymptomatic. Symptomatic infections often present as gingivostomatitis in children or as pharyngitis and a mononucleosis-like syndrome in young adults which is always caused by HSV-1. The mouth and lips are the most common sites of involvement, with lesions typically appearing on the buccal mucosa and gingivae. Edema and painful oropharyngeal ulcerations can lead to dysphagia and drooling. The duration, untreated, is 1~2 weeks.

70% neonatal herpes simplex infections are caused by HSV-2. 85% neonatal herpes simplex infections occur at delivery, 10%~15% occur from nonmaternal sources after 5% occur in utero with intact membranes. In utero infection may result in fetal anomalies, including skin lesions and scars, limb hypoplasia, microcephaly, microphthalmos and intracerebral calcifications. It is either fatal or complicated by permanent neurologic sequelae.

Eczema herpeticum is also named as Kaposi Varicelliform eruption (KVE), which is presented as eczema or atopic dermatitis in children. In its severest form, hundreds of vesicles or pustules may be present at the onset, with fever and adenopathy. Although the cutaneous eruption is alarming, the disease is often self-limited in healthy individuals. In patients with systemic immunosuppression in addition to an impaired barrier, KVE can be fatal.

A painful vesicle or pustule is found on a finger in, for example, a children while thumb sucking or nail biting during their initial herpes outbreak or by touching an infectious lesion of an adult ('herpetic whitlow')(Fig. 23-1). Similar direct inoculation is sometimes seen in sportsmen such as wrestlers ('herpes gladiatorum').

HSV-2 primary infection is normally seen after sexual contact in young adults, who develop acute vulvovaginitis or penile or perianal lesions. Culture-positive genital herpes simplex in a pregnant woman at the time of delivery is an indication for caesarean section, as neonatal infection can be fatal.

When patients have their first clinical lesion, this is usually a recurrence, because the initial clinical presentation is not associated with a new infection, the previous terminology of primary infection has been abandoned.

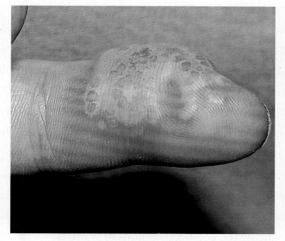

Fig. 23-1   **Primary herpes simplex occurring as a herpetic whitlow on a finger.**

Recurrent type

Recurrence is a hallmark of herpes simplex infection; it occurs at a similar site each time, usually on the lips, face (Fig. 23-2) or genitals (Fig. 23-3). Rarely, herpes simplex may appear in a zosteriform dermatomal distribution. The outbreak of groups of vesicles is often preceded for a few hours by tingling or burning. Crusts form within 24~48h, and the infection fades after a week. Attacks may be precipitated by respiratory infection (hence 'cold' sore), sunlight or local trauma.

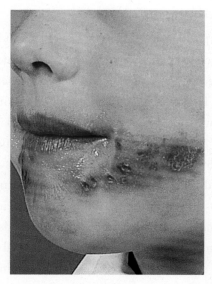

Fig. 23-2   **Herpes simplex on the cheek of a child.**

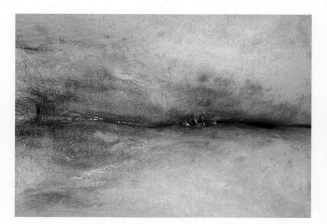

Fig. 23-3   **Genital lesions of recurrent herpes simplex.**

Differential diagnosis

Herpetic lesions are composed of grouped tense, small vesicles which can be confused with impetigo and herpes zoster. Whereas in bullous impetigo, the blisters are unilateral, occur at the periphery of a crust, and are flaccid. Herpes zoster presents with clusters of lesions along a dermatome, but if the number of zoster lesions is limited early on, it can be relatively indistinguishable from herpes simplex. And in recurrent type, the recurrent nature usually indicates the diagnosis.

Complications

Complications are infrequent but can be serious. They include the following:

- *Secondary bacterial infection.* This is usually due to *Staphylococcus aureus.*
- *Eczema herpeticum.* Widespread herpes simplex infection is a serious and potentially fatal complication seen in patients with atopic eczema or Darier's disease.
- *Disseminated herpes simplex.* Widespread herpetic vesicles may occur in the newborn or in immunosuppressed patients.
- *Chronic herpes simplex.* Atypical and chronic lesions may be seen in patients with HIV infection.
- *Herpes encephalitis.* This is a serious complication of herpes simplex, not always accompanied by skin lesions.
- *Carcinoma of the cervix.* This is more common in women with serological evidence of infection

with type 2 herpes simplex, which may be a predisposing factor.

- *Erythema multiforme*. Herpes simplex infection is the most common cause of recurrent erythema multiforme.

Lab test

Viral culture is regarded as the golden standard of diagnosis of HSV infection. A Tzanck smear of scrapings from early lesions (e.g. the base/edges of a freshly unroofed vesicle) reveals multinucleated epithelial giant cells in the majority of HSV outbreaks. Polymerase chain reaction (PCR) is increasingly being used as a rapid, sensitive and specific method to detect HSV DNA in specimens from the skin and other organs. Serum HSV-IgM antibody detection have assisted diagnostic value, however, IgG antibody is of little value in diagnosis, which is often used for epidemiological investigation.

Management

Therapeutic principles is to shorten the duration of symptoms, prevent secondary bacterial infections and systemic spread, reduce the chance of recurrence.

Mild herpetic lesions may not require any medication. The treatment of choice for recurrent mild facial or genital herpes simplex is acyclovir cream (applied five times a day for 5 days), which reduces the length of the attack and the duration of viral shedding, and should preferably be started at the first indication of a recrudescence. More severe episodes warrant oral treatment with acyclovir (200mg five times a day for 5 days), which shortens the attack. Long-term oral administration is useful in those with frequent recurrent attacks. Intravenous aciclovir may be life-saving in the immunosuppressed and in infants with eczema.

Herpes zoster

Herpes zoster (shingles) is an acute, self-limiting, vesicular eruption occurring in a dermatomal distribution; it is caused by a recrudescence of varicella zoster virus (VZV).

Aetiopathogenesis and pathology

VZV has a worldwide distribution and 98% of the adult population is seropositive. Airborne droplets are the usual route of transmission of varicella, and direct contact with vesicular fluid is another mode of spread. The incubation period ranges from 11 to 20 days, and 80%~90% of susceptible household contacts develop a clinically evident infection. The affected individual is infectious from 1 to 2 days before skin lesions appear until all of the vesicles have crusted. The virus always lies dormant in the sensory root ganglion of the spinal cord but, when reactivated, the virus replicates and migrates along the nerve to the skin, producing pain and ultimately inducing the cutaneous lesions of shingles.

Herpes zoster appears upon reactivation of VZV, which may occur spontaneously or be induced by stress, fever, radiation therapy, local trauma or immunosuppression (especially that due to HIV infection, allogeneic hematopoietic stem cell transplantation). During a herpes zoster outbreak, the virus continues to replicate in the affected dorsal root ganglion and produces a painful ganglionitis. Neuronal inflammation and necrosis can result in a severe neuralgia that intensifies as the virus spreads down the sensory nerve. There is only one serotype of VZV, so the infection after a lifelong immunity can be obtained.

Clinical presentation

Typical performance of herpes zoster include pain, tenderness or paraesthesia in the dermatome which may precede the eruption by 3~5 days. The lesions tend to locate along unilateral nerve in zonal distribution, such as intercostal nerve (55%), cranial nerves (25%), lumbar sacral nerve (15%) and sacral nerve (5%). The eruption initially presents as papules and plaques of erythema in the dermatome (Fig. 23-4). Within hours the plaques develop blisters. Lesions continue to appear for several days. The eruption may have few lesions or reach total confluence in the dermatome. Lesions may become hemorrhagic, necrotic or bullous. In typical cases, new vesicles appear for 1~5 days, become pustular, crust, and heal.

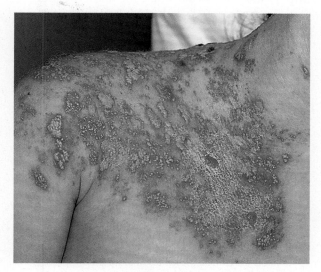

Fig. 23-4 **Herpes zoster of the C4 dermatome**.

The total duration of the eruption depends on patient age, severity of eruption and presence of underlying immunosuppression. The total duration is 2~3 weeks in younger patients, whereas the cutaneous lesions may require 6 weeks or more to heal in elderly patients.

Differential diagnosis

A unilateral and painful lesions of grouped vesicles along a dermatome, with hyperesthesia and on occasion regional lymph node enlargement, is typical. The prodromal pain of herpes zoster can mimic cardiac or pleural pain, or an acute abdominal emergency. But once the eruption has appeared, the diagnosis is usually obvious, although herpes simplex may infrequently occur in a dermatomal fashion.

Complications

Serious complications may occur in herpes zoster. These include the following:

- *Ophthalmic zoster*. Corneal ulcers and scarring with severe pain may result from shingles of the first trigeminal division, the elder are mostly involved.
- *Herpes zoster oticus*. Ear canal or periosteum herpes may result from shingles of the facial nerve and the auditory nerve. When geniculate ganglion is involved and the motor and sensory nerve fibers of facial nerve are violated at the same time, facial paralysis, earache, and external auditory canal herpes can appear, which is called Ramsay-Hunt syndrome.

- *Disseminated herpes zoster*. It is defined as more than 20 lesions outside the affected dermatome. It occurs chiefly in the old or individuals, such as immunosuppressed subjects, and patients with Hodgkin's disease in particular, can develop confluent haemorrhagic involvement, which spreads and may become necrotic or gangrenous.

- *Post-herpetic neuralgia* (PHN).It is characterized by dysesthetic pain that persists after the skin lesions have healed (often four weeks later), three basic types have been described: the constant, monotonous, usually burning or deep, aching pain; the shooting, lancinating pain; and triggered pain. This affects 10%~20% of all herpes zoster patients and increases in both incidence and severity with age.

Lab test

A Tzanck smear and/or direct fluorescent antibody (DFA) can help to rapidly confirm the diagnosis. The latter (but not the former) can differentiate between HSV and VZV. Varicella and herpes zoster have the same histologic findings as HSV infections, but immunohistochemical staining can distinguish between the two viruses.

Additional laboratory tests include viral culture, serology and PCR. Viral culture is not very sensitive and results may not be available for >1 week. Serologic assays are diagnostic of VZV if the convalescent serum has at least a fourfold increase in the VZV titer relative to the acute serum. As a result, serology is only useful in retrospect. PCR is a highly sensitive and rapid technique, and its use for the detection of VZV is increasing.

Management

As this disease is self-limiting, the therapeutic principles is antiviral, relieving pain, antiphlogosis, prevention of complications.

In mild shingles, treatment is symptomatic, with rest, analgesia and bland drying preparations such as calamine lotion. More severe cases may be treated, if seen within 48 h of onset, with oral aciclovir (800mg five times a day for 7 days) or famciclovir (750mg once daily for 7 days), which promotes resolution, reduces the viral shedding time and may reduce PHN. Immunosuppressed patients often require intravenous aciclovir. Oral prednisolone, given early in the course of herpes zoster for 14 days, reduces the incidence of post-herpetic neuralgia, but must not be used if the patient is immunosuppressed.

The management of PHN is unsatisfactory. There are three classes of medication which are used as standard therapies to manage PHN: tricyclic antidepressants (TCAs), antiseizure medications and long-acting opiates.

Herpes simplex and herpes zoster

Herpes simplex
- HSV-1 infection: usually orofacial, childhood onset. Vesicles become eroded.
- HSV-2 infection: mostly genital, adult onset.
- Characterized by recurrent bouts at the same locus.
- Aciclovir is an effective topical or systemic treatment.

Herpes zoster
- Recrudescence of dormant *Varicella zoster* virus. Grouped vesicles form crusts.
- Dermatomal, especially thoracic and trigeminal distributions.
- Neuralgia may complicate, mainly in the elderly.
- Dissemination suggests underlying immunosuppression.

Web resource

http://www.herpes-coldsores.com/std/herpes.htm

Key words

Kaposi varicelliform eruption　卡波西水痘样疹
herpetic whitlow　疱疹性瘭疽
herpes gladiatorum　外伤性疱疹
herpes encephalitis　疱疹性脑炎
ophthalmic zoster　眼带状疱疹
herpes zoster oticus　耳带状疱疹
disseminated herpes zoster　播散性带状疱疹
post-herpetic neuralgia　疱疹后神经痛

Review questions

1. What is the clinical presentation of herpes simplex?
2. What is post-herpetic neuralgia and its treatment?
3. What is the difference between HSV-1 and HSV-2 infection?
4. How to explain the life long immunity after the VZV infection?

(Weimin Shi)

Chapter 24   Human immunodeficiency virus disease and immunodeficiency syndromes

Immunodeficiency results from absence or failure of one or more elements of the immune system. It may be acquired, e.g. acquired immune deficiency syndrome (AIDS), or inherited, e.g. chronic mucocutaneous candidiasis.

Human immunodeficiency virus (HIV) disease

Infection with HIV is a progressive process that mostly leads to the development of AIDS.

Aetiopathogenesis

HIV1 and HIV2 (the latter mainly found in West Africa) are retroviruses containing reverse transcriptase, which allows incorporation of the virus into a cell's DNA. The virus infects and depletes helper/inducer CD4 T lymphocytes, leading to loss of cell-mediated immunity and opportunistic infection, e.g. with Pneumocystis jiroveci, mycobacteria or cryptococci. HIV is spread by infected body fluids, e.g. blood or semen. High-risk groups for HIV infection include men who have sex with men, intravenous drug users and haemophiliacs who have received infected blood products. From mother to child transmission is also an important way, it has not found the evidence that HIV can be infected by respiratory tract, food, sweat, tears, shaking hands, sharing the swimming pool.

Clinical presentation

The acute infection may be symptomless but, in a variable proportion of cases, seroconversion is accompanied by a non-specific glandular fever-like illness with a maculopapular exanthem on the trunk. HIV infection may be asymptomatic for several years, although most infected individuals will eventually develop symptoms. In the early stages of symptomatic infection, skin changes, fatigue, weight loss, generalized lymphadenopathy, diarrhoea and fever are present without the opportunistic infections that define AIDS. Opportunistic organisms include the ubiquitous *Mycobacterium avium* complex and *Cryptococcus neoformans*, and toxoplasmosis and cytomegalovirus.

As the disease progresses, the number of CD4$^+$ lymphocytes falls and, when the blood count is below 50cells/ml in the late phase of HIV infection (AIDS), *M. avium* complex infection, tuberculosis, Pneumocystis jiroveci, lymphoma and encephalopathy may develop. The mean latent period between infection and the development of AIDS is 8~10 years. Skin signs include the following (Table 24-1).

■ *Dry skin.* Skin dryness, often with asteatotic eczema, and seborrhoeic dermatitis (Fig. 24-1) are common and early findings. Their severity increases as the disease advances.

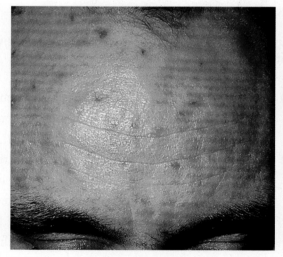

Fig. 24-1 **Seborrhoeic dermatitis, often seen in early and intermediate HIV infection.**

■ *Fungal and papillomavirus infections.* Tinea infections and perianal and common viral warts are seen in early disease.

Table 24-1	Skin signs and the progressive stages of HIV infection (Centers for Disease Control)			
Group	I (Primary phase)	II (Early phase: asymptomatic)	III (Persistent generalized lymphadenopathy)	IV (Symptomatic: AIDS)
Skin signs	Transient maculo-papular eruption on trunk	Hypersensitivity reactions, onset or worsening of eczemas, psoriasis or folliculitis, wart virus and fungal infections	Herpes zoster, eczemas worsen, candidiasis, Kaposi's sarcoma	Candidiasis, opportunistic infections, Kaposi's sarcoma, lymphoma

- *Acne and folliculitis.* These worsen in early and mid-stage disease.
- *Other infections.* Oral candidiasis, oral hairy leukoplakia (thought to be associated with Epstein-Barr virus; Fig. 24-2) and infection with herpes simplex, herpes zoster, molluscum contagiosum and *Staphylococcus aureus* are increased in advanced disease.

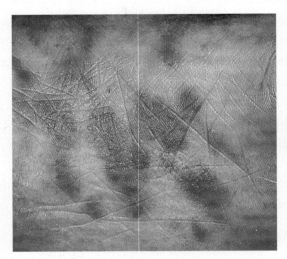

Fig. 24-3 **Kaposi's sarcoma, found in intermediate and late HIV infection.**

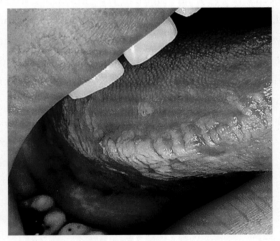

Fig. 24-2 **Oral hairy leukoplakia, seen in late HIV infection (AIDS).**

- *Other dermatoses.* Drug eruptions, hyperpigmentation and basal cell carcinomas are more common; psoriasis can get worse and syphilis may coexist.
- *Kaposi's sarcoma.* Kaposi's sarcoma is a multicentric tumour of vascular endothelium seen in a third of patients with AIDS or AIDS-related complex, particularly in male homosexuals. It presents as purplish nodules or macules on the face, limbs, trunk or in the mouth (Fig. 24-3), but often also involves the internal organs and lymph nodes. Kaposi's sarcoma is due to co-infection with herpes virus 8. A more benign sporadic form, seen in elderly East European Jewish men, is not associated with HIV.

- *Lymphoma.* Lymphomas seen with late-phase HIV infection are often extranodal and sometimes cutaneous.

Management

Clinical diagnosis of HIV infection is confirmed by a blood test for the virus by enzyme-linked immunosorbent assay (ELISA), western blot test (WB), and the disease is staged by measurement of $CD4^+$ count and viral load by polymerase chain reaction (PCR). Other co-transmitted diseases (including syphilis and hepatitis C) and tuberculosis should be tested for. Patients should be managed in departments with special experience in HIV disease. Infected individuals are counselled and sexual contacts are traced. Without anti-retroviral therapy, 5 years after HIV infection, 15% will have progressed to AIDS, but two-thirds of the remainder will be asymptomatic. Ten years after infection, 50% will have developed AIDS, of whom 80% will have died. After AIDS has developed, mortality is high, with 50% dying in 1 year and 85% in 5 years. About 20%~50% of infants born to HIV-infected women have HIV disease.

The best predictors of progression are the CD4 count (<250cells/ml predicts a 66% chance of developing AIDS within 2 years), HIV RNA viral load and the development of oral candidiasis.

Medical intervention is by highly active anti-retroviral therapy (HAART, with reverse transcriptase and protease inhibitors). The prophylaxis of opportunistic infection and general support including early treatment of infections. Aerosol pentamidine or oral co-trimoxazole is effective in preventing *P. jiroveci* pneumonia, and ganciclovir is used to control cytomegalovirus infection. Kaposi's sarcoma may be treated with radiotherapy, cytotoxic agents or interferon-α.

Congenital immune deficiency syndromes

Congenital immune deficiency syndromes are divided into:

- *B cell deficiency*: immunoglobulin deficit; sometimes combined with infection, malignant tumor and autoimmune diseases.
- *T cell deficiency*: impairment of cell-mediated immunity.
- *Defects in effector mechanisms* such as complement or neutrophils.

Many of these conditions are very rare and present in infancy with failure to thrive. Opportunistic or pyogenic infections that often involve the skin are a feature. Examples of these include the following:

- *X-linked agammaglobulinaemia.* Infections occur in infancy once maternal antibodies run out.
- *IgA deficiency.* Affects 1 in 700 caucasians; half have recurrent infections.
- *Severe combined immune deficiency.* Fatal in infancy because of overwhelming infection unless treated by bone marrow transplant.
- *Wiskott-Aldrich syndrome.* X-linked with T cell defects, thrombocytopenia and an associated eczema.
- *Chronic mucocutaneous candidiasis.* Seen with severe immune deficiencies, multiple endocrine

dysfunction or occurring sporadically; mainly due to a T cell defect. Candidiasis usually involves the mouth, skin or nails (Fig. 24-4).

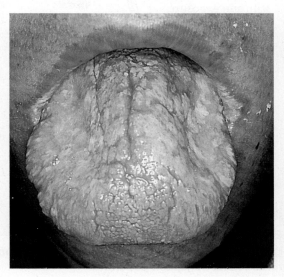

Fig. 24-4   **Chronic mucocutaneous candidiasis, mainly due to a T cell defect.**

- *Chronic granulomatous disease.* Phagocytosis is defective.

Skin signs of immunosuppression for allografts

The use of corticosteroids, azathioprine and ciclosporin for the suppression of allograft rejection is well established. Cutaneous side-effects include not only drug eruptions and side-effects from the drugs but also infections and tumours, which develop as a result of impairment of immune surveillance, and graft-versus-host disease, which is a manifestation of an immune reaction against the host's body by the grafted tissue. Recipients of renal allografts seem to be at particular risk of developing skin cancers. Specific skin problems in immunosuppressed allograft recipients include the following:

- *Infections and infestations.* Herpes zoster, herpes simplex and cytomegalovirus infection may be reactivated with immunosuppressive therapy. Boils and cellulitis are common, and crusted 'Norwegian' scabies may occur.
- *Human papillomavirus infection.* About 50% of renal transplant patients have viral warts (Fig. 24-5).

These may be associated with actinic keratoses or other dysplastic lesions on sun-exposed sites. The human papillomavirus acts as a carcinogen along with sun exposure.

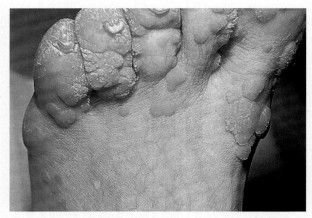

Fig. 24-5 **Extensive viral warts in an immunosuppressed renal transplant patient.**

■ *Skin cancers.* The risk of skin cancer in renal transplant recipients is increased 20-fold compared with the normal population. Squamous cell carcinomas (Fig. 24-6) are more common than basal cell carcinomas. The tumours may look clinically and histologically banal but behave aggressively. Malignant melanoma is also more common.

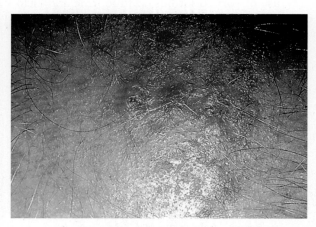

Fig. 24-6 **Squamous cell carcinoma associated with immunosuppression in a renal transplant recipient.**

■ *Graft-versus-host disease.*

> ### *HIV disease and immunosuppression*
> ■ **HIV infection** may be asymptomatic for several years. Skin signs of early HIV disease include dry skin and seborrhoeic dermatitis; signs of late disease are extensive infections, oral candidiasis and Kaposi's sarcoma, Cardiovascular disease and tumors. HAART and the prevention of opportunistic infection have transformed the outlook for patients with HIV.
> ■ **Congenital immune deficiency syndromes** are rare, often present with failure to thrive in infancy and are associated with opportunistic or pyogenic infections.
> ■ **Immunosuppression for allografts** is particularly associated with human papillomavirus infection, squamous cell carcinomas or dysplastic lesions, and graft-versus-host disease.

Web resource

http://www.tht.org.uk/informationresources/hivan-daids/

http://www.aidsmap.com/

Key words

human immunodeficiency virus　人类免疫缺陷病毒
Pneumocystis jiroveci　耶氏肺孢子虫病
oral candidiasis　口腔念珠菌病
Kaposi's sarcoma　卡波西肉瘤
highly active anti-retroviral therapy (HAART)　高效抗逆转录病毒治疗
structured intermittent therapy　结构性间歇治疗
graft-versus-host disease　移植物抗宿主病

Review questions

1. What are the clinical presentations of HIV?
2. How to treat and prevent HIV?
3. What kinds of skin signs of immunosuppression for allografts?

(Nan Yu)

Chapter 25   Fungal infections

The skin constitutes the main site of recognizable fungal infections in humans which can be divided into superficial and deep mycoses. When restricted to the skin, most mycotic infections are superficial and are limited to a depth of 1mm to 2mm. Fungal infections in human skin is common and is mainly due to two groups of fungi. The infections are usually confined to the stratum corneum.

■ *Dermatophytes*: multicellular filaments or hyphae.

■ *Yeasts*: unicellular forms that replicate by budding.

Pityriasis versicolor due to the yeast *Malassezia* (previously *Pityrosporum ovale*).

Dermatophyte infections

The mycoses caused by dermatophytes are called dermatophytosis. Dermatophyte fungi reproduce by spore formation. They infect the stratum corneum, nail and hair, and induce inflammation by delayed hypersensitivity or by metabolic effects. There are three asexual genera:

■ *Microsporum* infect skin and hair.

■ *Trichophyton* infect skin, nail and hair.

■ *Epidermophyton* infect skin and nail.

Forty-five species are pathogenic in humans. Zoophilic species (transmitted to humans from animals), e.g. *Trichophyton verrucosum* (*T. verrucosum*) (Fig. 25-1), produce more inflammation than anthropophilic (human only) species.

Pathology

Dermatophytes inhabit keratin as branching hyphae, identifiable on microscopy. Skin scrapings, placed on a slide with 10% aqueous potassium hydroxide (to separate the keratinocytes) and a coverslip, are examined microscopically for hyphae. The dermatophyte is identified by culturing the scrapings on medium (e.g. Sabouraud's) for 3 weeks.

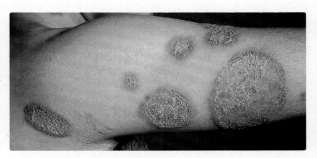

Fig. 25-1   **Tinea corporis.** The infection is due to animal ringworm (*T. verrucosum*) and shows intense inflammation.

Clinical presentation

■ Tinea (Latin: *worm*) denotes a fungal skin infection which is often annular. The exact features depend on the site. The various presentations include the following: **Tinea corporis** (trunk and limbs). Tinea corporis includes all superficial dermatophyte infections of the skin other than those involving the scalp, beard, face, hands, feet, and groin. They are single or multiple plaques, with scaling and erythema especially at the edges, characterize this presentation. The lesions enlarge slowly, with central clearing, leaving a ring pattern, hence 'ringworm' (Figs. 25-1 and. 25-2). Pustules or vesicles may be seen.

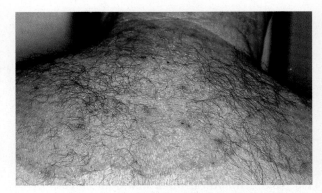

Fig. 25-2   **Tinea corporis showing a well-defined edge.**

■ **Tinea cruris** (groin). This is more common in men and is often seen in athletes ('jock itch'), who may also have tinea pedis. It spreads to the

Table 25-1 **Superficial mycoses: causative organisms and differential diagnosis**

Area	Commonest organism	Differential diagnosis
Body/limbs (corporis)	T. verrucosum, M. canis, T. rubrum	Discoid eczema, psoriasis, pityriasis rosea
Feet (pedis)	T. rubrum, T. interdigitale, E. floccosum	Contact dermatitis, psoriasis, pompholyx, erythrasma
Groin (cruris)	T. rubrum, E. floccosum, T. interdigitale	Intertrigo, candidiasis, erythrasma
Hand (manuum)	T. rubrum	Chronic eczema, psoriasis, granuloma annulare
Nail (unguium)	T. rubrum, T. interdigitale	Psoriasis, trauma, candidiasis
Scalp (capitis)	M. canis, M. audouinii, T. tonsurans, T. schoenleinii	Alopecia areata, psoriasis, seborrhoeic eczema, furunculosis

upper thigh but rarely involves the scrotum. The advancing edge may be scaly, pustular or vesicular. Causative organisms are shown in Table 25-1.

■ **Tinea incognito.** Tinea incognito is a fungal infection of the skin masked and often exacerbated by application of a topical immunosuppressive agent. The usual agent is a topical corticosteroid. As the skin fungal infection has lost some of the characteristic features due to suppression of inflammation, it may have a poorly defined border and florid growth. Occasionally, secondary infection with bacteria occurs with concurrent pustules and impetigo.

■ **Tinea manuum** (hand). Typically, this appears as a unilateral, diffuse powdery scaling of the palm (Fig. 25-3). *Trichophyton rubrum* (*T. rubrum*) is often the cause. It is usual to find unilateral infection in tinea of the hand, coexisting with tinea pedis, hence the expression "two-foot, one-hand disease".

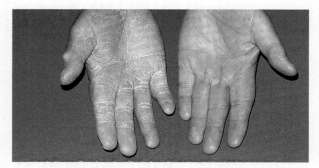

Fig. 25-3 **Unilateral tinea manuum caused by** *T. rubrum.*

■ **Tinea capitis** (scalp/hair).
■ **Tinea unguium** (nails).
■ **Tinea pedis** (athlete's foot).

Athlete's foot is common in adults (especially young men), rare in children and predisposed to by communal washing, swimming baths, occlusive footwear and hot weather. Itchy interdigital maceration, usually of the fourth/fifth toeweb space, is most frequent, but diffuse 'moccasin' involvement is seen. Recurrent vesicles also occur, sometimes with pompholyx as an id reaction. The commonest organisms are *T. rubrum*, *T. mentagrophytes* var. *interdigitale* and *Epidermophyton floccosum.*

The differential diagnoses of superficial mycoses are shown Table 25-1. Microscopy and culture of skin scrapings are often helpful. Wood's ultraviolet light examination is used for tinea capitis, especially for screening during outbreaks. Hair infected by *Microsporum audouinii* and *M. canis* fluoresces green, but *Trichophyton tonsurans* does not fluoresce.

Management

Humid and sweaty conditions, including occlusive footwear, should be minimized, and dusting powder may help to keep the feet or body folds dry. Minor fungal infections respond to topical treatments, but widespread involvement or diseases of the nails or scalp requires systemic therapy.

Topical therapy

Tinea corporis, tinea pedis and tinea cruris respond to topical imidazole (e.g. clotrimazole and miconazole) creams, sprays or powders. Terbinafine cream once daily is often effective. Amorolfine, applied once weekly, produces a 40-50% cure for tinea unguium of one or two nails; similarly tioconazole may be used topically.

Systemic therapy

Tinea capitis, tinea manuum, tinea unguium and extensive tinea corporis often require systemic treatment. Griseofulvin is still the licensed choice for tinea capitis in children (10mg/kg daily for 1~2 months) but, for other indications, it has largely been superseded by the newer antifungals, terbinafine (Lamisil, often used off-licence) and itraconazole (Sporanox), which show greater efficacy, have fewer side-effects and require shorter treatments.

Terbinafine 250mg daily or itraconazole 100mg daily may be used for tinea capitis, corporis, cruris, manuum and pedis, given for 2~4 weeks. In tinea unguium, terbinafine (250mg daily for 6~12 weeks) is the drug of choice; itraconazole (200mg daily for 12 weeks or as 'pulsed' courses) is an alternative. In the elderly, uncomplicated fungal toenail infection may not require any therapy. Itraconazole can potentially cause hepatotoxicity and requires cautious use in heart failure.

Ketoconazole (Nizoral) by mouth, although effective, is limited in use by hepatotoxicity.

Candida albicans infection

Candida albicans (*C. albicans*) may cause different types of lesions of the skin, nails, mucous membranes, and viscera. It is a ubiquitous commensal of the mouth and gastrointestinal tract that can produce opportunistic infection. Predisposing factors include:

- moist and opposing skin folds
- obesity or diabetes mellitus
- immunosuppression
- pregnancy
- poor hygiene
- humid environment
- wet work occupation
- use of broad-spectrum antibiotic.

Clinical presentation

In infection, hyphal forms of *C. albicans* are seen in the stratum corneum. Infection may present as the following:

- **Genital.** Thrush commonly appears as an itchy, sore vulvovaginitis. White plaques adhere to inflamed mucous membranes, and a white vaginal discharge may occur. Males develop similar changes on the penis. It can be spread by sexual intercourse.
- **Intertrigo.** Superinfection with *C. albicans*, and often also with bacteria, gives a moist, glazed and macerated appearance to the submammary, axillary or inguinal body folds. The interdigital clefts are involved (Fig. 25-4) in wet workers who do not dry their hands properly.

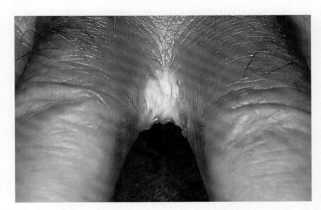

Fig. 25-4 **Intertrigo of the interdigital cleft due to *C. albicans*.**

- **Mucocutaneous candidiasis.** This rare, sometimes inherited disorder of immune deficiency starts in infancy. Chronic *C. albicans* intertrigo with nail and mouth infections is seen.
- **Oral.** Grayish white plaques are found on the surface of the mucous membrane. The base of these plaques is moist, reddish, and macerated. Broad-spectrum antibiotics, false teeth and poor oral hygiene predispose. Angular stomatitis may coexist.
- **Paronychia.**
- **Systemic.** *C. albicans* is capable of causing a severe, destructive, disseminated disease, and mostly occur in immunosuppressed patients. Red nodules are seen in the skin.

Management

C. albicans infections must be differentiated from other conditions (Table 25-2). General measures are important. Body folds are separated and kept dry with dusting powder. Hands are dried carefully and oral hygiene improved. Systemic antibiotics may need to be stopped. Specific agents against *Candida* are used topically and systemically.

Table 25-2 **Differential diagnosis: *C. albicans* infections**	
Variant	**Differential diagnosis**
Genital	Psoriasis, lichen planus, lichen sclerosus
Intertrigo	Psoriásis, seborrhoeic dermatitis, bacterial secondary infection
Oral	Lichen planus, epithelial dysplasia
Paronychia	Bacterial infection, chronic eczema

Topical therapy

Imidazoles are effective and available as creams, powders, pessaries and lotions. For oral *candida*, use amphotericin, nystatin or miconazole as lozenges, suspension or gels.

Systemic therapy

Bowel carriage may be reduced in recurrent candidiasis by oral nystatin. Itraconazole 100mg daily or fluconazole 50mg daily, but not griseofulvin, can be given as a short course for persistent *C. albicans* infections and in the long term for mucocutaneous candidiasis. Vaginal candidiasis is treated by a single dose of 500mg clotrimazole or 150mg econazole as a pessary, or with itraconazole or fluconazole by mouth. *C. glabrata* is increasingly identified and is frequently resistant to fluconazole.

> *Fungal infections*
> - Dermatophytes infect the feet, groin, body, nails, hands and scalp. The commonest dermatophyte pathogens are *Trichophyton rubrum*, *T. mentagrophytes* var. *interdigitale* and *Epidermophyton floccosum*.
> - Topical imidazoles and oral terbinafine or itraconazole are effective for most dermatophyte infections.
> - *C. albicans* produces opportunistic infection of the body folds, mouth, genitals and nail fold. These are predisposed to by humidity, obesity, diabetes and oral antibiotic therapy.
> - Topical imidazoles are usually effective for candidiasis.

Key words

pityriasis versicolor　花斑糠疹

tinea corporis　体癣

tinea cruris　股癣

tinea incognito　难辨认癣

tinea manuum　手癣

tinea capitis　头癣

tinea unguium　甲癣

tinea pedis　足癣

mucocutaneous candidiasis　皮肤黏膜念珠菌病

Review questions

1. What are the main fungi which cause infections in human skin?

2. What are the typical clinical presentations of dermatophyte infections in skin such as Tinea corporis?

3. What are the indications of systemic treatment for dermatophyte infections?

(Houmin Li)

Chapter 26 Tropical infections and infestations

Infections constitute one of the biggest problems in dermatology in tropical countries of the developing world. Leprosy, for example, despite being a treatable disease, continues to ravage in many parts of the globe.

However, tropical infections may also be seen in countries in which they are non-endemic - among visitors and immigrants, or when acquired abroad by the indigenous population.

Leprosy

Leprosy is a chronic disease caused by *Mycobacterium leprae* (*M. leprae*). This is an acid- and alcohol-fast bacillus that has not been successfully cultured in vitro. It requires temperature of ~35℃ to grow, and thus has a preference for cooler regions of the body (e.g. the nose, testicles and ear lobes) as well as regions where the peripheral nerves are close to the skin. Nasal and oral droplets spread the infection, and the incubation period varies widely, from months to over 30 years, but it is usually 4~10 years. Leprosy affects all races and ages; however, it speak incidence occurs in individuals between 10~15 and 30~60 years of age. Most cases are found in India, Brazil, Indonesia, Myanmar, Madagascar and Nepal. The manifestation of the disease depends on the delayed (type Ⅳ) hypersensitivity response in the infected individual. Those with intact cell-mediated immunity develop tuberculoid leprosy, whereas those with the least cell-mediated immunity develop lepromatous leprosy. Borderline lesions are seen in those whose immune state is intermediate.

M. leprae has a predilection for nerves and the dermis but, in the lepromatous type, infection may be much more widespread. Tuberculoid leprosy is characterized by a granulomatous reaction in the nerves and dermis with no acid-fast bacilli demonstrated using the Ziehl-Neelsen stain. In contrast, bacilli are plentiful in the dermis of the lepromatous type, and large numbers of macrophages are seen on microscopy.

Clinical presentation

The clinical manifestations of leprosy involve primarily the skin and the nervous system.

In *Tuberculoid leprosy*, the lesions are solitary or few in number (five or less).The typical lesion is the large, erythematous plaque with a sharply defined and elevated border, which is usually dry and hairless (Fig. 26-1). The most common locations are the face, limbs, or trunk. A tuberculoid lesion is anesthetic or hypesthetic and anhidrotic, and superficial peripheral nerves serving or proximal to the lesion are enlarged, tender, or both. Nerve involvement is early and prominent, leading to characteristic changes in the muscle groups served.

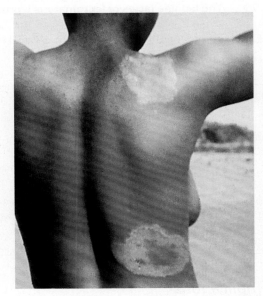

Fig. 26-1 **Hypopigmented plaques of tuberculoid leprosy.**

Lepromatous leprosy is characterized initially by multiple, poorly defined, erythematous macules, papules, nodules and plaques. They are diffusely and symmetrically distributed. The most common sites of involvement are the face, buttocks and lower extremities. Infiltration of the skin of the forehead can lead to a leonine facies with loss of eyebrows (Fig. 26-2). There is little or no loss of sensation over the lesions. Anesthesia in a stocking or glove distribution may develop.

Borderline leprosy, as its name implies, shows features that are intermediate between *lepromatous leprosy* and *tuberculoid leprosy*.

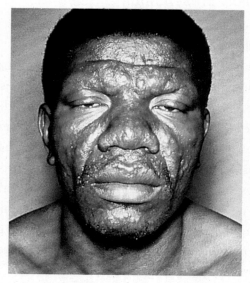

Fig. 26-2 **The leonine facies of lepromatous leprosy.**

Leprosy must be distinguished from a variety of other dermatological conditions (Table 26-1).

Table 26-1	**Differential diagnosis of leprosy**
Type of leprosy	**Differential diagnosis**
Tuberculoid	Vitiligo, pityriasisversicolor, pityriasis alba, sarcoidosis, lupus vulgaris, granuloma annulare, post-inflammatory hypopigmentation
Lepromatous	Disseminated cutaneous leishmaniasis, yaws, guttate psoriasis, discoid lupus erythematosus, mycosis fungoides

Complications

As a result of the nerve damage, muscular paralysis and atrophy generally affect the small muscles of the hands and feet or some of the facial muscles. The fingers develop contractures, with the formation of a clawhand, and owning to resorption of phalangeal bones, fingers and toes become shorter. Trophic ulceration usually manifests as a perforating ulcer on the foot. In *lepromatous leprosy*, late sequelae include saddle nose, testicular atrophy and acquired ichthyosis on the lower extremities. Reactions are a characteristic and clinically important aspect of Hansen's disease, especially during treatment. These are characterized by acute inflammation that appears suddenly. The reactions are due to a change in the immunologic state of the patient.

Management

Lepromatous (multibacillary) leprosy is treated with rifampicin, dapsone and clofazimine. Treatment is for at least 2 years, continued until skin smears are negative. Tuberculoid (paucibacillary) leprosy responds to rifampicin and dapsone, given for 6 months. The complications of leprosy may require the skills of rehabilitation specialists and orthopaedic and plastic surgeons.

In countries where leprosy is endemic, the education of the public about the disease is important in reducing the stigma attached to sufferers. Public health programmes aimed at leprosy control are active in several countries.

Leishmaniasis

Leishmaniasis is a disease caused by *Leishmania* protozoa, which are transmitted by sand fly bites. It exists in tropical and subtropical areas in a cutaneous, mucocutaneous or visceral form. Three protozoa cause disease:

1. *Leishmaniatropica* causes the cutaneous 'oriental sore' and is seen around the Mediterranean coast, in the Middle East and in Asia.
2. *L. braziliensis*, endemic in Central and South America, leads to cutaneous and mucosal disease.
3. *L. donovani* is widely distributed in Asia, Africa and South America, and causes visceral disease (kala-azar) with associated skin lesions.

Clinical presentation

Oriental sore is a common infection in endemic areas normally affecting children, who subsequently develop immunity. In non-endemic regions, it is not infrequently seen in travellers after a Mediterranean holiday. The face, neck or arms are usually affected. At the site of inoculation, a red or brown nodule appears, which either ulcerates or spreads slowly to form a crust-topped plaque (Fig. 26-3). Untreated, the lesion will heal in 6~12 months, although a chronic form is seen. In *mucocutaneousleishmaniasis*, the skin lesion resembles an oriental sore but, subsequently, necrotic ulcers affect the nose, lips and palate with deformity. *Kala-azar* principally affects children and has a significant mortality. It causes hepatomegaly, splenomegaly, anaemia and debility. The cutaneous signs are patchy pigmentation on the face, hands and abdomen.

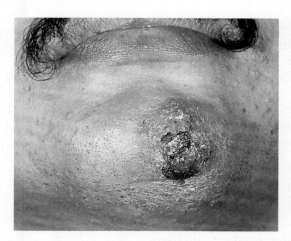

Fig. 26-3 **The oriental sore of cutaneous leishmaniasis.** Small lesions may respond to cryotherapy. Otherwise, intravenous sodium stibogluconate may be given.

Leishmaniasis must be distinguished from some other disorders (Table 26-2).

Table 26-2	**Differential diagnosis of leishmaniasis**
Variant	**Differential diagnosis**
Cutaneous	Lupus vulgaris, leprosy, discoid lupus erythematosus
Mucocutaneous	Syphilis, yaws, leprosy, blastomycosis
Kala-azar	Leprosy

Management

Cutaneous leishmaniasis may heal spontaneously, and small areas respond to cryotherapy. When specific treatment is needed, it is usual to give sodium stibogluconate (Pentostam) intravenously, usually for 15~21 days. The treatment for the mucocutaneous and visceral forms is similar.

Larva migrans

Larva migrans is a 'creeping' eruption due to penetration of the skin by the larval stage of animal hookworms. Larva migrans is often acquired from tropical beaches where ova from the hookworms of dogs and cats have hatched into larvae that are able to penetrate the human skin. Penetration usually occurs on the feet. The larvae advance at the rate of a few millimetres a day in a serpiginous route causing red intensely itchy tracks to appear (Fig. 26-4). They eventually die spontaneously after a few weeks, as they cannot complete their life cycle in humans.

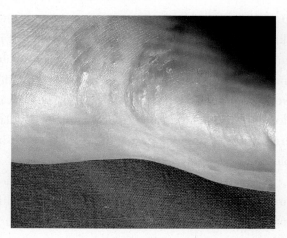

Fig. 26-4 **Larva migrans seen in a child who had just visited the beaches of the West Indies.** Treatment is with oral ivermectin or topical thiabendazole.

Topical 10% thiabendazole cream or a single oral dose of ivermectin (200mcg/kg) is usually effective.

Deep mycoses

Deep mycoses are defined as the invasion of living tissue by fungi, causing systemic disease. Brief details are given in Table 26-3.

Filariasis

Filariasis is seen in the tropics and is often due to the nematode worm *Wuchereria bancrofti*. Lymphatic damage ultimately results in gross oedema of the legs and scrotum ('elephantiasis'). Treatment is with diethylcarbamazine.

Table 26-3   **The deep mycoses**

Mycosis	Clinical features	Management
Actinomycosis (filamentous bacteria)	A chronic suppurating granulomatous infection with multiple sinuses discharging yellow granules, particularly around the jaw, chest and abdomen	Long-term high-dose penicillin, surgical excision
Blastomycosis	Ulcerated discharging nodules that show central clearing with scarring; may spread from pulmonary infection	Oral itraconazole, systemic amphotericin B or ketoconazole
Histoplasmosis	Seen in immunosuppressed patients who develop lung disease with granulomatous skin lesions	Oral itraconazole or ketoconazole, or systemic amphotericin B
Mycetoma	A chronic granulomatous infection usually of the foot, involving skin, subcutaneous tissue and bones, due to several types of fungi or actinomycetes; nodules with abscesses, sinuses, ulceration and tissue necrosis result	Depends on the organism; surgical excision, dapsone with co-trimoxazole, and itraconazole may help
Sporotrichosis	An abscess forms with nodules subsequently occurring proximally along the line of lymphatic drainage	Potassium iodide, itraconazole or terbinafine

Onchocerciasis

Onchocerciasis is a disease affecting the eyes and skin, caused by the worm *Onchocerca volvulus*. It is endemic in Africa and Central America and is an important cause of blindness. A gnat transmits the worm to humans. Dermal nodules with lichenification and pigmentary change follow an itchy papular eruption. Microfilariae invade the eye and result in blindness.

Ivermectin, as a single dose, is the drug of choice for onchocerciasis. Retreatment at 6- or 12-month intervals may be needed until the worms die out.

Tropical infections

- **Leprosy:** tuberculoid and lepromatous forms mainly affect the skin and nerves; treatment is with dapsone, rifampicin and clofazimine.
- **Leishmaniasis:** cutaneous, mucocutaneous and visceral types; treatment is with sodium stibogluconate.
- **Larva migrans:** creeping eruption due to animal hookworms; responds to thiabendazole cream or oral ivermectin.
- **Deep mycoses:** serious infections that may be difficult to eradicate.
- **Onchocerciasis:** an important cause of blindness; skin shows lichenified nodules and pigmentary changes. Treatment is with oral ivermectin.

Web resources

http://www.who.int/lep/en/
http://www.cdc.gov/ncidod/dpd/

Key words

leprosy   麻风
hypersensitivity response   超敏反应
tuberculoid leprosy   结核样型麻风
lepromatous leprosy   瘤型麻风
borderline leprosy   中间界线类麻风
leishmaniasis   利什曼病

Review questions

1. What are the clinical types of leprosy?
2. What are the typical clinical manifestations of different types of leprosy?
3. What are the possible complications of leprosy?

(Houmin Li)

Chapter 27   Infestations

Infestation is defined as the harbouring of insect or worm parasites in or on the body. Worms - on or in the skin - are infrequent except in tropical countries. Insect life on the skin is usually transient in temperate climes, although a mite (*Demodex folliculorum*) may live harmlessly in facial hair follicles.

Insects cause a variety of skin reactions (Table 27-1). Contact with an insect or an insect bite can produce a chemical effect, such as a bee sting, or an irritant effect, such as dermatitis from contact with a caterpillar or blistering due to cantharadin released from a crushed beetle. Contact may also cause an immune-mediated response.

Table 27-1	**Insect effects on the skin**
Insect	**Effect**
Animal ticks	Bites, disease vector
Ants, bedbugs, fleas	Bites
Bees, wasps	Stings
Caterpillars	Dermatitis
Cheyletiella	Papular urticaria
Demodex folliculorum	Normal inhabitant
Food and harvest mites	Bites
Lice	Infestation (bites), disease vector
Mosquitoes	Bites, myiasis, disease vector
Sarcoptes scabei	Scabies

Insects act as vectors of skin disease, as in Lyme disease, when animal ticks transmit *Borrelia burgdorferi*. They involve the skin directly by burrowing (e.g. scabies) or by laying eggs that hatch into larvae (myiasis).

Insect bites

The cutaneous reaction following the bite of an insect is due to a pharmacological, irritant or allergic response to the introduced foreign material.

Clinical presentation

The lesions of insect bites vary from itchy wheals (Fig. 27-1) through papules to quite large bullae (Fig. 27-2). The morphology will depend on the insect (Table 27-1) and the type of response elicited. Insect bites are usually grouped or track up a limb. Papular urticaria defines recurrent itchy urticated papules on the limbs or trunk, quite often in a child. The culprits, which may be difficult to trace, include garden insects, fleas or mites on household pets. Bedbugs cause bites on the face, neck and hands. They lie inactive in crevices in furniture during the day and emerge at night. Secondary bacterial infection of excoriated insect bites is common.

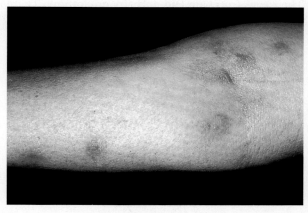

Fig. 27-1 **Papular urticaria, showing grouped and linear lesions.**

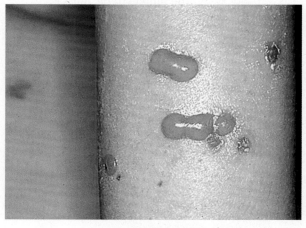

Fig. 27-2 **Grouped blisters due to insect bites.**

Differential diagnosis

The linear or grouped nature of the lesions is usually suggestive, but sometimes urticaria, scabies, atopic eczema or dermatitis herpetiformis may need to be considered.

Management

Elimination of the cause is often not easy, as the insects are difficult to trace. Household pets must be inspected and treated if necessary. Cat fleas exist for months on carpets without a cat being present. Birds nesting or perching by a window can introduce *Cheyletiella* into a house. An individual with insect bites can be helped by Eurax-Hydrocortisone cream or calamine lotion.

Lice infestation (pediculosis)

Lice are flat, wingless, blood-sucking insects (Fig. 27-3). Their eggs (nits) are laid on hairs or clothing. There are two anthropophilic species:

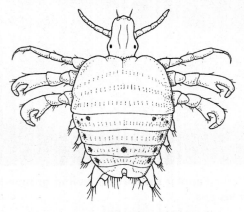

Fig. 27-3 **The female pubic louse.**

1. Pubic louse.
2. Body louse (the head louse is a variant).

   Head lice are common among schoolchildren and spread by head-to-head contact. The nits are often easier to see than the lice. The body louse is mainly seen in vagrants who live in unhygienic or poor social conditions. Spread is by infested bedding or clothing. The pubic louse is sexually transmitted and is mostly found in young adults. Lice induce intense itching which, through scratching, results in excoriation and secondary infection.

Clinical presentation

The itching of head lice usually starts at the sides and back of the scalp. Scratching results in secondary infection that may cause matted hair. Body lice result in excoriations on the trunk and, in chronic infestation, lichenification and pigmentation. The lice are found in the seams of clothes. Pubic lice, known colloquially as 'crabs', result in severe pruritus with secondary eczema and infection. They may involve the eyelashes. Lice infestation should not be confused with other conditions (Table 27-2).

Table 27-2	**Differential diagnosis of pediculosis**
Louse infestation	**Differential diagnosis**
Body louse	Scabies, chronic eczema
Head louse	Impetigo, eczema
Pubic louse	Scabies, eczema
Pubic louse	Scabies, eczema

Management

Head lice are treated with malathion or phenothrin lotion, applied to the scalp for 12h, washed out and repeated in 7 days. Dimeticone is an alternative. Nits are removed by wet combing. Contacts are also treated. Body lice are eradicated by treating the clothing with tumble drying, laundering or dry cleaning. Malathion or permethrin lotions may be used on the skin. Infestation with pubic lice requires the application of malathion or permethrin aqueous lotions to all the body. Sexual partners should be treated.

Scabies

The scabies mite, *Sarcoptes scabei* var. *hominis*, is 0.4mm in length (Fig. 27-4) and is spread by direct physical transfer, including sexual contact. The fertilized female mite burrows through the stratum corneum at the rate of 2mm/day, laying two or three eggs each day. The eggs hatch after 3 days into larvae, which form shallow pockets in the stratum corneum where they moult and mature within about 2 weeks. The mites mate in the pockets; the male dies, but the fertilized female burrows and continues the cycle. After first being infested, it takes 3~4 weeks for the hypersensitivity reaction to the mite, and the intense itching that it causes, to develop. On average, about 12 mites are present at the itching stage, but it can be many more.

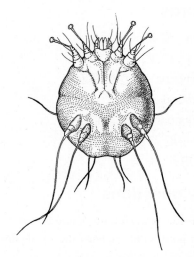

Fig. 27-4 **The female scabies mite.**

Clinical presentation

The irregular, tortuous and slightly scaly burrows measure up to 1cm long. They are commonest on the sides of fingers (Fig. 27-5), wrists, ankles and nipples, and on the genitalia where they form rubbery nodules. Small vesicles are often seen. Itching induces excoriations (Fig. 27-6). In infants, the feet are frequently involved and the face can be affected. The mite is occasionally visible as a white dot at the end of a burrow. If extracted with a needle and viewed under a microscope, the diagnosis is irrefutable.

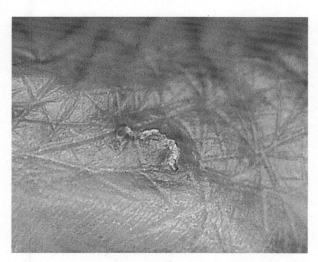

Fig. 27-5 **A scabetic burrow on the side of the finger in an elderly patient.**

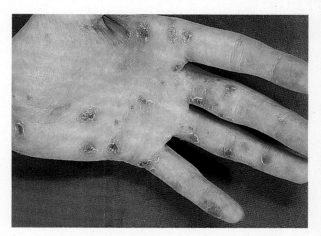

Fig. 27-6 **Multiple excoriations on the hand due to scabies infestation.**

Scabies is often accompanied by an ill-defined eczematous urticated papular hypersensitivity reaction on the trunk. Untreated, scabies becomes chronic.

Differential diagnosis

Other intensely itchy eruptions, such as lichen planus, dermatitis herpetiformis, papular urticaria and eczema, may need to be considered, but only scabies shows burrows. Animal scabies, due to animal mites, causes an itchy eruption, but burrows are absent.

Complications

Scabies commonly becomes secondarily infected. In institutionalized or immunosuppressed patients, very large numbers of mites proliferate to produce an extensive crusted eruption known as 'Norwegian' scabies

Patients commonly feel itchy for some days even after adequate treatment, and pruritic non-infested 'post-scabetic' nodules may persist for weeks. Scabicides often cause an irritant dermatitis, and care must be taken to distinguish this from persistent or recurrent infestation.

Management

An adequate application technique and the treatment of all contacts are most important in the treatment of scabies. If either is lacking, persistence or re-infestation may result. An instruction leaflet for patients is helpful. The aqueous preparations of permethrin

(Lyclear Dermal) and malathion (Derbac-M) are effective. Benzyl benzoate, crotamiton (Eurax) and 10% sulphur ointment are alternatives. Oral ivermectin (200mcg/kg) two doses 1 week apart may be used when topical therapy alone is ineffective, e.g. in crusted scabies. For topical treatment, the suggested technique is as follows:

■ Apply the lotion or cream to the entire body surface including scalp, face, neck and ears.

■ Pay special attention to fingerweb and toeweb spaces, and under the nails.

■ Leave the lotion on for 12~24h and then wash off in the bath or shower.

■ If the hands are washed during this period, reapply the lotion or cream.

■ Repeat the treatment after 1 week.

Recently infested individuals do not itch, and close contacts (such as the whole family) and sexual partners need treatment. Scabies often breaks out in old people's homes or geriatric wards and presents the problem of how far to extend the therapeutic net. The safe rule is to treat all members of a ward or home, including nurses, who have contact with the index case. Clothing and bedding is laundered. The mite dies within a few days away from the skin.

Infestations

■ **Insect bites** present on the trunk and limbs as groups of itchy, often blistering, papules; secondary infection is common.

■ **Head lice** infestation is transmitted between schoolchildren by head contact. Secondary infection is common. Repeated treatment is often necessary.

■ **Body lice** occur in those living in poor social conditions and produce excoriation and lichenification.

■ **Pubic lice** are sexually transmitted and present with pruritus and secondary infection.

■ **Scabies** is spread by direct transfer and is intensely itchy. All contacts need treatment. Outbreaks are frequently seen in nursing homes where there is quite often an 'index' case with crusted scabies.

Web resources

http://www.cdc.gov/lice/
http://www.cdc.gov/scabies/

Key words

Infestation　侵袭
insect bite　虫咬
papular urticaria　丘疹性荨麻疹
lice infestation　虱病
blood-sucking insect　吮血昆虫
scabies　疥疮
burrow　虫孔 / 潜洞

Review questions

1. What are the clinical features of insect bites?
2. In what position of the body the female mites mainly living?

(Weihua Pan)

Chapter 28   Sebaceous and sweat glands - Acne, rosacea and other disorders

Acne

Acne is a chronic inflammation of the pilosebaceous units, producing comedones, papules, pustules, cysts and scars on the face, back and chest. It affects nearly every adolescent. Acne has an equal sex incidence and tends to affect women earlier than men, although the peak age for clinical acne is 18 years in both sexes. Acne results from:

- increased sebum excretion - seborrhoea (greasy skin)
- pilosebaceous duct hyperkeratosis and comedone formation
- colonization of the duct with *Propionibacterium acnes*
- release of inflammatory mediators (including cytokines).

In acne, the androgen-sensitive pilosebaceous unit shows a hyper-responsiveness that results in increased sebum excretion. Factors in sebum and pilosebaceous duct hyperkeratosis induce comedones, and *P. acnes* initiates inflammation through chemical mediators inducing enzymes (e.g. lipase) and prostaglandins (Fig. 28-1).

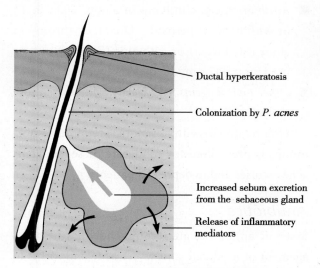

Fig. 28-1   **Aetiopathogenesis of acne.**

Ductal hyperkeratosis

Colonization by *P. acnes*

Increased sebum excretion from the sebaceous gland

Release of inflammatory mediators

Clinical presentation

The clinical features of acne include seborrhea, non-inflammatory lesions, inflammatory lesions, and various degrees of scarring. Seborrhea causes greasy skin. Non-inflammatory lesions mainly mean comedones. Comedones are either open (blackheads: dilated pores with black plugs of melanin-containing keratin) or closed (whiteheads: small cream-coloured, dome-shaped papules). They appear at about the age of 12 years and evolve into inflammatory papules (Fig. 28-2), pustules or cysts (Fig. 28-3). The sites of predilection - the face, shoulders, back and upper chest - have the highest density of pilosebaceous units. Inflammatory lesions include papules and pustules. The severity of acne depends on its extent and the type of lesion, with cysts being the most destructive.

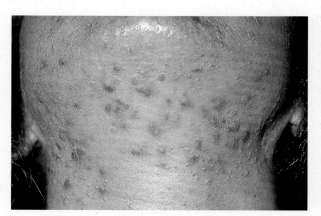

Fig. 28-2   **Papular-pustular acne of the chin, with some whiteheads.**

Acne usually persists until the early twenties, although in a few patients, particularly women, the disease continues into the fifth decade. Scars may follow healing, especially of cysts or abscesses. Scars may be 'ice-pick', atrophic (Fig. 28-4) or keloidal.

Some variants of acne are seen:

- *Acné excoriée*: due to squeezing, affects depressed or obsessional young women.

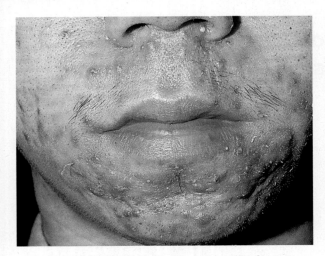

Fig. 28-3   **Pustulocystic acne on the face**.

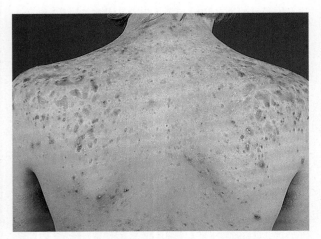

Fig. 28-4   **Scarring acne on the back**.

- *Chloracne*: caused by systemic toxicity of certain aromatic halogenated industrial chemicals.
- *Conglobate*: a mass of burrowing abscesses and sinuses with scarring.
- *Cosmetic*: pomade and cosmetic-induced comedonal and papular acne (mainly seen in the USA).
- *Drug-induced*: by systemic steroids, androgens and topical steroids.
- *Infantile*: mostly found on the faces of male infants; cause unknown.
- *Physical*: occlusion by the back of a wheelchair or on a violinist's chin.

Complications and differential diagnosis

Embarrassment, social withdrawal and depression and suicidal ideation are important sequelae of acne. These can improve with effective treatment. The rare and severe acne fulminans, seen in adolescent males, is associated with fever, arthritis and vasculitis. Long-term antibiotic treatment may induce a Gram-negative folliculitis.

Rosacea can usually be differentiated from acne (see below). Rosacea is more common in adults, the sites of predilection is in the middle of the face. Erythema, telangiectasia, flushing, papules, pustules, phymas and ocular signs and symptoms can be present, but comedones won't appear and sebum excretion is normal. Additionally, bacterial folliculitis is more acute than acne, but the two may coexist.

Management

Treatment depends on the type and extent of acne and the patient's psychological state. 'Over-the-counter' creams have often already been used.

Local treatment is adequate for mild acne and is used with systemic drugs for more severe cases.

- *Benzoyl peroxide* (Panoxyl, Brevoxyl) cream or gel, applied twice a day, works by reducing the number of *P. acnes* and preventing bacterial resistance. It may cause irritation, contact allergy and bleach clothing.
- *Tretinoin* (Retin-A gel) is good at reducing the number of comedones, it's recommended as monotherapy in primary comedonal acne, or in combination with topical or oral antibiotics in patients with mixed or primary inflammatory acne lesions. But it's irritant.
- *Antibiotics*, e.g. clindamycin alone (Dalacin T) or with benzoyl peroxide (Duac), erythromycin alone (Stiemycin) or with zinc (Zineryt), can be used for mild or moderately severe acne.
- *Other topical agents*, e.g. azelaic acid, isotretinoin and adapalene.

Oral treatment with antibiotics, retinoid or hormones is prescribed for moderate or severe acne, acné excoriée and in depressed patients.

Antibiotics

Systemic antibiotics are recommended in the management of moderate and severe acne and forms of inflammatory acne that are resistant to topical treatments. The first-line systemic antibiotic drug is oxy-tetracycline, 500mg twice daily (taken half an hour before food with water), given for a minimum of 4 months. Tetracyclines are contraindicated in children and in pregnancy, and may cause *Candida albicans* infection or photosensitivity. Lymecycline (Tetralysal, 408mg daily) and doxycycline (Vibramycin, 100mg once daily) are alternative tetracyclines that are better absorbed.

The second-choice antibiotics are erythromycin (500mg twice daily) and trimethoprim. Women on oral contraceptives who take an antibiotic are advised that, if diarrhoea develops, additional contraception is needed for the rest of the menstrual cycle.

Antiandrogen

The combination of an antiandrogen and an oestrogen (co-cyprindiol-cyproterone acetate, 2mg, and ethinylestradiol, 35mcg: Dianette) is used in females (not males) with moderate to severe acne that is resistant to conventional therapy. The antiandrogen suppresses sebum production. Co-cyprindiol is given for 6~12 months and is also a contraceptive.

Retinoid

Isotretinoin (Roaccutane), which reduces sebum excretion, inhibits *P. acnes* and is anti-inflammatory, is a very effective treatment for acne. It is used if acne is severe or unresponsive to conventional treatment, or if acne relapses quickly once antibiotics are stopped. A course lasts 4 months and requires the monitoring of liver function and fasting lipids. Isotretinoin is teratogenic. Women given the drug must not be pregnant and need to take the oral contraceptive throughout treatment and one month before and after. Side-effects include cracked lips, dry skin, nose bleeds, hair loss, muscle aches and mood change.

Other therapies

Acne cysts may require injection with triamcinolone acetonide (a steroid), or sometimes excision or cryotherapy. Comedones can be removed using an extractor. Diet has no effect on acne.

Rosacea

Rosacea is a chronic inflammatory facial dermatosis with a variety of clinical manifestations such as erythema and pustules. The cause of rosacea is unknown. Histologically, dilated dermal blood vessels, sebaceous gland hyperplasia and an inflammatory cell infiltrate are seen, however, skin biopsy findings in rosacea are usually nonspecific, therefore, the diagnostic value is limited. Also, Sebum excretion is normal.

Clinical presentation

Rosacea has an equal sex incidence. Although commonest in middle age, it also affects young adults and the elderly. The earliest symptom is flushing. Erythema, telangiectasia, papules, pustules (Fig. 28-5) and, occasionally, lymphoedema involve the cheeks, nose, forehead and chin. Rhinophyma, hyperplasia of the sebaceous glands and connective tissue of the nose (Fig. 28-5), and eye involvement by blepharitis and conjunctivitis are complications. Sunlight and topical steroids exacerbate the condition. Rosacea persists for years, but usually responds well to treatment. Rosacea lacks the comedones of acne and occurs in an older age group. Contact dermatitis, photosensitive eruptions, seborrhoeic dermatitis and lupus erythematosus often involve the face but are more acute or scaly, or lack pustules.

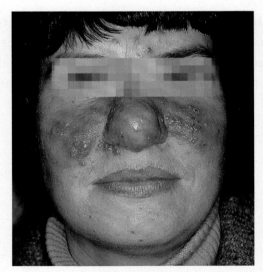

Fig. 28-5   **Rosacea with rhinophyma in a woman.** Rhinophyma usually affects men.

Management

Topically, metronidazole 0.75% cream (Rozex) or azelaic acid may be helpful. If this is ineffective, the usual oral treatment is oxytetracycline, initially 1g daily, reducing to 250mg daily after a few weeks and continued for 2~3 months. Erythromycin is an alternative. Repeated treatment is often needed. Isotretinoin can be used but is less effective than in acne. Plastic surgery is required for rhinophyma.

Other disorders

Perioral dermatitis is characterized by papulovesicular eruption that may occur around the mouth and chin of a woman who has used topical steroids. They will clear with steroid cessation and oral tetracycline therapy. Close follow-up is necessary in the initial treatment period, because the rebound phenomenon usually develops after cessation of previous topical treatment.

Hidradenitis suppurativa is an unpleasant chronic inflammatory condition of the infundibulum of hair follicles in the apocrine sweat gland areas of the axillae, groin and perineum. Skin signs include nodules, abscesses, cysts and sinuses. Finally, scars are left. Treatment is with topical antiseptics, a prolonged course of a systemic antibiotic or retinoid, surgical excision or infliximab. Conglobate acne may coexist.

Hyperhidrosis (excess sweating) due to eccrine gland overactivity is usually emotional in origin. Twenty per cent aluminium chloride in alcohol is often effective. Iontophoresis is used for the hands and Botox injection for the axillae.

> *Sebaceous and apocrine disorders*
> **Acne**
> - *Due to* increased sebum excretion, comedone formation, *P. acnes* and inflammation.
> - *Presentation*: comedones, pustules, cysts and scars seen over the face, chest and trunk.
> - *Treatment*: topical treatments include benzoyl peroxide and tretinoin; systemic treatments include antibiotics, e.g. tetracyclines or erythromycin, antiandrogen and isotretinoin.
> **Rosacea**
> - *Affects* the middle-aged or elderly. Often starts with facial flushing.
> - *Presentation*: facial erythema, telangiectasia and pustules; rhinophyma and conjunctivitis.
> - *Treatment*: topical metronidazole 0.75% cream, oral oxytetracycline.
> **Hidradenitis suppurativa**
> - *Presentation*: chronic nodules or abscesses of axillae and groin, resulting in scarring.
> - *Treatment*: local antiseptics, prolonged course of oral antibiotic or retinoid, excision.

Web resource

http://www.skincarephysicians.com/acnenet/

Key words

acne　痤疮
acne conglobate　聚合性痤疮
pilosebaceous unit　毛囊皮脂腺单位
comedo/comedones　粉刺
rosacea　酒渣鼻
telangiectasia　毛细管扩张
rhinophyma　肥大型酒渣鼻
perioral dermatitis　口周皮炎
hidradenitis suppurativa　化脓性汗腺炎
hyperhidrosis　多汗症

Review questions

1. What are the causes of acne?
2. How to differentiate rosacea from acne?
3. What are the manifestations of hidradenitis suppurativa?

(Xian Jiang)

Chapter 29   Disorders of hair

Hair loss (alopecia)

The division of alopecia into diffuse, localized and scarring or non-scarring helps in diagnosis (Table 29-1).

Table 29-1 **Causes of hair loss**	
Type of hair loss	**Causes**
Diffuse non-scarring	Male pattern/female pattern, hypothyroid, hypopituitary, hypoadrenal, drug induced, iron deficiency, telogen and anagen effluvium, diffuse alopecia areata
Localized/non-scarring	Alopecia areata, ringworm, traumatic, hair pulling, traction, secondary syphilis
Localized/diffuse scarring	Burns, radiation, shingles, kerion, tertiary syphilis, lupus erythematosus, morphoea, pseudopelade, lichen planus

Diffuse non-scarring

With diffuse non-scarring alopecia, patients usually notice excessive numbers of hairs on the pillow, brush or comb, and after washing their hair. The scalp shows a diffuse reduction in hair density. The causes are described below.

Male and female patterns (androgenetic alopecia)

Clinically, male pattern baldness is characterized by the gradual substitution of frontal and parietal hairs by vellus hair of less than 1 cm in length, a total reduction in the number of hairs, and an increase in the telogen hair ratio. Male pattern baldness is inherited (the exact mode is unclear) and androgen dependent. Over several cycles, the androgen-sensitive follicles miniaturize from terminal to vellus hairs. Males are affected from the second decade and, by the seventh decade, 80% have involvement. Patterned balding also occurs in females, the majority of whom are hormonally normal. It becomes more pro-

nounced after the menopause and is present in 70% of 80-year-old women. In men, bitemporal recession followed by a bald crown is the usual pattern (Fig. 29-1); women may show this but more commonly exhibit a diffuse thinning. Two medications, minoxidil (topical use) and finasteride, have been demonstrated efficacy and high tolerability as first-line agents to treat male pattern balding in men. Women can be treated with topical minoxidil.

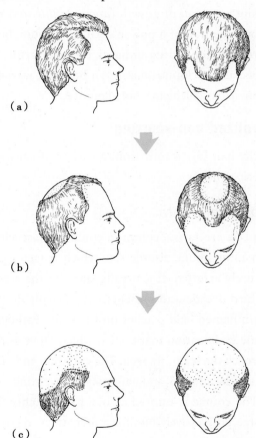

Fig. 29-1   Male pattern baldness. Hair loss may progress from bitemporal recession **(a)** to vertex involvement **(b)** to the most severe form **(c)**, where only a horseshoe of hair runs from the ears to the occiput.

Endocrine and nutrition related

Endocrine disorders often present with hair loss. Underactivity of the thyroid, pituitary or adrenals can cause diffuse alopecia, as may hyperthyroidism.

Androgen-secreting tumours in women produce male pattern baldness with virilization. Malnutrition induces dry brittle hair that becomes pale or red in kwashiorkor (protein deficiency). Diffuse hair loss is also seen with iron or zinc deficiency.

Telogen effluvium

Hair follicles are not usually in phase but, if synchronized into the telogen-resting mode, they will be shed in unison about 3 months later. Such an *effluvium* can be a response to high fever, childbirth, surgery, drug reaction or other stress.

Drug induced

Abrupt cessation of growth (*anagen effluvium*) may follow ingestion of a poison such as thallium, but is more commonly drug induced, e.g. with cytotoxics (especially cyclophosphamide), heparin, warfarin, carbimazole, colchicine and vitamin A.

Localized non-scarring

Patchy hair loss results from a variety of causes, as described below.

Alopecia areata

Alopecia areata is a common condition, associated with autoimmune disorders, in which anagen is prematurely arrested. It generally starts in the second or third decade and presents with sharply defined non-inflamed bald patches on the scalp. Pathognomonic exclamation mark hairs, which taper as they approach the scalp, are seen. The eyebrows and beard can also be affected, and nails may show pitting.

The course is unpredictable: bald patches may enlarge progressively but, for a first attack, regrowth (often initially with white hairs) is usual (Fig. 29-2). Prepubertal onset, extensive involvement (especially of the posterior scalp) and atopy signal a poor prognosis. Complete scalp alopecia (totalis) or loss of all bodily hair (universalis) is seen occasionally. Rarely, diffuse scalp alopecia occurs.

Treatment depends on the extent: if localized, spontaneous regrowth is probable, and intralesional steroid (e.g. triamcinolone acetonide) may accelerate

this. If extensive, therapy is less successful. Contact immunotherapy by the application of the sensitizer diphencyprone is effective but not widely available. Wigs are often necessary.

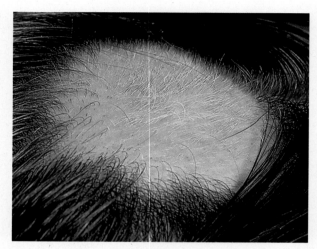

Fig. 29-2　**Alopecia areata showing some exclamation mark (!) hairs and growth of white hair.**

Trauma and traction

Constantly rubbing or pulling the hair can result in its loss. Traction from tight rollers or pulling hair into a bun causes alopecia at the scalp margins. Hair straightening, bleaching and permanent waving produces a damaged hair shaft that is easily broken.

Localized/diffuse scarring alopecia

In scarring (cicatricial) alopecia, hair follicles are destroyed. This condition can result from the following:

- *Burns or irradiation.* Chemical or thermal burns will scar the scalp, as may X-irradiation, which was used in the past to induce epilation in the treatment of scalp ringworm.
- *Infection.* Shingles of the first trigeminal dermatome, kerion (see below) and tertiary syphilis may leave a scarred scalp.
- *Lichen planus/lupus erythematosus.* Scarring alopecia of the scalp is seen, with erythema, scaling and follicular changes (Fig. 29-3). Lesions may exist elsewhere. Topical or intralesional steroids or systemic therapies are prescribed. Female frontal fibrosing alopecia may be a lichen planus variant.

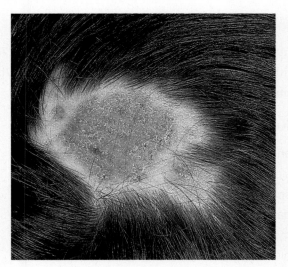

Fig. 29-3   **Scarring alopecia due to discoid lupus erythematosus, which involves the scalp with erythema and scaling.**

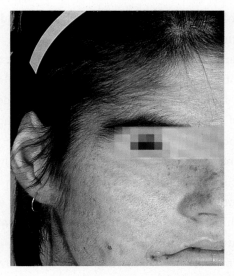

Fig. 29-4   **Hypertrichosis due to ingestion of minoxidil.**

■ *Pseudopelade.* Pseudopelade describes a scarring alopecia, the end stage of an idiopathic or unidentified destructive inflammatory process in the scalp.

Excess hair (hirsutism and hypertrichosis)

Hirsutism is the growth of terminal hair in a male pattern in a female. It is quite common and presents with hair growth in the beard area, around the nipples and in the male pubic pattern. It frequently causes a lot of anxiety, even if mild. Hirsutism in many women is racial or idiopathic (Table 29-2) but some will have the polycystic ovary syndrome (PCOS) in which there may be associated acne, raised blood androgens, irregular periods and ovarian cysts on ultrasound. Few cases are due to an androgen-secreting tumour, although it is important to identify virilizing features such as cliteromegaly, male pattern baldness and a deep voice that might indicate this. In hirsutism, endocrine investigations are usually indicated. *Hypertrichosis* is less common and is defined as excessive terminal hair growth in a non-androgenic distribution, in which fine terminal hair appears on the face, limbs and trunk (Fig. 29-4). It is mostly drug induced (Table 29-3).

Table 29-2	**Causes of hirsutism**
Type	**Example**
Pituitary	Acromegaly
Adrenal	Cushing syndrome, virilizing tumours, congenital adrenal hyperplasia
Ovarian	Polycystic ovaries, virilizing tumours
Iatrogenic	Androgens, progestogens
Idiopathic	End-organ hypersensitivity to androgens

Table 29-3	**Causes of hypertrichosis**
Type	**Example**
Localized	Melanocytic naevi, faun tail (associated with spina bifida occulta), chronic scarring or inflammation
Generalized	Malnutrition in children, anorexia nervosa, porphyria cutanea tarda, underlying malignancy, drugs, e.g. minoxidil, phenytoin, ciclosporin

Laser hair removal is widely available and effective for the treatment of hirsutism. Treatment with an antiandrogen (cyproterone acetate), usually with ethinylestradiol, is occasionally effective. PCOS can be treated with metformin and spironolactone. Hypertrichosis requires investigation to find the underlying cause.

Other disorders

Hair shaft defects are rare, usually inherited, conditions of the hair shaft (e.g. monilethrix) that result in broken hairs that are brittle, beaded and look abnormal.

Dandruff is an exaggerated physiological exfoliation of fine scales from an otherwise normal scalp. More severe forms merge with seborrhoeic dermatitis of the scalp. Psoriasis produces scaling and may give localized alopecia.

Tinea capitis usually affects children. Anthropophilic species cause defined scaly areas with slight inflammation and alopecia with broken hair shafts. Zoophilic infection with *Trichophyton verrucosum* produces an inflamed boggy, pustular swelling known as a kerion. Scarring may result. Infection with *T. schoenleinii* causes favus - a chronic crusted scarring alopecia.

Common hair disorders

- **Male pattern baldness:** the commonest cause of hair loss; if treatment is required, topical minoxidil or oral finasteride may help.
- **Alopecia areata:** common; discrete bald patches may show exclamation mark (!) hairs. Early cases recover spontaneously.
- **Scarring alopecia:** needs investigation to establish the underlying cause.
- **Hirsutism:** may be due to polycystic ovary disease. Endocrine investigations are indicated. Androgen-secreting virilizing tumors are uncommon.

Web resources

http://www.mayoclinic.com/health/hair-loss/DS00278
http://www.merck.com/mmhe/sec18/ch207/ch207b.html

Key words

androgenetic alopecia　雄激素性脱发
alopecia areata　斑秃
scarring alopecia　瘢痕性脱发
dandruff　头皮屑
hypertrichosis　多毛症
hirsutism　妇女多毛症

Review questions

1. What's the clinical feature of alopecia areata?
2. Please describe symptoms of male pattern hair loss.
3. What is hirsutism?

(Shanshan Li)

Chapter 30   Disorders of nails

Congenital disease

A number of usually rare congenital conditions can affect the nails.

- *Nail-patella syndrome* (NPS). In the NPS, the nails (and patellae) are absent or rudimentary. NPS is due to mutations of the *LMX1B* gene of chromosome 9.
- *Pachyonychia congenita*. Pachyonychia congenita is a kind of autosomal dominant genetic disease, the nails are thickened and discoloured from birth, always combined with hyperkeratosis on hands and feet.
- *Congenital nail dystrophy*. A feature of *dystrophic epidermolysis bullosa*.
- *Racket nails*. Racket nails is characterized by a broad short thumbnail, is the commonest congenital nail defect. It is dominantly inherited and more common in women.

Trauma

Trauma, especially from sport, commonly causes nail abnormalities. *Subungual haematomas* usually occur when a fingernail has been trapped or a toenail stood on or stubbed, but the possibility of a subungual malignant melanoma must always be considered. *Splinter haemorrhages* are induced by trauma, although they also occur with infective endocarditis. Ill-fitting shoes contribute to *ingrowing toenails*, and chronic trauma predisposes to *onychogryphosis* - in which the big toenails become thickened and grow like a horn. Trauma may also induce onycholysis (separation of the nail from the nail bed). Constant picking of the thumbnail will produce *a habittic dystrophy* with transverse ridges and grooves. *Brittle nails* are a common complaint, usually due to repeated exposure to detergents and water, although

iron deficiency, hypothyroidism and digital ischaemia are other causes.

Dermatoses

The nails are commonly involved in skin disease (Figs 30-1 and 30-2), and are routinely assessed in a dermatological examination. Details are given in Table 30-1, and a differential diagnosis of the changes is shown in Table 30-2. Treatment is aimed at the associated dermatosis; care of the hands is especially important.

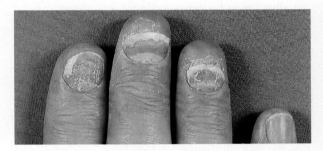

Fig. 30-1   **Psoriasis of the nails.** Pitting, onycholysis and brownish discoloration are apparent.

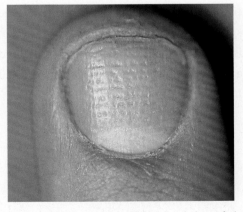

Fig. 30-2   **Alopecia areata.** Thimble pitting of the nail is seen.

Infections

Bacterial or fungal infection may involve the nail fold (paronychia) or the nail itself.

Table 30-1 **Nail involvement in common dermatoses**	
Dermatosis	**Nail changes**
Alopecia areata	Fine pitting, roughness of nail surface
Darier's disease	Longitudinal ridges, triangular nicks at distal nail edge
Eczema	Coarse pitting, transverse ridging, dystrophy, shiny nails due to rubbing
Lichen planus	Thinned nail plate, longitudinal grooves, adhesion between distal nail fold and nail bed (pterygium), complete nail loss
Psoriasis	Pitting, nail thickening, onycholysis (separation of nail from nail bed), brown discoloration, subungual hyperkeratosis

Onychomycosis (tinea unguium)

Fungal infection of the nails (onychomycosis) is usually caused by dermatophytes, but sometimes by yeasts and non-dermatophyte molds. The risk factors include tinea pedis, airtight shoes, immunocompromise and nail trauma. Fungal infection of the nails (onychomycosis) increases with age - children are seldom affected. Toenails, especially the big toenails (Fig. 30-3), are involved more than fingernails. The process usually begins at the distal nail edge and extends proximally to involve the whole nail. The nail separates from the nail bed (onycholysis), the nail plate becomes thickened, crumbly and yellow, and subungual hyperkeratosis occurs. Several - but almost never all - of the toenails may be involved. Tinea pedis often coexists and, if the fingernails are

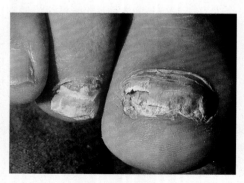

Fig. 30-3 **Fungal infection of toenails.** The nails are thickened, crumbly and discoloured. An adjacent nail is not affected. Dermatophytes, *C. albicans* and, occasionally, moulds such as *Fusarium* or *Scopulariopsis brevicaulis* are causative.

diseased, *Trichophyton rubrum* infection of the hand is usually seen. Treatment is with oral terbinafine (Lamisil) or itraconazole (Sporanox).

Chronic paronychia

Chronic paronychia of the fingernails due to *Candida albicans* is often seen in wet workers. The cuticle is lost, the proximal nail fold becomes boggy and swollen (Fig. 30-4) and light pressure may extrude pus. The nail plate becomes irregular and discoloured. Gram-negative bacteria may be co-pathogens and turn the nail a blue-green colour. Management is directed towards keeping the hands dry, applying an imidazole lotion or cream to the nail fold twice daily, or oral itraconazole for 14 days.

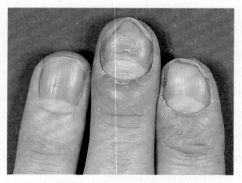

Fig. 30-4 **_C. albicans_ is the commonest pathogen in chronic paronychia.** The nail fold is inflamed and swollen, and the nail is ridged transversely.

Acute paronychia

Acute paronychia is usually bacterial, and staphylococci are often the cause. Oral flucloxacillin or erythromycin is required.

Systemic disease

Nail changes not infrequently indicate an underlying internal medical disorder. Table 30-2 shows some systemic associations.

Tumours

Cancers of the nail and nail bed are rare, but it is not uncommon to see benign tumours around the nail fold. Examples of both include the following:

Table 30-2   **Differential diagnosis of nail changes in dermatoses and systemic disease**

Change	Description of nail	Differential diagnosis
Beau's lines	Transverse grooves	Any severe systemic illness that affects growth of the nail matrix
Brittle nails	Nails break easily, usually at distal margin	Effect of water and detergent, iron deficiency, hypothyroidism, digital ischaemia
Colour change	Black transverse bands	Cytotoxic drugs
	Blue	Cyanosis, antimalarials, haematoma
	Blue-green	*Pseudomonas* infection
	Brown	Fungal infection, stain from cigarette smoke, chlorpromazine, gold, Addison's disease
	Brown 'oil stain' patches	Psoriasis
	Brown longitudinal streak	Melanocytic naevus, malignant melanoma, Addison's disease, racial variant
	Red ('splinter haemorrhages')	Infective endocarditis, trauma
	White spots	Trauma to nail matrix (not calcium deficiency)
	White transverse bands	Heavy metal poisoning
	White/brown 'half and half' nails	Chronic renal failure
	White (leuconychia)	Hypoalbuminaemia (e.g. associated with cirrhosis)
	Yellow	Psoriasis, fungal infection, jaundice, tetracycline
	Yellow nail syndrome (Fig. 30-5)	Defective lymphatic drainage - pleural effusions may occur
Clubbing	Loss of angle between nail fold and nail plate, bulbous fingertip, nail matrix feels spongy	*Respiratory*: bronchial carcinoma, chronic infection, fibrosing alveolitis, asbestosis *Cardiac*: infective endocarditis, congenital cyanotic defects *Other*: inflammatory bowel disease, thyrotoxicosis, biliary cirrhosis, congenital
Koilonychia	Spoon-shaped depression of nail plate	Iron deficiency anaemia; also lichen planus and repeated exposure to detergents
Nail fold telangiectasia	Dilated capillaries and erythema at nail fold	Connective tissue disorders including systemic sclerosis, systemic lupus erythematosus, dermatomyositis
Onycholysis	Separation of nail from nail bed	Psoriasis, fungal infection, trauma, thyrotoxicosis, tetracyclines (*photo-onycholysis*)
Pitting	Fine or coarse pits may be seen in nail bed	Psoriasis, eczema, alopecia areata, lichen planus
Ridging	Transverse (across nail) Longitudinal (up/down)	Beau's lines (see above), eczema, psoriasis, tic-dystrophy, chronic paronychia Lichen planus, Darier's disease

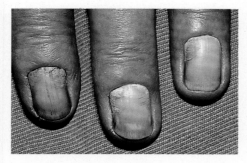

Fig. 30-5 **Yellow nail syndrome.** The nails grow very slowly, lymphatic drainage is abnormal, and pleural effusions may occur.

■ *Subungual glomus tumors.* A rare hamartoma originated from glomus. Blue or purple change under the nail usually accompanied by local emi-

nence. The patient feels an intolerable pain spontaneously or on touching the affected nail.

■ *Periungual fibromas.* These are seen in patients with tuberous sclerosis and appear at or after puberty.

■ *Myxoid (mucous) cysts.* The cysts appear adjacent to the proximal nail fold, usually on the fingers. They are fluctuant, semitranslucent papules that contain a clear gel and may arise from folds of synovium. Treatment is by cryotherapy, injection with triamcinolone acetonide (a steroid) or excision.

■ *Malignant melanoma.* A subungual malignant melanoma should be excluded by biopsy if a pigmented longitudinal streak appears and progresses in a nail. An acral malignant melanoma may be amelanotic and can resemble a pyogenic granuloma or even chronic paronychia. Any atypical or ulcerating lesion around the nail fold requires a biopsy to exclude a malignant melanoma.

Disorders of nails

- **Congenital nail problems** are uncommon except for racket nails.
- **Sports trauma** often results in subungual haematoma, onychogryphosis or onycholysis.
- **Common dermatoses**, e.g. psoriasis, lichen planus and eczema, have distinctive nail changes.
- **Fungal infection** of the big toenails is common, especially in the elderly. Oral terbinafine or itraconazole is prescribed if needed.
- **Chronic paronychia** of fingernails is due to *C. albicans*. Improved skin care, topical imidazole or oral itraconazole are suggested.
- **Acute paronychia** is usually bacterial: antibiotics are given.
- **Systemic diseases** may cause nail changes that help in diagnosis.
- **Malignant melanoma** of the nail bed must be considered with any subungual pigmentation or nail destruction.

Web resource

http://www.hooked-on-nails.com/naildisorders.html

Key words

nail-patella syndrome (NPS) 指甲髌骨综合征
pachyonychia congenita 先天性甲肥厚
onycholysis 甲剥离
onychomycosis 甲癣
paronychia 甲沟炎

Review questions

1. Which kind of fungi cause nail fungal infection?
2. What are the common malignant tumors of nail?

(Shanshan Li)

Chapter 31 Vascular and lymphatic diseases

Blood vessel disorders

Erythema

Erythema is redness of the skin, usually due to vaso-dilatation (Table 31-1). It may be localized, e.g. with pregnancy or liver disease (on palms), fixed drug eruption and infection (e.g. Lyme disease), or generalized, as with drug eruption, toxic erythema (e.g. viral exanthem) and connective tissue disease.

Flushing

Flushing is erythema due to vasodilatation. The causes are:

- physiological (autonomic response to emotion, heat or exercise)
- menopause (hormonal; often with associated sweating)
- foods (e.g. spices - gustatory; alcohol - aldehyde related)
- drugs (angiotensin-converting enzyme (ACE) inhibitors, 5-hydroxytryptamine ($5-HT_3$) antagonists, nifedipine)
- rosacea (mechanism unknown)
- carcinoid syndrome (serotonin - 5-HT)
- phaeochromocytoma (catecholamine).

Flushing is common and affects the face, neck and upper trunk. It is usually benign. A sudden onset and systemic symptoms (e.g. diarrhoea or fainting) mean that carcinoid syndrome or phaeochromocytoma must be excluded. In treatment, first remove the cause, e.g. spices or alcohol. Embarrassing physiological flushing may improve with a small dose of propranolol.

Telangiectasia

Telangiectasia is a visible dilatation of dermal venules or, in spider naevi (Fig. 31-1), an arteriole. It results from:

- *congenital* (e.g. hereditary haemorrhagic telangiectasia)
- *skin atrophy* (topical steroids, ageing skin, radiation dermatitis)
- *excess oestrogen* (e.g. liver disease, pregnancy, 'the pill')
- *connective tissue disease* (systemic sclerosis, lupus erythematosus, dermatomyositis)
- *rosacea* (on the face)
- *venous disease* (lower leg).

Isolated spider naevi are common and of little significance, but their number may increase with pregnancy and liver disease. A venous lake - acquired

Table 31-1	**Classification of blood vessel and lymphatic disorders**	
Vessel	**Process**	**Resulting lesion**
Small blood vessels	Dilatation (and/or increased flow)	Erythema, flushing, telangiectasia
	Release of extracellular fluid	Urticaria, oedema
	Release of blood	Purpura, capillaritis
	Reduced flow	Livedo reticularis, chilblains, Raynaud's phenomenon
	Inflammation damage	Vasculitis, erythema ab igne
Arteries	Atherosclerosis, Buerger's disease	Ischaemia and ulceration
	Inflammation	Vasculitis
Veins	Inflammation, flow reduction, clotting abnormalities	Thrombosis, skin changes, ulceration
	Dilatation	Venous lake
Lymphatics	Congenital hypoplasia	Lymphoedema (primary)
	Blockage or inflammation	Lymphoedema (secondary)
	Infection	Lymphangitis

venous ectasia - is often seen on the lower lip of the elderly. Telangiectasia is treated by fine-needle cautery, hyfrecation or laser.

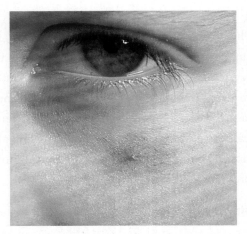

Fig. 31-1 **A spider naevus on the cheek of a child.**

Purpura

Purpura is a blue-brown discoloration of the skin due to the extravasation of erythrocytes (Fig. 31-2). It results from a variety of mechanisms:

- Vessel wall defects:
  1. vasculitis (e.g. due to immune complexes), paraproteinaemia (e.g. cryoglobulinaemia)
  2. infection (e.g. meningococcaemia)
  3. raised vascular pressure (e.g. venous disease).
- Defective dermal support:
  1. dermal atrophy (ageing, steroids, disease, e.g. lichen sclerosus)
  2. scurvy (vitamin C deficiency).
- Clotting defects:
  1. coagulation factor deficiency (e.g. disseminated intravascular coagulation) or inherited
  2. anticoagulant (heparin, warfarin)
  3. thrombocytopenia of any cause
  4. abnormal platelet function.
- Idiopathic pigmented purpuras.

Petechiae are small dot-like purpura, whereas ecchymoses are more extensive. Purpura is often seen in the elderly or those on steroids, and develops spontaneously or after minor trauma. Idiopathic pigmented purpura is seen as brownish punctate lesions (capillaritis) on the legs.

Mostly, there is no specific therapy. Underlying causes, e.g. blood disorders or vasculitis, are treated as necessary.

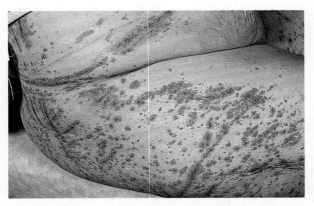

Fig. 31-2 **Purpura in a patient with thrombocytopenia.**

Raynaud's phenomenon

Raynaud's phenomenon is characterized by a paroxysmal vasoconstriction of the digital arteries, usually provoked by cold, in which the fingers turn white (due to ischaemia), cyanotic blue (due to capillary dilatation with a stagnant blood flow) and then red (due to reactive hyperaemia). When no cause is found, it is known as 'Raynaud's disease'. Causes include:

- *arterial occlusion*: atherosclerosis, Buerger's disease
- *connective tissue disease*: systemic sclerosis (including CREST syndrome), systemic lupus erythematosus
- *hyperviscosity syndrome*: polycythaemia, cryoglobulinaemia
- *neurological defects*: syringomyelia, peripheral neuropathy
- *reflux vasoconstriction*: with use of vibration tools
- *toxins/drugs*: ergot, vinyl chloride, beta-blockers.

Raynaud's phenomenon mostly affects women. It may be the forerunner of a connective tissue disease. The hands should be kept warm and protected from the cold. Smoking must be stopped. A calcium channel blocker (e.g. nifedipine) or naftidrofuryl may help. In resistant cases, prostacyclin infusions are given.

Livedo reticularis

Livedo reticularis is a marble-patterned cyanosis of the skin, due to reduced arteriole blood flow, usually in women. The condition has the following causes:

■ *Physiological,* i.e. cold induced.

■ *Vasculitis* due to connective tissue disease, e.g. systemic lupus erythematosus and polyarteritis nodosa.

■ *Hyperviscosity* due to cryoglobulinaemia, polycythaemia.

■ *Sneddon syndrome,* which consists of livedo vasculitis with cerebrovascular disease and circulating antiphospholipid antibodies.

Cold-induced livedo reticularis gives a mottled meshwork pattern on the outer thighs of children and is reversible. Fixed livedo (Fig. 31-3) is due to vasculitis and requires investigation. Treatment is aimed at the underlying disease.

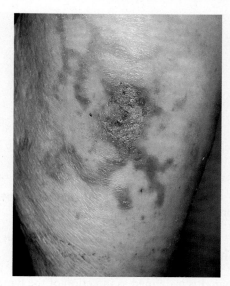

Fig. 31-4 **Erythema ab igne on the upper outer shin from sitting in front of a fire.**

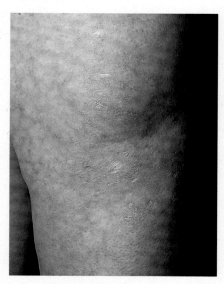

Fig. 31-3 **Livedo reticularis.** In this case, the condition was associated with systemic lupus erythematosus.

Erythema ab igne

Erythema ab igne is a reticulate pigmented erythema (Fig. 31-4) due to heat-induced damage. It is usually seen on the inner thighs and shins of persons (mostly women) who highly rely on heater during the winter or with the use of heat pads or laptop computers.

Chilblains

Chilblains are inflamed and painful purple-pink swellings on the fingers, toes or ears that appear in response to cold. Chilblains result from an overcompensatory cold-induced vasoconstriction of cutaneous arterioles and venules. They occur in the winter and usually affect women. Warm housing and clothing are advised. Oral nifedipine may help.

Lymphatic disorders

Lymphoedema

Lymphoedema is oedema, often of a limb, due to inadequate lymphatic drainage. The condition may be primary or secondary. Primary lymphoedema is the result of a congenital developmental defect. Secondary causes include:

■ recurrent infection - lymphangitis

■ blockage - filariasis, tumour

■ destruction - surgery, radiation.

Primary lymphoedema presents in adolescence and may follow infection. The lower legs are commonly affected. In chronic lymphoedema, the oedema is non-pitting and fibrotic, and the overlying epidermis hyperkeratotic (Fig. 31-5). Radiolabelled lymphoscintigraphy (or X-ray or magnetic resonance imaging (MRI) lymphangiography) shows the defect.

A lymphoedematous limb is at risk of repeated infection (particularly erysipelas), and long-term prophylaxis with oral phenoxymethylpenicillin is recommended. Exercise, compression support and massage can help. Surgical reconstruction is rarely possible.

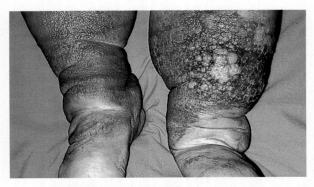

Fig. 31-5 **Chronic lymphoedema of the legs with papillomatosis.**

Lymphangitis

Lymphangitis is defined as infection of the lymphatic vessels, usually due to streptococci. It presents as a tender red line extending proximally up a limb, usually from a focus of infection. Hospital admission is usually necessary. Therapy is with a suitable intravenous antibiotic (e.g. benzylpenicillin).

Vascular and lymphatic diseases

■ **Erythema:** can be localized, e.g. liver palms, or generalized, e.g. toxic erythema.

■ **Flushing:** usually emotional; rarely carcinoid syndrome or phaeochromocytoma.

■ **Telangiectasia:** commonly seen with skin atrophy, but lesions can occur with oestrogen excess or connective tissue disease. Treatment is by hyfrecation or laser.

■ **Purpura:** caused by defects of the vessel wall, supporting dermis or clotting mechanism, or 'idiopathic'. Treat the underlying disorder.

■ **Livedo reticularis:** physiological or due to underlying hyperviscosity or connective tissue disorder.

■ **Chilblains:** describes cold-induced perniosis of the fingers, toes and ears.

■ **Raynaud's phenomenon:** vasoconstriction of the digital arteries with colour changes.

■ **Lymphoedema:** results from absence of or damage to lymphatics. Long-term prophylaxis with antibiotics prevents recurrent infection in chronic cases.

Key words

erythema　红斑

flushing　阵发性潮红

telangiectasia　毛细血管扩张

Raynaud's phenomenon　雷诺现象

livedo reticularis　网状青斑

purpura　紫癜

Erythema ab igne　火激红斑

lymphoedema　淋巴水肿

chilblain　冻疮

Review question

Please comment on classification of blood vessel and lymphatic disorders.

(Jianyun Lu)

Chapter 32 Leg ulcers

Leg ulcers affect 1% of the adult population and account for 1% of dermatology referrals. They are twice as common in women as in men and are a major burden on the health service. One half is venous, a tenth arterial and a quarter 'mixed' - due to venous *and* arterial disease. The remainder are due to rare causes.

Venous disease

Damage to the venous system of the leg results in pigment change, eczema, oedema, fibrosis and ulceration.

Aetiopathogenesis

The superficial low-pressure venous system of the leg is connected to the deep higher pressure veins by perforating veins. Blood flow relies on the pumping action of surrounding muscles and the integrity of valves. Throughout the superficial, communicating and deep veins, one-way bicuspid valves ensure unidirectional flow toward the deep system, thus allowing blood to flow in a cephalad direction and preventing reflux. It is primarily the contraction of calf muscles that drives blood from the leg toward the heart. Valve incompetence, occasionally congenital but usually due to damage by thrombosis or infection, results in a rise in capillary hydrostatic pressure and permeability (Fig. 32-1). Fibrin is deposited as a pericapillary cuff, interfering with diffusion of nutrients and resulting in disease.

Clinical presentation

Venous disease usually starts in middle age and continues into later life. It is commoner in women and is predisposed to by obesity and venous thrombosis. Varicose veins are often present, but are not essential. The syndrome progresses through stages:

- *Heaviness and oedema*: early symptoms. The legs feel heavy and swell.

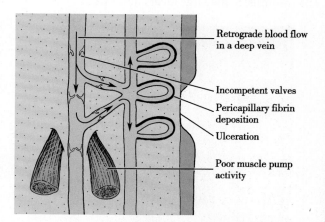

Fig. 32-1 **The aetiopathogenesis of venous ulceration.**

- *Discoloration*: brown haemosiderin deposits from extravasated red cells. Telangiectasia and white lacy scars (atrophie blanche) occur at the ankle (Fig. 32- 2).

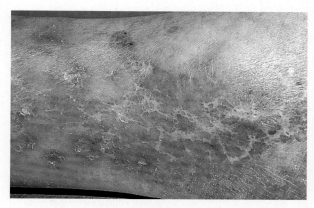

Fig. 32-2 **Atrophie blanche with white lace-like scarring and haemosiderin deposition.**

- *Eczema*: commonly occurs, often complicated by allergic or irritant contact dermatitis.
- *Lipodermatosclerosis*: fibrosis of the dermis and subcutis around the ankle results in firm induration.
- *Ulceration*: often follows minor trauma, and typically affects the medial and, to a lesser extent, the lateral malleolus (Fig. 32-3). Neglected ulcers enlarge and may encircle the lower leg. Initially, venous ulcers are exudative but, under favour-

able conditions, they granulate and enter a healing phase in which the epidermis grows in from the sides and from small epithelial islands in the middle. Healing is invariably slow, often taking months. Some large ulcers never heal.

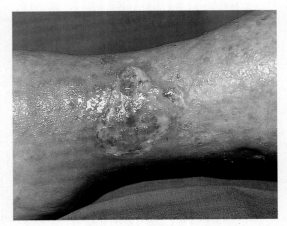

Fig. 32-3 **A venous ulcer at the lateral malleolus.**

- *Post-ulcer leg*: fibrosis may lead to a slender sclerosed ankle.

Differential diagnosis and complications

Venous ulcers can be differentiated from other ulcers (Table 32-1) by history, position and additional signs. Arterial ulcers are deep, painful and gangrenous, and situated on the foot or mid-shin. Complications of venous ulcers are common and include the following:

Table 32-1	**Causes of leg ulceration**
Division	**Condition**
Venous disease	Damaged valves (e.g. deep vein thrombosis), clotting disorder, congenital valve incompetence
Arterial disease	Atherosclerosis, Buerger's disease, polyarteritis nodosa
Small vessel disease	Diabetes mellitus, rheumatoid arthritis, vasculitis, sickle cell disease, hypertension
Infection	Tuberculosis, Buruli ulcer (p. XXX), mycetoma, syphilis
Neuropathy	Diabetes mellitus, leprosy, syphilis, syringomyelia
Neoplasia	Squamous cell carcinoma, Kaposi's sarcoma, malignant melanoma
Trauma	Direct injury, artefact
Unknown	Pyoderma gangrenosum, necrobiosis lipoidica

- *Infections.* Bacteria invariably colonize ulcers. Systemic antibiotics are needed only for overt infection, as suggested by a purulent discharge, a rapidly advancing ulcer edge, cellulitis or septicaemia.
- *Lymphoedema.* Lymphatic drainage is impaired in legs with chronic venous ulcers, adding to the oedema.
- *Contact dermatitis.* Contact sensitivity to topical medicaments and bandages frequently develops, especially to lanolin, neomycin, rubber chemicals and preservatives. Allergic contact dermatitis can resemble an exacerbation of venous eczema and is suspected if there is generalized secondary spread. Some local therapies, and the ulcer exudate itself, are irritant.
- *Malignant change.* Rarely, squamous cell carcinoma develops in an ulcer.

Management

Treatment of a leg ulcer is long term and progress usually slow. The initial examination includes palpation of peripheral pulses and an assessment of contributing factors such as obesity, anaemia, cardiac failure and arthritis. Doppler studies, to exclude coexisting arterial disease, are essential when compression bandaging is proposed. Treatments are as follows:

- *Compression bandages.* These reduce oedema and promote venous return. Bandages are applied from the toes to the knee. Self-adhesive bandages (e.g. Coban) are preferred, and are left on for 2~7 days. Arterial disease precludes compression bandaging. Once an ulcer has healed, a toe-to-knee compression stocking maintains venous return.
- *Elevation, exercise and diet.* Some doctors recommend rest with leg elevation. Walking is encouraged, as is dieting for obese individuals and ankle exercises to maintain joint mobility.
- *Topical therapy.* Table 32-2 shows what to use and when to use it. Venous eczema is treated with a mild to moderate potency steroid or an emollient.
- *Oral therapy.* Adequate analgesia is vital. Diuretics are given for cardiac oedema, and antibiotics for overt infection. An anabolic steroid, stanozolol,

Table 32-2	**Topical therapy for venous ulcers**		
Type of wound	**Role of dressing**	**Examples of dressing**	**Qualities of dressing**
Dry, necrotic, black, yellow, sloughy	Moisture retention or rehydration, especially if dry; if moist, fluid absorption; removal of excess slough; possibly absorption of odour; possibly antimicrobial activity; infrequent changes so as not to disturb wound	Irrigation fluid, e.g. physiological saline Hydrocolloid, e.g. Comfeel Plus, Granuflex, DuoDERM Extra Thin or Aquacel Larval therapy may be considered in suitable casesO-dour-absorbing dressing, e.g. Actisorb Silver 220, Lyofoam C	Use of irritant cleansers may be harmful; debris and dressing remnants can be removed with saline irrigation Absorbent layer on vapour-permeable film. Occlusive; facilitates rehydration/autolytic debridement of dry slough or necrotic wounds; promotes granulation; change daily or less frequently Absorbs odour; may bind bacteria; change daily or less frequently as dictated by clinical response
Clean, exudating, granulating	Fluid absorption; thermal insulation to give optimal temperature for healing; possibly odour absorption; possibly antimicrobial activity; optimal pH for wound healing	Alginate, e.g. Kaltostat, Sorbsan or SeaSorb Foam, e.g. Allevyn Thin or Lyofoam Low adherent tulle, e.g. Jelonet or Neotulle	Highly absorbent; suitable for moderate/heavily exudating wounds; not for dry wound or eschar; change daily or less frequently Suitable for exudative wound; useful for overgranulation resulting from occlusive dressing; used as secondary dressing Used as interface layer under a secondary absorbent dressing; medicated tulle dressings are not generally recommended
Dry, low exudate, epithelializing	Moisture retention or rehydration; low adherence; thermal insulation	Hydrogel, e.g. Aquaform, Intrasite Conformable	Amorphous cohesive material; takes shape of wound; needs secondary dressing; moisturizes/debrides dry wound

may help lipodermatosclerosis, but side-effects (fluid retention, jaundice) limit its use. Oxerutins reduce capillary permeability, relieving oedema.

■ *Surgery*. Vein surgery may prevent problems in younger patients, but is rarely applicable in the elderly. Split skin grafts or pinch grafts (from the thigh) are of limited use. However, experimental culturing of keratinocytes in a 'skin equivalent', to use as a graft, is promising and gives rapid pain relief.

Arterial disease

Lower leg ischaemia and ulceration can result from arterial disease. Up to 25% of patients with leg ulcers have peripheral arterial disease and a significant number of patients have a combination of arterial and venous insufficiencies. Ischaemia presents with claudication, coldness of the foot, loss of hair, toenail dystrophy and dusky cyanosis. Deep, sharply defined ulcers occur on the foot or mid-shin (Fig. 32-4). Pulses in the legs are absent or reduced. Buerger's

disease, seen in young male smokers, is a severe form of arterial disease.

Doppler studies and contrast angiography define the arterial lesions, which may be amenable to vascular reconstruction or angioplasty. Compression bandaging is contraindicated if the ABPI is <0.5, but reduced compression may be used under supervision for ABPIs of 0.6~0.8.

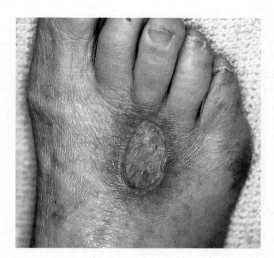

Fig. 32-4   **An arterial ulcer on the dorsal aspect of the foot.**

Other causes of leg ulceration

Vasculitic ulcers start as purpura, but become necrotic and punched out (Table 32-1). *Peripheral neuropathic ulcers* and diabetes can produce ulcers on the feet (Fig. 32-5). *Buruli ulcer* and deep mycoses are important in the tropics.

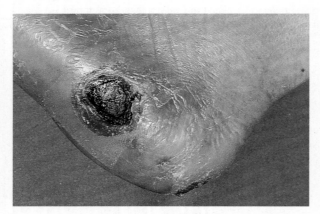

Fig. 32-5 **A necrotic neuropathic ulcer on the side of the foot.**

> *Leg ulcers*
> **Venous ulcers**
> - Result from venous hypertension.
> - Show associated skin discoloration, eczema and fibrosis.
> - Occur at the medial or lateral malleolus.
> - Require compression bandaging after checking Doppler pressures.
> - May coexist with arterial disease.
> - May be complicated by contact allergy.
>
> **Arterial ulcers**
> - Are associated with other symptoms and signs of leg ischaemia.
> - Occur on the foot or mid-shin.
> - Are usually deep and painful.
> - Prohibit most compression bandaging.
>
> **Other causes**
> - Vasculitis, trauma, neuropathy, diabetes, and some types of infection can also cause leg ulceration.

Web resource

http://www.nhs.uk/Conditions/Leg-ulcer-venous/Pages/Treatment.aspx

Key words

leg ulcer　腿部溃疡病
venous ulcer　静脉性溃疡
arterial ulcer　动脉性溃疡

Review questions

1. What stages do leg venous ulcers develop through?
2. What is the most effective treatment for leg venous ulcers?
3. What are the typical manifestations of arterial ulcers?

(Xiaodong Li)

Chapter 33   Pigmentation

Skin colour is due to a mixture of the pigments melanin, oxyhaemoglobin (in blood) and carotene (in the stratum corneum and subcutaneous fat). Pigmentary diseases are common and particularly distressing to those with darker skin. Skin pigmentation disorders are generally divided into two types: hypopigmentation and hyperpigmentation.

Hypopigmentation

Pigment loss may be generalized or patchy. Generalized hypopigmentation occurs with albinism, phenylketonuria and hypopituitarism; patchy loss is seen in vitiligo, after inflammation, following exposure to some chemicals and with certain infections (Table 33-1).

Table 33-1	**Causes of hypopigmentation**
Cause	**Example**
Chemical	Substituted phenols, hydroquinone
Endocrine	Hypopituitarism
Genetic	Albinism, phenylketonuria, tuberous sclerosis, piebaldism
Infection	Leprosy, yaws, pityriasis versicolor
Postinflammatory	Cryotherapy, eczema, psoriasis, morphoea, pityriasis alba
Other	Vitiligo, lichen sclerosus, halo naevus, scarring

Vitiligo

Vitiligo is an acquired idiopathic disorder showing white non-scaly macules. Melanocytes are absent from affected skin on histology. The prevalence rate in China is about 0.1%~0.2%. The association with thyroid disease, pernicious anemia and Addison's disease suggests an autoimmune etiology in some cases. About 30% of patients give a family history of the disorder.

Pathogenesis

The pathogenesis is complex and involves the interplay of multiple factors. However, the cause is typically unknown. It is believed to be due to genetic susceptibility that is triggered by an environmental factor such that an autoimmune disease occurs. This results in the destruction of melatocytes.

Clinical presentation

Vitiligo is seen in all races and is most troublesome in those with a dark skin. The sex incidence is equal, and the onset, usually between 10 and 30 years of age, may be precipitated by injury or sunburn. The only sign of vitiligo is the presence of pale patchy areas of depigmented skin which tend to occur on the extremities. The patches are initially small, but often grow and change shape. When skin lesions occur, they are most prominent on the face, hands and wrists. The loss of skin pigmentation is particularly noticeable around body orifices, such as the mouth, eyes, nostrils, genitalia and umbilicus. Some lesions have increased skin pigment around the edges. The sharply defined white macules are often symmetrical (Fig. 33-1). Patients who are stigmatized

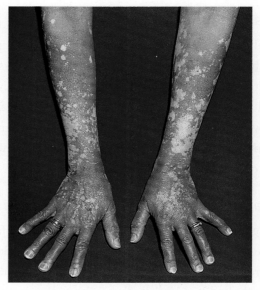

Fig. 33-1 **Vitiligo showing symmetrical involvement of the forearms in a patient with pigmented skin.**

for their condition may experience depression and similar mood disorders. Occasionally, vitiligo is segmental (e.g. down an arm), generalized or universal. The course is unpredictable, areas may remain static, spread or (infrequently) repigment. In light-skinned individuals, vitiligo may be discernible only in summer, when the non-vitiliginous areas become suntanned.

According to the location and distribution of lesions, three types are classified: localized vitiligo, generalized vitiligo and universal vitiligo.

- Localized vitiligo.
  1. Segmental vitiligo: It tends to affect areas of skin that are associated with dorsal roots from the spinal cord and is most often unilateral.
  2. Mucosal vitiligo: depigmentation of only the mucous membranes.
- Generalized vitiligo: the most common pattern, wide and randomly distributed areas of depigmentation.
  1. Vulgaris vitiligo: white patches are spread in several parts of body.
  2. Acrofacial vitiligo: fingers and periorificial areas.
  3. Mixed vitiligo: this type is the mixture of vitiligo types mentioned above.
- Universal vitiligo: depigmentation encompasses most of the body.

Histopathology

Vitiligo is characterized mainly by typical findings in the dermal-epidermal junction. While borders of white macules still demonstrate residual melanocytes and a few granules of melanin, the rest of the lesion show no melanocytes and the absence of melanin. Sometimes, a lymphoid infiltrate may be evident in the outer active part of the lesion.

Diagnosis and Differential Diagnosis

Diagnosis is mainly based on clinical features. In fact, there are no particular tests to identify vitiligo. However, evaluation of the presence of organ-specific autoantibodies, especially those directed against thyroid and adrenal glands could be useful. A Wood's lamp could be used for the optimal evaluation of some uncertain lesions.

Differential diagnosis includes some acquired hypopigmented disorders, like pityriasis versicolor, pityriasis alba, lichen sclerosus et atrophicus, leprosy, tertiary stage of pinta, morphea, and sarcoidosis. Obviously, chemical leukoderma and post-inflammatory hypopigmentation should be excluded. However, a variety of congenital diseases could be included in differential diagnosis, including tuberous sclerosis, piebaldism, nevus depigmentosus Vogt-Harada-Koyanagi syndrome, Waardenburg's syndrome and Ziprkowski-Margolis syndrome.

Management

The aim of the treatment is to obtain skin repigmentation.

Topical steroids

Topical corticosteroids (TCs) are still the mainstay of treatment for localized forms of vitiligo. Although they have several widely known side effects, such as atrophy or telangiectasia, TCs are considered as first-line therapy because of their wide availability, low cost and efficacy. Regarding the high power TCs, it has been reported that they should be used for no longer than 2~4 months.

Calcineurin inhibitors

This class of drugs includes two topical immunosuppressants, namely tacrolimus and pimecrolimus. Compared to TCs, topical calcineurin inhibitors (TCIs) do not provoke skin atrophy.

Systemic therapy

Although some different approaches have been attempted in cases of disseminated vitiligo lesions, steroids still remain the principle therapy.

Physical therapy

There are three main types of physical therapy for vitiligo, namely narrow band UVB, phototherapy with UVA and psoralens (PUVA therapy) and monochromatic excimer light (MEL).

NB-UVB (311nm) is now considered one of the

most effective and safest types of therapy for vitiligo It has been widely reported that NB-UVB reached the same or better results in repigmentation compared to PUVA. In addition, NB-UVB was not found to increase the risk of melanoma and non melanoma skin cancers, while PUVA slightly increases the risk of both melanoma and non melanoma skin cancers. NB-UVB alone reaches repigmentation rates between 41.6% and 100%.

Surgical therapy

Surgical therapy could be useful in patients in whom medical therapy has failed. Several surgical techniques are usually employed. The blister graft technique, involving the creation of a subepidermal bulla from the donor site, is the most widely applied therapy.

Hyperpigmentation

Hyperpigmentation is mostly hypermelanosis (Table 33-2), but sometimes other pigments colour the skin, e.g. iron deposition (with melanin) in haemochromatosis, and carotene (causing an orange discoloration) in carotenaemia, usually due to eating too many carrots.

Table 33-2	**Causes of hyperpigmentation**
Cause	**Example**
Drugs	Photosensitizers, psoralens, oestrogens, phenothiazines, minocycline, amiodarone
Endocrine	Addison's disease, Cushing syndrome, Graves' disease
Genetic	Racial, freckles, neurofibromatosis, Peutz-Jeghers syndrome
Metabolic	Biliary cirrhosis, haemochromatosis, porphyria
Nutritional	Carotenaemia, malabsorption, malnutrition, pellagra
Postinflammatory	Eczema, lichen planus, systemic sclerosis, lichen amyloidosis
Other	Acanthosis nigricans, naevi, malignant melanoma, argyria, chronic renal failure

Melasma

Melasma is a patterned macular facial pigmentation

occurring with pregnancy and in women on oral contraceptives. The pigmentation is symmetrical and often involves the forehead (Fig. 33-2). Pregnancy stimulates melanocytes generally, and also increases pigmentation of the nipples and lower abdomen and in existing melanocytic naevi. Melasma may improve spontaneously. Topical tretinoin, azelaic acid or hydroquinone can reduce pigmentation. Sunscreens and camouflage cosmetics can help.

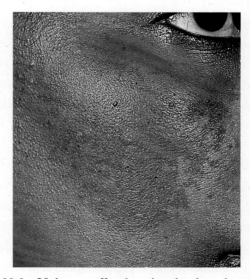

Fig. 33-2   **Melasma affecting the cheek and causing a cosmetic disability.**

Pathogenesis

Melasma is thought to be the stimulation of melanocytes by the female sex hormones estrogen and progesterone to produce more melanin pigments when the skin is exposed to sun. Women with a light brown skin type who are living in regions with intense sun exposure are particularly susceptible to developing this condition. Genetic predisposition is also a major factor in determining whether someone will develop melasma. The incidence of melasma also increases in patients with thyroid disease. It is thought that the overproduction of melanocyte-stimulating hormone (MSH) brought on by stress can cause outbreaks of this condition. Other rare causes of melasma include allergic reaction to medications and cosmetics.

Clinical presentation

The symptoms of melasma are dark, irregular well

demarcated hyperpigmented macules to patches commonly found on the upper cheek, nose, lips, upper lip and forehead. These patches often develop gradually over time. Melasma does not cause any other symptoms beyond the cosmetic discoloration. Melasma is also common in pre-menopausal women. It is thought to be enhanced by surges in certain hormones.

Histopathology

The staining intensity and number of epidermal melanocytes increased in melasma lesions. Lesional skin showed more prominent solar elastosis compared with normal skin. Melanosomes increased in number and were more widely dispersed in the keratinocytes of the lesional skin.

Diagnosis and Differentiation Diagnosis

Melasma is usually diagnosed visually or with assistance of a Wood's lamp. Under Wood's lamp, excess melanin in the epidermis can be distinguished from that of the dermis. Differential diagnosis includes post inflammatory hyperpigmentation, actinic lichen planus and hydroquinone-induced exogenous ochronosis.

Management

The discoloration usually disappears spontaneously over a period of several months after giving birth or stopping the oral contraceptives or hormone replacement therapy. Treatments are often ineffective as it comes back with continued exposure to the sun. Treatments to hasten the fading of the discolored patches include:

- Topical depigmenting agents, such as hydroquinone (HQ) either in over-the-counter (2%) or prescription (4%) strength. HQ is a chemical that inhibits tyrosinase, an enzyme involved in the production of melanin.
- Azelaic acid (20%), thought to decrease the activity of melanocytes.
- Oral Tranexamic acid has shown to provide rapid and sustained lightening in melasma by decreasing melanogenesis in epidermal melanocytes.
- Chemical peels.
- Microdermabrasion to dermabrasion.

In all of these treatments the effects are gradual and a strict avoidance of sunlight is required. The use of broad-spectrum sunscreens with physical blockers, such as titanium dioxide and zinc dioxide is preferred over that with only chemical blockers. This is because UVA, UVB and visible lights are all capable of stimulating pigment production. Patients should avoid other precipitants including hormonal triggers. Cosmetic camouflage can also be used to hide melasma.

Freckles

Freckles are small, light brown macules, typically facial, which darken on sun exposure. The formation of freckles is triggered by exposure to sunlight. The exposure to UVB radiation activates melanocytes to increase melanin production, which can cause freckles to become darker and more visible.

Clinical presentation

Freckles are predominantly found on the face, although they may appear on any skin exposed to the sun, such as arms or shoulders. Heavily distributed concentrations of melanin may cause freckles to multiply and cover an entire area of skin, such as the face. Freckles are rare on infants, and more commonly found on children before puberty. Upon exposure to the sun, freckles will reappear if they have been altered with creams or lasers and not protected from the sun, but do fade with age in some cases.

Histopathology

Freckles have normal basal layer melanocyte numbers but increased melanin. Freckles do not have an increased number of the melanin-producing cells melanocytes, but instead have melanocytes that overproduce melanin granules (melanosomes) changing the coloration of the outer skin.

Management

Avoiding sunshine and unblocks application is necessary. Topical depigmenting agents, such as hydroquinone and chemical peels are effective in freckles. Laser is very useful in pigmentation removal, but pigment macules may reappear.

Riehl's Melanosis

Riehl's melanosis is a form of contact dermatitis, beginning with pruritus, erythema, and pigmentation that gradually spreads which, after reaching a certain extent, becomes stationary. In Riehl's melanosis, facial hyperpigmentation, most pronounced on the forehead and in the zygomatic and/or temporal regions is the dominant symptom.

Pathogenesis

The pathogenesis of Riehl's melanosis is believed to be sun exposure following the use of some perfumes or creams. It is thought to be a kind of photocontact dermatitis.

Clinical Presentation

The dark brown pigmentation engaged the entire face, but was most pronounced on the forehead and in the zygomatic and temporal regions. The pigmentation was generally more pronounced laterally on the face than in the middle. It extended to the ears, neck, and nape of the neck, and onto the scalp for a varying distance. The skin surface looked as though it were covered with flour or was slightly scaly, and on the forehead, cheeks, and ears horny plugs were seen in widened follicular orifices. The diseased skin was thickened and slightly rough. There was no atrophy, no exudation, and almost no hyperaemia. The areas of pigmentation were not demarcated sharply. The uniform discoloration of the head and neck gradually diminished towards the thorax, breaking up into small pigmented macules or discrete papules, usually follicular. New, isolated efflorescences were to start with reddish brown, only later becoming dark brown. The hands, forearms, axillae, and submammary and umbilical skin were less commonly involved, and here the pigmentation was also less pronounced. The patients had no signs of general disease.

Histopathology

Histologic examination showed thick infiltrates of round cells in the dermis and strongly pigmented cells in the infiltrates. The epidermis contained little pigment. Some edema was present in rete malpighii, and the horny layer was thickened. Follicular keratosis was seen.

Diagnosis and Differentiation Diagnosis

The disease can be diagnosed according to the typical skin lesions in combination with the history. The differential diagnosis includes melanosis and chloasma, pigmentation in Addison's disease, poikiloderma of Civatte.

Management

Complete avoidance of the suspected allergen is necessary, and removal of these agents often leads to gradual improvement. Consider Use of allergen-free apparel, soaps, cosmetics and sun-protection is essential. Topical treatments as used for melasma, hydroquinone, retinoids, and azelaic acid or light chemical peels such as glycolic acid can also be considered. Cosmetic camouflage makeup may be suggested if the cosmetic disability is distressing to the patient. The use of intense pulsed light therapy or Q-switched Nd: YAG lasers can improve pigmentation.

Disorders of pigmentation
- **Vitiligo:** common, autoimmune; well-defined depigmented macules.
- **Freckles:** brown macules darken with sun; normal number of melanocytes.
- **Melasma:** facial pigmentation; related to pregnancy and 'the pill'.
- **Riehl's Melanosis:** facial hyperpigmentation, most pronounced on the forehead and in the zygomatic and/or temporal regions.

Web resources

http://www.vitiligosociety.org.uk/
http://emedicine.medscape.com/article/1068640-overview

Key words

hypopigmentation　色素减退

Wood's lamp　伍氏灯

NB-UVB　窄波紫外线

hyperpigmentation　色素沉着

topical corticosteroids　局部糖皮质激素药物

hydroquinone　氢醌

blister graft technique　吸疱移植术

Review questions

1. What is the classification of skin pigmentation disorders?
2. What are the clinical features of vitiligo?
3. Can you talk about the phototherapy of vitiligo?
4. Can you list several hyperpigmentation diseases?
5. What is the possible reason of Riehl's melanosis?

(Weimin Shi)

Chapter 34   Disorders due to Physical factors

Clavus

Clavus (corn) are circumscribed, horny, conical thickenings produced by pressure. The hyperkeratosis occurs on parts subject to intermittent pressure, particularly on the palms and soles, with the base on the surface and the apex pointing inward and pressing upon subjacent structures.

Clinical presentation

There are two varieties in clavus. The hard clavus, which occur on the external surfaces of the soles and toes, and the soft clavus, which are present between the toes and are softened by the macerating action of sweat. In hard clavus, the surface is shiny and polished. When the upper layer are shaved away, a core is noted in the densest part of the lesion (Fig. 34-1). When press on the underlying sensory nerves in the papillary layer, the core causes dull, boring or sharp pain. The soft clavus usually occurs in the forth interdigital space of the foot. They are soft, soggy, and macerated so that they appear white. By the result of pressure, a bony spur or exostosis is present beneath both hard and soft clavus of long duration. Unless this exostosis is removed, cure is impossible. Clavus arise at sites of friction or pressure, when these caus-ative factors are removed, they may spontaneously disappear.

Differential diagnosis

Clavus must be differentiated from warts. In most cases, the differentiation can be done with confidence only by paring off the surface keratin until either the pathognomonic elongated dermal papillae of the wart, or the clear horny core of the corn, can be clearly seen.

Management

The relief of pressure or friction by corrective footwear is required. However, this step alone frequently does not cure the clavus. In the case of the soft clavus, it may be necessary to remove the underlying exostosis. For the hard clavus, salicylic acid and dichloracetic acid have been favorite methods of treatment. Soaking the feet in hot water and paring the surface by means of a razor or sharp knife to remove the corn.   After paring of the corn with emphasis on removing the center core carefully, 40% salicylic acid plaster is applied. 48 hours later, the corn is removed, the white macerated skin is rubbed off, and a new plaster is reapplied. The operation is continued until the corn is gone. Use a salicylic acid-lactic acid in collodion is another option. The collodion medication is painted on the pared site of the corn and allowed to dry. This is done everyday for a week, when the foot is soaked for a half hour and the collodion peeled off the corn site. The pain of a corn on the dorsum of a toe may be greatly alleviated by the injection just under it of 0.01 to 0.02ml of triamcinolone suspension, 40mg per ml.

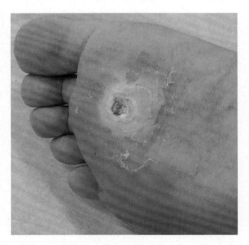

Fig. 34-1   **Clavus showing core on the soles**

Frostbite

Frostbite is a kind of skin disorder caused by low temperature, which result in frozen and locally deprived of blood supply on soft part. Various degrees of tissue destruction similar to those caused by burns are encountered.

Clinical presentation

Frostbite most often affected ears, nose, cheeks, fingers, and toes. The frozen part becomes pale and waxy but there is scarcely any pain or discomfort. Erythema and edema, vesicles and bullae, superficial gangrene, deep gangrene are common presentations on frozen part (Fig. 34-2). Sometimes the injury is deep to muscles, tedons, periosteum, and nerves. After swelling and hyperemia have developed, the patient should be kept in bed with the injured limb slightly flexed, elevated, and at rest.

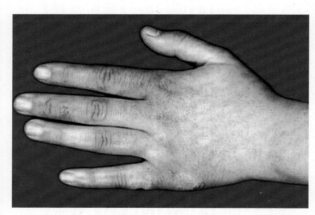

Fig. 34-2 **Frostbite**

Management

Early dispose of frostbite before swelling develops is to maintain a slightly warm temperature so that adequate blood circulation can be maintained. Treatment consists of covering the part with clothing or with the warm hand or other body surface. Any bubbing of the affected part should avoided, gentle massage of proximal portions of the extremity that not numb may be helpful. After swelling and hyperemia have developed, the patient should be kept in bed with the affected limb slightly flexed, and at rest. Protection by a heat cradle may be desirable. Papaverine or nicotinic acid may be given to reduce vasospasm. Antibiotics should be given as a prophylactic measure against infection.

> *Disorders due to Physical factors*
> - **Clavus:** circumscribed, horny, conical thickenings produced by pressure. If treatment is required, the relief of pressure or friction by corrective footwear is necessary.
> - **Frostbite:** it is a kind of skin disorder caused by low temperature, any bubbing of the affected part should avoided.

Web resources

http://www.ncbi.nlm.nih.gov/books/NBK10757/

Key words

clavus　鸡眼

sole　足底

hyperkeratosis　角质过度

frostbite　冻伤

low temperature　低温

Review questions

1. Where is the place clavus present commonly?
2. What's the management principle of frostbite?

(Weihua Pan)

Chapter 35 Urticaria and angioedema

Urticaria (hives) is a common eruption characterized by transient, usually pruritic, wheals due to acute dermal oedema from extravascular leakage of plasma. Angioedema signifies a larger area of oedema involving the dermis and subcutis. A classification is shown in Table 35-1.

Aetiopathogenesis

Urticaria is mediated through immune (allergic) or non-immune mechanisms. Lesions result from the release from mast cells of biologically active substances, particularly histamine, which produce vasodilatation and increased vascular permeability. Several pathways are recognized:

- *IgE-mediated (type I) hypersensitivity* is the best understood mechanism; antigen cross-links immunoglobulin (Ig) E molecules on the surface of mast cells, resulting in degranulation with release of vasoactive agents.
- *Complement activation* can produce dermal oedema, as in hereditary angioedema or urticaria associated with circulating immune complexes.
- *Direct release of histamine* from mast cells, in a non-immune manner, is caused by some drugs, e.g. opiates and contrast media.
- *Blocking of the prostaglandin pathway* from arachidonic acid, by some drugs such as aspirin and non-steroidal anti-inflammatory agents, promotes urticaria by accumulating vasoactive leukotrienes.
- *Anti-IgE receptor (anti-FcεR1) antibodies* have been shown to be present in 40% of cases of 'chronic' urticaria, which is capable of inducing autoimmune mast cell degranulation.

Pathology

The dermis is oedematous with dilatation of vessels and mast cell degranulation. Vessel damage and a lymphocytic infiltrate may be seen with urticarial vasculitis.

Clinical presentation

Urticaria is commonly defined as the sudden appearance of wheals with central swelling and surrounding erythema which are typically pruritic and resolve within about 24h without scarring, although some lesions may last up to 48h before resolving. Urticaria is traditionally classified into acute and chronic. When urticaria is present daily for less than 6 weeks it is called acute. If urticaria occurs continuously on most days for langer than 6 weeks it is called chronic. Three-quarters of cases of urticaria fall into the 'chronic idiopathic' or acute categories. Another 20% are due to dermographism, cholinergic urticaria or physical factors. Other causes are rare.

Table 35-1	Classification of urticaria and angioedema	
Allergic (IgE mediated) mast cell degranulation	Systemic	Food, drugs, latex (aerosols)
	Skin contact	Animal saliva, pollen, latex
Non-allergic (non-IgE mediated) mast cell degranulation	Chronic ordinary	No cause identifiable (commonest subtype)
	Physical	Dermographism, cholinergic, cold, solar, heat, delayed pressure
	Pharmacological	Aspirin, opiates, non-steroidal drugs, food additives, ACE inhibitors
	Autoimmune disease	Systemic lupus erythematosus, thyroid antibodies, anti-IgE receptor antibodies, urticarial vasculitis
	Genetic	C1 esterase inhibitor deficiency, mastocytosis
	Other	Infection, paraneoplastic, skin contact (nettle sting)

Chronic idiopathic urticaria

Itchy pink wheals appear as papules or plaques anywhere on the skin surface (Fig. 35-1). Typically, they last for less than 24h and disappear without a trace. Wheals may be round, annular or polycyclic, and vary in diameter from a few millimetres to several centimetres. Their number ranges from a few to many appearing each day, depending on the severity of the condition. Angioedema, usually with swelling of the tongue or lips, may occur (Fig. 35-2). Pharmacological agents often act as provoking factors, but normally no underlying cause is found. The condition may troubled for months or years.

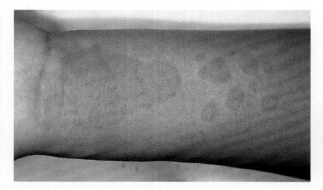

Fig. 35-1 **Chronic urticaria.** Typical wheals are seen on the forearm.

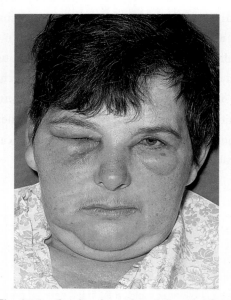

Fig. 35-2 **Angioedema involving the face.**

Acute urticaria

The sudden onset of urticaria or angioedema may be due to an IgE-mediated type I reaction. The patient can often identify the offending allergen. Commonly, it is a food (e.g. egg, fish or peanuts), a drug (e.g. an antibiotic) or contact with latex. Sometimes no cause is found.

Physical urticarias

Cold, heat, sun exposure, pressure and even water can all induce urticaria at the stimulated site. Dermographism, found in 5% of normal people, describes whealing induced by firm stroking of the skin (Fig. 35-3). In a few individuals, it is exaggerated and symptomatic. The wheals in cholinergic urticaria are small, intensely itchy papules that appear in response to sweating, as induced by exercise, heat, emotion or spicy food. The eruption lasts for a few minutes to an hour. In solar urticaria, wheals develop at the site of exposure within minutes of visible light or ultraviolet and usually fade within 2h.

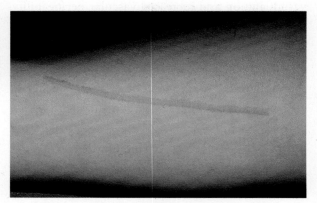

Fig. 35-3 **Dermographism.** This was induced by stroking the forearm.

C_1 esterase inhibitor deficiency

Hereditary angioedema is a rare and potentially fatal autosomal dominant condition with angioedema symptoms only (no urticaria). It usually presents in childhood, with episodes of angioedema often with vomiting and abdominal pain. A deficiency of C1 esterase inhibitor allows complement activation (e.g. caused by trauma) to go unchecked, with an accumulation of vasoactive mediators. Individuals will have low levels of C4 during attacks. Acute attacks are treated with intravenous infusion of C1 esterase inhibitor concentrate. Novel synthetic peptide blockers of bradykinin B2 receptors or kallikrein can also be utilized in acute attacks. Acquired deficiency of C1 esterase inhibitor will present later in life with identical features to the inherited form, except genetic testing will be negative.

Differential diagnosis

Urticaria is usually differentiated from urticarial vasculitis. Urticarial vasculitis often has an acute onset with widespread urticarial lesions that are unusual as they persist for more than 24h and fade leaving purpura (Fig. 35-4). Systemic abnormalities and low complement levels may be found. Toxic erythema and erythema multiforme may be urticated at first but, when the lesions persist for over 48h, urticaria can be excluded. Facial erysipelas sometimes resembles angioedema but has a sharper margin and the patient is unwell with a fever.

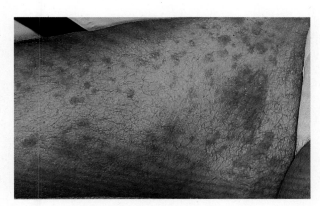

Fig. 35-4 **Urticarial vasculitis.** Resolving areas have left bruising.

Investigation

Underlying causes or provoking factors are better revealed by a careful history and examination than by laboratory tests. However, a full blood count, liver function tests, antinuclear antibody test, erythrocyte sedimentation rate (ESR) and urinalysis are often done to exclude systemic conditions (Table 35-1). Dermographism is demonstrated by firmly stroking the skin, and cold urticaria induced by holding an ice cube on the arm for up to 20 min. If C1 esterase inhibitor deficiency is suspected, C4 levels can be used as a screening test prior to C1 esterase inhibitor level assay.

Management

Any underlying cause should be eliminated. Provoking factors, e.g. aspirin ingestion, swimming (for those with cold urticaria) or sun exposure, are to be avoided. Desensitization may be possible for some physical urticarias; for example, individuals with cold urticaria can build up tolerance by gradual immersion of progressively more of the body in cold water. However, the mainstay of treatment is with antihistamines.

Antihistamines

Histamine type 1 receptor blockers (H_1 blockers) are usually effective. The second generation of potent, specific, low-sedation H_1 antihistamines is now the treatment of choice. Non-sedative antihistamines, such as cetirizine 10mg daily, fexofenadine 180mg once daily, desloratadine 5mg once daily or acrivastine 8mg three times daily, are now preferred unless the sedative qualities of the older preparations are desired.

Corticosteroids

Systemic steroids are very occasionally used to control severe acute urticaria or angioedema and urticarial vasculitis, but are not indicated for chronic urticaria.

Adrenaline (epinephrine)

Acute airway obstruction or anaphylactic shock is treated with adrenaline as an intramuscular injection (500 micrograms; 0.5ml adrenaline injection 1 in 1000), repeated 5 min later if necessary. An antihistamine such as chlorphenamine (Piriton), 10~20mg given by slow intravenous injection, is a useful adjunct. Intravenous steroids are often given, although their onset of action is delayed by several hours.

Diet

Salicylates in food aggravate chronic urticaria in up to a third of cases, and dietary azo dyes and benzoic acid preservatives produce an exacerbation in 10%.

Diets low in these compounds are tried if routine measures are ineffective.

Urticaria

■ Urticaria is a common eruption of transient pruritic wheals that typically clear within 1 day.

■ Associated dermal oedema is usually the result of mast cell degranulation and the release of vaso-active amines.

■ No cause is usually found, but urticaria may result from histamine-releasing IgG autoantibodies, IgE-mediated allergy, physical stimuli, the pharmacological effect of drugs or food additives, or complement deficiencies.

■ Causative or provoking factors should be eliminated, and non-sedating antihistamines prescribed.

■ Systemic steroids are rarely used in treatment. Aspirin is avoided. Intramuscular adrenaline is given for an anaphylactic reaction.

Key words

urticaria　荨麻疹

angioedema　血管性水肿

dermographism　皮肤划痕症

cholinergic urticaria　胆碱能性荨麻疹

urticarial vasculitis　荨麻疹性血管炎

cold urticaria　寒冷性荨麻疹

antihistamines　抗组胺药

anaphylactic shock　过敏性休克

Review questions

1. What is the aetiopathogenesis of urticaria?
2. What is the classification and clinical presentation of urticaria?
3. What is the drug of choice for urticaria?
4. How to treat anaphylactic shock?

(Meng Pan)

Chapter 36   Blistering disorders

Blistering is often seen with skin disease. It is found with common dermatoses such as acute contact dermatitis, pompholyx, herpes simplex, herpes zoster and bullous impetigo, and it also occurs after insect bites, burns and friction or cold injury. The type of blister depends on the level of cleavage: subcorneal or intraepidermal blisters rupture easily, but subepidermal ones are not so fragile (Fig. 36-1). The primary acquired autoimmune bullous disorders, dealt with here, are rare but important.

Pemphigus

Pemphigus is an uncommon, severe and potentially fatal autoimmune blistering disorder affecting the skin and mucous membranes.

Aetiopathogenesis

Over 80% of patients have circulating immunoglobulin (Ig) G autoantibodies detectable in the serum by indirect immunofluorescence, which bind with desmoglein 3 and desmoglein 1, a desmosomal cadherin involved in epidermal intercellular adhesion. The antibodies, possibly with complement activation and protease release, result in loss of adhesion and an intraepidermal split. Direct immunofluorescence shows the intercellular deposition of IgG in the suprabasal epidermis.

Clinical presentation

In Europe, pemphigus is much less common than pemphigoid, and tends to affect middle-aged or young adults. According to the clinical features, pemphigus is divided into four major forms: *pemphigus vulgaris, pemphigus vegetans, pemphigus foliaceus, and pemphigus erythematosus. Pemphigus vulgaris* is the most frequent representative of group of pemphigus diseases. Oral erosions signal the onset of *pemphigus vulgaris* in 50%~70% of patients and often precede cutaneous blistering by months. Flaccid superficial blisters develop over the scalp, face, back, chest and flexures. The blistering is not always obvious, and lesions may consist of crusted erosions. Untreated, the blistering is progressive and, prior to the introduction of steroids, three out of four patients died within 4 years, usually from uncontrolled fluid and protein loss or secondary infection.

Less common variants include *pemphigus foliaceus*, in which shallow erosions appear on the scalp, face and chest (Fig. 36-2). *Pemphigus erythematosus* is simply a localized benign variant of *pemphigus foliaceus. Pemphigus vegetans* is a rare vegetative variant of pemphigus vulgaris, in which pustular and vegetating lesions affect the axillae and groins. In Brazil, an endemic form of pemphigus foliaceus, *fogo selvagem*, seems to be induced by an infective agent.

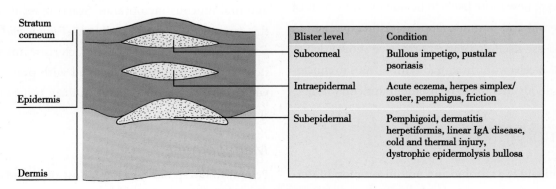

Blister level	Condition
Subcorneal	Bullous impetigo, pustular psoriasis
Intraepidermal	Acute eczema, herpes simplex/ zoster, pemphigus, friction
Subepidermal	Pemphigoid, dermatitis herpetiformis, linear IgA disease, cold and thermal injury, dystrophic epidermolysis bullosa

Fig. 36-1   **The level of cleavage in blistering disorders.**

Paraneoplastic pemphigus describes a variant associated with underlying malignancy.

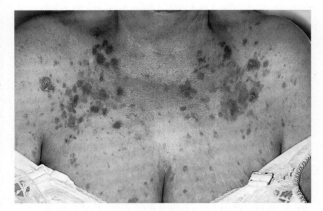

Fig. 36-2 **Pemphigus foliaceus showing blisters and erosions on the chest.**

Differential diagnosis

Aphthous ulcers or Behçet's disease can simulate the oral erosions of pemphigus. Cases with rapid onset need to be differentiated from toxic epidermal necrolysis. Widespread skin erosions may suggest epidermolysis bullosa or pemphigoid. The diagnosis relies on the histological examination of a bulla and direct immunofluorescence.

Management

Systemic steroids and other immunosuppressive agents are required. Prednisolone is given initially in a high dose (1.0~1.5mg/kg daily), often with azathioprine or cyclophosphamide. Once blistering is controlled, the steroid dosage can be lowered. Treatment usually needs to be continued for years, although remission occurs occasionally. Mortality and morbidity are now more likely to be due to side-effects of the steroid and immunosuppressive therapy than to the disease itself. Recent reports have shown depletion of B cells with rituximab (anti-CD20) monoclonal antibody therapy to be useful in this condition.

Pemphigoid

Pemphigoid is a chronic and not uncommon blistering eruption of the elderly.

Aetiopathogenesis

IgG autoantibodies to bullous pemphigoid antigens BP230 and BP180 in the hemidesmosomes at the basement membrane zone bind complement, which induces inflammation and protease release, leading to subepidermal bulla formation. The IgG and C3 are detected by direct immunofluorescence. Indirect methods demonstrate circulating autoantibodies in 75% of cases.

Clinical presentation

Bullous pemphigoid usually affects the elderly. Tense large blisters arise on red or normal-looking skin, often of the limbs, trunk and flexures (Fig. 36-3). Oral lesions occur in only 10% of cases. A pruritic urticarial eruption may precede the onset of blistering. Pemphigoid is sometimes localized to one site, often the lower leg. The differential diagnosis of pemphigoid may include dermatitis herpetiformis, linear IgA disease or pemphigus. Immunofluorescence and histology reveal the diagnosis.

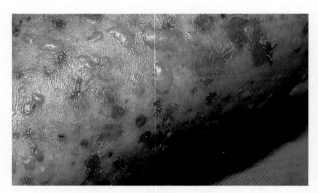

Fig. 36-3 **Bullous pemphigoid.** Tense blisters on an arm.

Cicatricial pemphigoid mainly affects the ocular and oral mucous membranes. Scarring results, and this can cause serious eye problems. *Pemphigoid (herpes) gestationis* is a rare but characteristic, intensely itchy bullous eruption associated with pregnancy, which remits after the delivery but can recur during subsequent pregnancies.

Management

Pemphigoid responds to a lower dose of steroids than pemphigus: 0.5mg/kg daily of oral prednisolone is usually sufficient, and this can normally be reduced to below 15mg within weeks. Azathioprine is sometimes also prescribed. The disease is self-limiting in many cases, and steroids can often be stopped after 2~3 years. Cicatricial pemphigoid does not respond so well, but pemphigoid gestationis is controlled by standard doses. Steroid-induced side-effects may be a problem, especially in the elderly.

Dermatitis herpetiformis

Dermatitis herpetiformis (DH) is an uncommon eruption of symmetrical itchy blisters on the extensor surfaces. Jejunal villus atrophy is an associated finding in most cases.

Aetiopathogenesis

DH is characterized by the finding of granular IgA at the dermal papillae on immunofluorescence, and by the response of the skin lesions (and the villus atrophy seen in over 75% of patients) to a gluten-free diet. Despite this, the cause of the eruption - and its relationship to the undoubted gluten sensitivity of both the gut and the skin - remains unclear. It is doubtful whether the IgA induces the itch, as it is present in asymptomatic patients.

Clinical presentation

DH usually presents in the third or fourth decade and is twice as common in males as in females. The classical onset is with groups of small, intensely itchy vesicles on the elbows, knees, buttocks and scalp (Fig. 36-4). The blisters are often broken by scratching to leave excoriations. Although most patients have small bowel villus atrophy, symptoms of gastrointestinal disturbance and malabsorption are uncommon.

Differential diagnosis

Distinction from scabies, eczema and linear IgA disease is important. Biopsy shows a subepidermal bulla, and direct immunofluorescence of normal-looking skin demonstrates granular IgA at the dermal papilla. The small bowel can be investigated by jejunal biopsy. Serum folate, vitamin B12 and ferritin estimates detect any biochemical malabsorption. Antiendomysial antibodies are present.

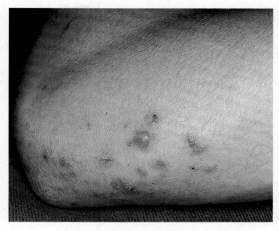

Fig. 36-4   **Dermatitis herpetiformis.** Itchy blisters on an elbow.

Management

A gluten-free diet is the treatment of choice, as this corrects both the bowel and the skin lesions. Dapsone (50~200mg daily) will control the eruption and is often given until the gluten-free diet has its beneficial effect. A haemolytic anaemia may occur with dapsone. Regular blood counts are necessary.

Linear IgA disease

Linear IgA disease is a rare heterogeneous condition of blisters and urticarial lesions on the back or extensor surfaces (Fig. 36-5). The disorder responds to dapsone and may resemble DH or pemphigoid. Direct immunofluorescence reveals linear IgA at the basement membrane. In the childhood variant, blisters occur around the genitalia. Linear IgA disease induced by medication (commonly vancomycin) is well recognized.

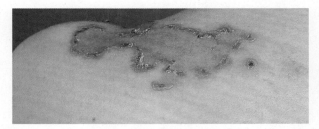

Fig. 36-5   **Linear IgA disease.** A figurate lesion with peripheral blisters.

Blistering disorders

Disorder	Clinical details	Direct (and indirect) immuno-fluorescence	Treatment
Bullous pemphigoid (BP)	Not uncommon, seen in elderly, limbs > trunk, oral lesions rare, tense blisters often seen	Linear IgG at basement membrane zone (to hemidesmosome BP antigens), indirect 75% positive	Modest dose of oral prednisolone with or without azathioprine
Pemphigus vulgaris	Rare, middle-aged affected, trunk > limbs, often starts with oral lesions, flaccid blisters may be seen	Intercellular epidermal IgG (to desmoglein in desmosomes), indirect 80% are positive	High dose of oral prednisolone and azathioprine or other immunosuppressive
Dermatitis herpetiformis	Young adults (M > F), extensor surfaces show itchy blisters, villus atrophy is usual	Granular IgA at dermal papilla (exact antigen is unknown), indirect test is negative	Gluten-free diet with or without dapsone

Web resources

http://www.pemphigus.org.uk/
http://www.pemphigus.org

Key words

blistering disorders　大疱病
desmoglein　桥粒芯蛋白
pemphigus vulgaris　寻常型天疱疮
pemphigus foliaceus　落叶型天疱疮
pemphigus vegetans　增殖型天疱疮
paraneoplastic pemphigus　副肿瘤性天疱疮
bullous pemphigoid　大疱性类天疱疮
cicatricial pemphigoid　瘢痕性类天疱疮

pemphigoid gestationis　妊娠型类天疱疮
dermatitis herpetiformis　疱疹样皮炎
linear IgA disease　线状 IgA 皮肤病

Review questions

1. How to differentiate pemphigus vulgaris from bullous pemphigoid?
2. What are the clinical features of subtypes of pemphigus?
3. What are the characteristics of direct immunofluorescence test in pemphigus vulgaris, bullous pemphigoid, dermatitis herpetiformis and linear IgA disease?
4. Is dapsone a major medicine for pemphigus or linear IgA disease?

(Liangchun Wang)

Chapter 37   Connective tissue diseases

The inflammatory disorders of connective tissue often affect several organs, as in systemic lupus erythematosus (LE), but they may also involve the skin alone (e.g. discoid LE). Autoantibodies are a feature of these diseases, which can thus be regarded as 'autoimmune'.

Lupus erythematosus

Lupus erythematosus represents a spectrum of cutaneous disease from scarring (discoid) to multisystem (systemic).

Aetiopathogenesis

There is increasing evidence that the induction of autoantibodies (such as anti-nuclear antibodies, ANA) against self-proteins derives from an impaired ability to clear dying (apoptotic) cells. Both genetic (human leucocyte antigen (HLA)) and environmental (toxins, drugs, UV radiation, viruses) factors have been implicated in disease pathogenesis.

Pathology

Discoid lesions show epidermal atrophy, hyperkeratosis and basal layer degeneration. Subacute lesions show greater atrophy but the other features are less evident. Systemic lesions have similar changes with dermal edema and fibrinoid change, inflammatory infiltrate and sometimes vasculitis. Direct immunofluorescence shows a 'lupus band' at the dermo-epidermal junction in lesional systemic and discoid LE, but this is also found in approximately 20% of healthy individuals on sun-exposed skin.

Clinical presentation

Systemic lupus erythematosus (SLE; 99% ANA, 50% Ro, 60% dsDNA positive)

Skin signs are found in 80%. The facial butterfly eruption (Fig. 37-1) is characteristic, but photosensi-

tivity, discoid lesions, diffuse alopecia, mouth lesions and vasculitis also occur. Multisystem involvement with serological or haematological abnormalities must be demonstrated to diagnose SLE (Table 37-1). Signs and symptoms such as fatigue, weight loss, fever, and lymphadenopathy are non-specific but common indicators of SLE. The female:male ratio is 8:1.

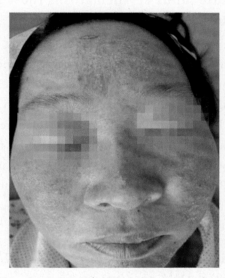

Fig. 37-1 **Systemic LE.** The typical butterfly eruption is present on the face.

Table 37-1	**Organ involvement in systemic LE**
Organ	**Involvement**
Skin	Photosensitivity, facial rash, vasculitis, hair loss, Raynaud's phenomenon
Blood	Anaemia, thrombocytopenia
Joints	Arthritis, tenosynovitis, calcification
Kidney	Glomerulonephritis, nephrotic syndrome
Heart	Pericarditis, endocarditis, hypertension
Central nervous system	Psychosis, infarction, neuropathy
Lungs	Pneumonitis, effusion

Criterion for SLE

Clinical criteria include acute cutaneous lupus, chronic cutaneous lupus, oral or nasal ulcers, non-scarring alopecia, synovitis, serositis, renal manifestation, neurologic manifestation, hemolytic anemia, leukopenia or lymphopenia, thrombocytopenia. Immunological criteria include ANA, anti-dsDNA, anti-Sm or antiphospholipid antibodies, low complement, and Direct Coombs' test.

Classify a patient as having SLE if the patient satisfies four of the criteria listed above, including at least one clinical criterion and one immunologic criterion, or the patient has biopsy-proven nephritis compatible with SLE and with ANA or anti-dsDNA antibodies.

Subacute lupus erythematosus (60% ANA, 80% Ro, <5% dsDNA positive)

The skin involvement is usually on the neck, trunk and arms. The erythema is non-scarring and may be papulosquamous or annular and resolves with hypopigmentation and telangiectasia. Mouth ulceration, livedo reticularis, periungal telangiectasia and Raynaud's phenomenon may also be noted. Multisystem involvement can be seen, but is usually mild. Photosensitivity is predominant in subacute LE patients, and anti-Ro52 antibody is detected in majority of them.

Discoid lupus erythematosus (35% ANA, 2% Ro, <5% dsDNA positive)

One or more round or oval plaques appear on the face, scalp or arms (Fig. 37-2), and may be distributed widely. The lesions are well demarcated, red, atrophic, scaly and show keratin plugs in dilated follicles. Scarring leaves alopecia on the scalp and

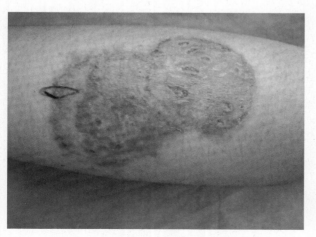

Fig. 37-2 **Discoid LE on the forearm.**

hypopigmentation in those with a pigmented skin. It is the most common type of chronic cutaneous LE. The relation between sun exposure and discoid lesion development remains unclear. Remission occurs in over 50%. Internal involvement is not a feature, and only 6% develop systemic LE. The risk is higher in patients with widespread lesions. Women outnumber men by 2:1.

Other forms

Neonatal LE is due to the placental transfer of anti-Ro antibodies and presents as an annular atrophic eruption, sometimes with heart block. Skin lesions usually develop within the first few weeks.

Differential diagnosis

Discoid LE can usually be differentiated from other facial rashes such as rosacea, seborrhoeic dermatitis, lupus vulgaris or psoriasis. A biopsy should be performed. The photosensitive eruption of systemic LE may resemble polymorphic light eruption, dermatomyositis or drug reaction.

Management

Immunological screening is important for diagnosis and to predict complications (e.g. anti-Ro and congenital heart block; anticardiolipin and thromboses and spontaneous abortions; antihistone and drug-induced lupus). Discoid LE usually responds to potent or very potent topical steroids which, in this instance, can be applied to the face. Sunblock creams are essential. Widespread disease may need systemic therapy with hydroxychloroquine; the small risk of retinopathy demands monitoring of visual acuity. The treatment of systemic LE depends on the type of involvement. Sunscreens reduce photosensitivity but, if there is internal disease, antimalarials and systemic steroids are required, often with immunosuppressive agents. Immune response modifiers may be promising for future therapeutic benefits.

Systemic sclerosis

Systemic sclerosis is an uncommon, progressive multisystem disease in which collagen deposition and fibrosis occur in several organs.

Aetiopathogenesis

The pathogenesis of systemic sclerosis is not clarified. Microvascular damage, autoantibody production, and tissue fibrosis are the key pathological processes. Dysregulated transforming growth factor (TGF)-β-induced fibroblast overproduction of collagen is central to tissue fibrosis. However, endothelial cell damage by T cells and macrophages may also be important.

Clinical presentation

Raynaud's phenomenon is frequently the presenting sign. The skin of the fingers, forearms and lower legs becomes tight, waxy and stiff, and the finger pulps are resorbed. Facial signs include perioral furrowing, telangiectasia and restricted mouth opening. Dyspigmentation, calcinosis cutis, and cutaneous ulcers are also found in systemic sclerosis patients (Fig. 37-3). Internal organ involvement, e.g. renal failure, may prove fatal (Table 37-2). Gastrointestinal tract, lung, kidney, and heart are the most commonly affected. Women are affected more than men (F:M ratio 4:1). Some 90%~95% of cases are ANA positive. The diagnosis is rarely in doubt in diffuse disease, although chronic graft-versus-host disease shows similar changes. Limited cutaneous systemic sclerosis has a better prognosis and usually affects only the

neck, forearms and lower legs. A subset described as CREST syndrome, is confined to *C*alcinosis, *R*aynaud's phenomenon, *E*sophageal dysmotility, *S*clerodactyly and *T*elangiectasia.

Table 37-2	**Organ involvement in systemic sclerosis**
Organ	**Involvement**
Skin	Raynaud's phenomenon, calcinosis, sclerodactyly, telangiectasia
Gut	Oesophageal dysmotility, malabsorption, dilated bowel
Lung	Fibrosis, pulmonary hypertension
Heart	Pericarditis, myocardial fibrosis
Kidney	Renal failure, hypertension
Muscle	Myositis, tendon involvement

Management

Treatment is mainly supportive. Nifedipine can help Raynaud's phenomenon. Hypertension is controlled. Systemic steroids, penicillamine and immune-suppressives have been used with little benefit. Photophoresis may be tried. Renal crises (associated with antiRNA polymerase I and III antibodies) should be managed aggressively with angiotensin converting enzyme (ACE) inhibitors. Cyclophosphamide may benefit the cutaneous diseases. While physical therapy is an important assistant.

Morphoea (localized scleroderma)

Morphoea consists of localized indurated plaques or bands of sclerosis on the skin. Internal disease is not found. The cause is unknown, although it may follow trauma. Histology shows bands of collagen with loss of appendages.

Morphoea presents with round or oval plaques of induration and erythema, often with a purplish edge (Fig. 37-4). These become shiny and white, eventually leaving atrophic hairless pigmented patches. The trunk or proximal limbs are affected. Morphoea is more common in women (F:M ratio 3:1). *Linear morphoea* may involve the face or a limb and, when seen in a child, can retard growth of the underlying tissues, including bone. The prognosis is usually good.

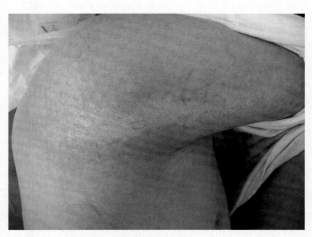

Fig. 37-3   **Systemic sclerosis.** Note the tightly bound waxy skin on the right shoulder with hypopigmented macules.

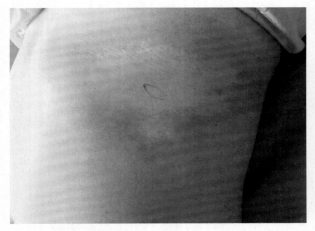

Fig. 37-4 **Morphoea.** Seen here on the left leg of a child. The white indurated plaque has an erythematous edge.

There is no well established treatment, although topical steroids, Calcipotriene, nonsteroidal anti-inflammatory drugs, psoralen with UVA, and UVA alone are often given. The disease usually resolves spontaneously within months to years.

Dermatomyositis

Dermatomyositis is an uncommon disorder in which inflammation of skin, muscle and blood vessels gives a distinctive eruption, with muscle weakness of varying severity. The cause is unknown but an underlying malignancy is found in a subgroup.

Clinical presentation

In dermatomyositis/polymyositis, skin changes or muscle weakness may predominate. Poikiloderma is the most common cutaneous feature. The typical eruption is a lilac-blue discoloration around the eyelids, cheeks and forehead, often with oedema. Bluish-red papules or streaks on the dorsal aspects of the hands (Fig. 37-5), elbows and knees are seen, known as Gottron's sign, sometimes with pigmentation and nail fold telangiectasia. Photosensitivity is common. There is no strong association with autoantibodies, although anti-Jo-1 antibodies predict lung involvement. An association with malignancy exists in patients over 40 years, 40% of whom have an underlying tumour, usually of the lung, breast or stomach.

A childhood variant mainly affects the muscles and causes calcinosis and contractures.

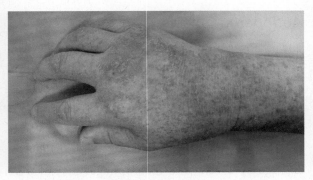

Fig. 37-5 **Dermatomyositis.** Bluish-red papules are seen on the dorsal aspects of the hands.

Management

Investigations must define the degree of myositis and, in adults, exclude the possibility of underlying neoplasia. Treatment is with systemic steroids in moderate to high dosage, often with an immunosuppressive such as azathioprine or methotrexate. Immunoglobulin infusion and possibly photophoresis may help.

Connective tissue diseases

- **Systemic LE** is an autoimmune, multisystem disease in which a butterfly rash, photosensitivity, vasculitis and alopecia may be seen. Treatment depends on the type and degree of involvement and often includes systemic steroids and immunosuppressive agents.
- **Subacute LE** is a less aggressive form of LE with predominantly cutaneous features.
- **Discoid LE** is confined to the skin. Scaly atrophic plaques and scarring alopecia are found. Topical steroids and sunscreens are helpful. Sometimes, systemic therapy, e.g. with hydroxychloroquine, is used.
- **Systemic sclerosis** is a serious multisystem disorder. Sclerodactyly, Raynaud's phenomenon, telangiectasia and calcinosis are seen.
- **Morphoea** is characterized by white indurated plaques, usually on the trunk and proximal limbs. In children, it may retard growth of underlying tissues, producing atrophy. In adults, the condition is generally self-limiting.
- **Dermatomyositis** is an autoimmune inflammation of skin and muscle. The skin signs are a lilac-blue discoloration around the eyelids and red streaks on the dorsa of the hands. Exclude underlying malignancy in those over 40 years of age.

Summary

The common connective tissue diseases include lupus erythematosus, systemic sclerosis, and dermatomyositis. Their pathogenesis involves autoimmunity and the production of autoantibodies. The clinical presentation varies largely in patients with lupus erythematosus. The diagnosis and management of connective tissue diseases depend on their subtypes.

Web resource

http://www.lupus-support.org.uk/
http://www.lupus.org/

Key words

discoid lupus erythematosus　盘状红斑狼疮

subacute lupus erythematosus　亚急性红斑狼疮
dystemic lupus erythematosus　系统性红斑狼疮
lupus band　狼疮带
photosensitivity　光敏感
Raynaud phenomenon　雷诺现象
CREST Syndrome　CREST 综合征
calcinosis　钙质沉着症
sclerodactylia　指（趾）硬化
morphoea　硬斑病
Gottron's sign　Gottron 征

Review questions

1. What are the diagnostic criteria of SLE?
2. What internal organs may be involved in dermatomyositis?
3. What is the classification of scleroderma?

(Yumin Xia)

Chapter 38 Vasculitis and the reactive erythemas

Vasculitis and the reactive erythemas are characterized by inflammation within or around blood vessels. This may result from a type III hypersensitivity response, with circulating immune complexes, but other mechanisms are also possible.

Vasculitis

Vasculitis is a disease process usually centred on small or medium-sized blood vessels. It is often due to circulating immune complexes (CICs).

Aetiopathogenesis

The CICs, which may be associated with several conditions (Table 38-1), lodge in the vessel wall where they activate complement and cytokine release, attract polymorphs and damage tissue. Inflammatory cells infiltrate vessels. Endothelial cells may show swelling, fibrinoid change or necrosis.

Table 38-1	Causes of vasculitis
Group	**Example**
Idiopathic	50% of cases (no cause found)
Blood disease	Cryoglobulinaemia
Connective tissue disease	Systemic lupus erythematosus, rheumatoid arthritis
Drugs	Antibiotics, diuretics, non-steroidals, anticonvulsants, allopurinol, cocaine
Infections	Hepatitis B, streptococci, *Mycobacterium leprae*, *Rickettsia*
Neoplasia	Lymphoma, leukaemia
Other	Wegener's granulomatosis, giant cell arteritis, polyarteritis nodosa

Clinical presentation

This depends on the size and site of the vessels involved. Vasculitis may be confined to the skin, or may be systemic and involve the joints, kidneys, lungs, heart, gut and nervous system. The skin signs

are of palpable purpura, often painful and usually on the lower legs or buttocks (Fig. 38-1). Specific types are as follows:

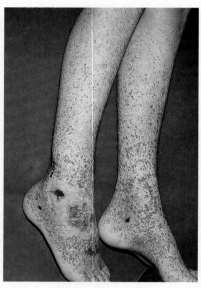

Fig. 38-1 **Vasculitis with purpura and impending skin necrosis.**

■ *Henoch-Schönlein purpura* describes these signs, with arthritis, abdominal pain and haematuria. Direct immunofluorescence studies on a skin biopsy will show the small vessel immunoglobulin (Ig) A-CIC vasculitis, which can be helpful diagnostically. Mainly affects children and often follows a streptococcal infection.

■ *Nodular vasculitis*, characterized by tender subcutaneous nodules on the lower legs, results when deeper dermal vessels are involved.

■ *Polyarteritis nodosa* is characterized by a necrotizing vasculitis in medium-sized arteries. It is uncommon and afflicts middle-aged men who, in addition to tender subcutaneous nodules along the line of arteries, may develop hypertension, renal failure and neuropathy.

■ *Wegener's granulomatosis* is a rare but potentially fatal granulomatous vasculitis of unknown cause. Malaise, upper and lower respiratory tract necrosis, glomerulonephritis and, in 40% of cases, a cutaneous vasculitis are found. Classical antineutrophil cytoplasm antibodies (c-ANCA) directed at proteinase 3 (PR3) are present.

■ *Giant cell arteritis* affects medium-sized arteries in the elderly. Visual loss may result if prednisolone is withheld. Patients present with scalp tenderness due to temporal artery involvement that can progress to scalp necrosis.

In vasculitis, a skin biopsy is helpful along with tests to look for internal organ involvement. Other causes of purpura need exclusion.

Management

The cause is identified and remedied if possible. Some idiopathic cases settle with bed rest but, if lesions continue to develop and if internal organs are involved, treatment is indicated. Dapsone, 100mg daily, is often effective for cutaneous vasculitis. Otherwise, prednisolone (sometimes with an immunosuppressive) is prescribed. Giant cell arteritis, polyarteritis nodosa and Wegener's granulomatosis nearly always require oral steroids and immunosuppression.

Erythema multiforme

Erythema multiforme is an immune-mediated disease, characterized by target lesions on the hands and feet. It has a variety of causes (Table 38-2).

Table 38-2	Causes of erythema multiforme
Group	**Cause**
Idiopathic	50% of cases (no cause found)
Viral	Herpes simplex, hepatitis B, orf, adenovirus, mumps, *Mycoplasma*
Bacterial	Streptococci, *Rickettsia*
Fungal	Coccidioidomycosis, histoplasmosis
Drugs	Antibiotics, phenytoin, non-steroidals
Other	Lupus erythematosus, pregnancy, malignancy

Aetiopathogenesis

Cell-mediated immunity seems to be involved. CICs are also present and can be demonstrated in blood vessels. No provoking factor is found in 50% of cases.

On histology, the epidermis is necrotic and the dermis shows oedema, an inflammatory infiltrate and vasodilatation.

Clinical presentation

Typical target lesions, seen on the hands and feet, consist of red rings with central pale or purple areas, which may blister (Fig. 38-2). Involvement of the oral, conjunctival and genital mucosae is not uncommon and, if extensive, is known as erythema multiforme major. Crops of new lesions appear for 2~3 weeks. The differential diagnosis includes toxic erythema, Stevens-Johnson syndrome, toxic epidermal necrolysis, Sweet's disease, urticaria and pemphigoid. A biopsy is often helpful. *Toxic epidermal necrolysis* may sometimes represent erythema multiforme in a severe form.

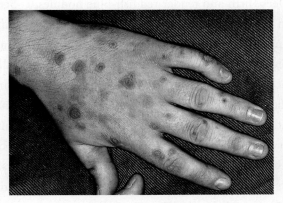

Fig. 38-2   **Erythema multiforme.** Target lesions are seen here on the dorsal aspect of the hand.

Management

Identification and treatment of the underlying cause is the ideal. Mild cases resolve spontaneously and require symptomatic measures only. Extensive involvement necessitates hospital admission for supportive therapy. Systemic steroids are often prescribed to moderate the acute symptoms, although it is debatable whether they affect the outcome.

Erythema nodosum

Erythema nodosum is a panniculitis (i.e. an inflammation of the subcutaneous fat) that usually presents as painful red nodules on the lower legs. It is believed to result from CIC deposition in vessels of the sub-cutis. Infection, drugs and some systemic diseases are underlying causes (Table 38-3).

Table 38-3	**Causes of erythema nodosum**
Group	**Cause**
Idiopathic	About 20% of cases
Bacterial	Streptococci, TB, leprosy, *Yersinia*, *Mycoplasma*, *Salmonella*
Fungal	Coccidioidomycosis, *Trichophyton*
Viral	Cat-scratch fever, chlamydiae
Drugs	Sulphonamides, oral contraceptives
Systemic disease	Inflammatory bowel disease, sarcoidosis, Behçet's disease, malignancy (rare)

Clinical presentation

Deep, firm and tender reddish-blue nodules, 1~5cm in diameter, develop on the calves (Fig. 38-3), shins and occasionally on the forearms. Joint pains and fever are common. Spontaneous resolution usually occurs within 8 weeks. Women are affected more than men (F:M ratio 3:1). Other causes of panniculitis (e.g. pancreatic disease, cold, trauma and lupus erythematosus), cellulitis and phlebitis need to be excluded. A skin biopsy is helpful. If tuberculosis or sarcoidosis is suspected, a chest radiograph and Mantoux test are indicated.

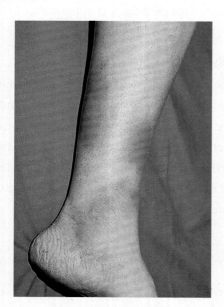

Fig. 38-3 **Erythema nodosum of the lower leg.**

Management

As spontaneous remission is usual, active therapy is rarely needed, although a non-steroidal anti-inflammatory drug, potassium iodide or dapsone may help.

Sweet's disease

Sweet's disease (*acute febrile neutrophilic dermatosis*) occurs as raised plum-coloured plaques on the face or limbs (Fig. 38-4), typically with fever and a raised neutrophil count. It is not a true vasculitis but results from polymorph infiltration of the dermis. Leukaemia, ulcerative colitis and other disorders may be associated and must be excluded. Drugs are another cause. Treatment with prednisolone is usually required.

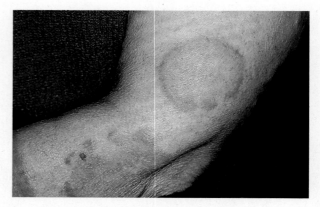

Fig. 38-4 **Sweet's disease.** A variant associated with rheumatoid arthritis is shown. Infiltrated annular plaques are seen on the arm.

Graft-versus-host (GVH) disease

GVH disease occurs when immunologically competent donor lymphocytes react against host tissues, principally the skin and gut. It is mostly associated with bone marrow transplantation, e.g. given for leukaemia or aplastic anaemia. Fever, malaise and a morbilliform eruption (Fig. 38-5), which may progress to toxic epidermal necrolysis, typify the acute GVH reaction. The acute type may be difficult to differentiate from a drug eruption, a viral infection or a cutaneous reaction to radiation therapy. Chronic GVH disease may resemble lichen planus or systemic sclerosis. A skin biopsy often helps, and treatment with systemic steroids is usually needed.

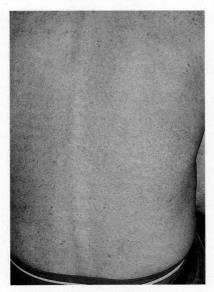

Fig. 38-5 **Graft-versus-host disease.** An acute eruption is shown in a patient following bone marrow transplant.

Behçet's disease

Behçet's disease, also called Behçet's syndrome, is a rare immune-mediated small-vessel systemic vasculitis. The disease was named after the Turkish dermatologist Hulusi Behçet, who first described the triple-symptom complex of recurrent oral aphthous ulcers, genital ulcers, and uveitis. The cause of Behcet's disease is unknown. This disease often presents with recurrent ulcers in the mouth and on the genitals, and eye inflammation. Behcet's disease may involve multiple systems, causing various types of skin lesions, arthritis, bowel inflammation, meningitis, and cranial nerve palsies. It may involve all organs and affect the central nervous system, causing memory loss and impaired speech, balance, and movement. In very rare situation, this syndrome can be fatal due to ruptured vascular aneurysms or severe neurological complications.

Pigmented purpuric dermatoses

Pigmented purpuric dermatoses (PPD) are a group of vascular disorders with varied manifestations. They are chronic, progressive, and are resistant to treatment. The key features of PPD are clustered petechial hemorrhage, often with a background of yellow-brown discoloration due to hemosiderin deposition. The location and pattern depends on the particular variant, including: ① Schamberg's disease or Progressive pigmentary dermatosis of Schamberg; ② Pigmented purpuric lichenoid dermatosis of Gougerot and Blum; ③ Purpura annularis telengiectoides or Majocchi's disease; ④ Lichen aureus; Itching purpura (Eczematid like purpura of Doucas and Kapetanakis).

Vasculitis and the reactive erythemas

■ **Vasculitis** is a circulating immune complex (CIC) disorder showing palpable purpura, sometimes with internal organ involvement. Investigations may reveal the underlying cause. Treatment with dapsone, prednisolone or other immunosuppressive drugs is often indicated.

■ **Erythema multiforme** is an immune-mediated reaction with target and mucosal lesions, often due to infection, commonly herpes simplex, or drugs. The underlying cause should be sought.

■ **Erythema nodosum** presents as painful red nodules on the lower legs and is regarded as a CIC response to infection (e.g. streptococcal), drugs or internal disease (e.g. sarcoidosis).

■ **Sweet's disease** is characterized by plum-coloured plaques on the face and limbs. Leukaemia or a systemic disorder may be associated. A course of prednisolone is often required.

■ **Behçet's disease** presents as recurrent ulcers in the mouth and on the genitals, and eye inflammation. Behçet's disease may involve multiple systems.

■ **Pigmented purpuric dermatoses (PPD)** are a group of vascular disorders with varied manifestations. The key features of PPD are clustered petechial hemorrhage, often with a background of yellow-brown discoloration due to hemosiderin deposition.

Web resource

https://www.vasculitisfoundation.org/

Key words

vasculitis   血管炎

circulating immune complexes   循环免疫复合物

purpura   紫癜

nodular vasculitis   结节性血管炎

polyarteritis nodosa   结节性多动脉炎

Wegener's granulomatosis　韦氏肉芽肿病

giant cell arteritis　巨细胞动脉炎

erythema multiforme　多形红斑

target lesions　靶形皮损

toxic epidermal necrolysis　中毒性表皮坏死松解症

erythema nodosum　结节性红斑

panniculitis　脂膜炎

acute febrile neutrophilic dermatosis　急性发热性嗜中性（细胞）皮肤病

graft-versus-host disease　移植物抗宿主病

Behçet's disease　白塞病

Behçet's syndrome　贝赫切特综合征

pigmented purpuric dermatoses　色素性紫癜性皮肤病

Review questions

1. What are the skin signs of vasculitis?
2. What are the clinical features of Henoch-Schönlein purpura, nodular vasculitis, polyarteritis nodosa, wegener's granulomatosis and giant cell arteritis?
3. What is the cause of erythema multiforme?
4. What is the treatment of Sweet's disease?
5. What is the triple-symptom of Behçet's disease?

(Yi Zhao)

Chapter 39 Skin changes in internal conditions

Skin signs are seen with many internal disorders and are not uncommonly their presenting feature. The astute dermatologist can recognize undiagnosed systemic disease.

Skin signs of endocrine and metabolic disease

Almost all endocrine diseases (and several metabolic defects) have cutaneous signs that depend on the over- or underproduction of a hormone or metabolite (Table 39-1).

Diabetes mellitus

Candida albicans or bacterial infection is more common with untreated or poorly controlled diabetes. The neuropathy or arteriopathy of diabetes may result in *ulcers* on the feet, and an associated secondary hyperlipidaemia can produce *eruptive xanthomas* (Fig. 39-4). *Diabetic dermopathy* describes depressed pigmented scars on the shins, associated with diabetic microangiopathy. *Necrobiosis lipoidica* (Fig. 39-1), characterized by shiny atrophic yellowish-red plaques on the shins, was associated with diabetes

in 65% of cases in one series, although others find a much lower figure. It affects less than 1% of all diabetics. Histologically, degenerate dermal collagen is seen with epithelioid cells and giant cells. The condition is chronic and may ulcerate. It is unresponsive to treatment. In contrast, *granuloma annulare* - recognized as palpable annular lesions on the hands, feet or face (Fig. 39-2) - is only rarely associated with diabetes and usually fades in 2 years. It must be differentiated from tinea corporis.

Thyroid disease

Both over- and underproduction of thyroxine result in skin and hair changes (Table 39-1). *Pretibial myxoedema* (Fig. 39-3), seen in 1%~10% of patients with hyperthyroidism, presents on the shins as raised erythematous plaques due to the deposition of mucin in the dermis. Topical steroids may be of benefit.

Flushing

Flushing may be physiological, drug/food induced or associated with *thyrotoxicosis*, but rarely with *carcinoid syndrome*, *mastocytosis* and *phaeochromocytoma*.

Table 39-1	**Skin signs of endocrine and metabolic disorders**
Disorders	**Skin signs**
Diabetes mellitus	Necrobiosis lipoidica, granuloma annulare, xanthomas, *Candida albicans* infection, 'dermopathy', neuropathic ulcers
Thyrotoxicosis	Pink soft skin, hyperhidrosis, alopecia, pigmentation, vitiligo, onycholysis, clubbing, pretibial myxoedema, palmar erythema
Myxoedema	Alopecia (including eyebrows), coarse hair, dry puffy yellowish skin (e.g. hands, face), asteatotic eczema, xanthomas
Addison's disease	Pigmentation, vitiligo, loss of axillary and pubic hair
Cushing's disease	Pigmentation, hirsutism, striae, acne, obesity, buffalo 'hump'
Acromegaly	Thickened moist greasy skin, pigmentation, skin tags
Phenylketonuria	Fair hair and skin, atopic eczema, photosensitivity
Hyperlipidaemia	Xanthomas (tuberous, tendinous, eruptive, plane), xanthelasma
Cutaneous porphyrias	Photosensitivity, blistering, skin fragility, atrophic scarring, thickening of skin, hypertrichosis, pigmentation

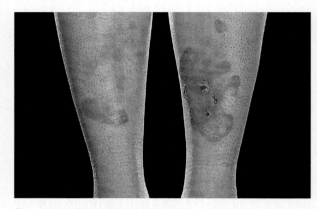

Fig. 39-1 **Necrobiosis lipoidica.** Yellowish-red atrophic areas are seen on the shins of a diabetic patient.

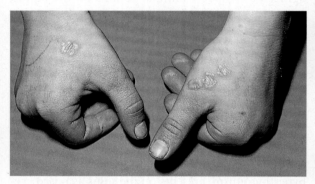

Fig. 39-2 **Granuloma annulare, seen on the dorsal aspects of the hands.**

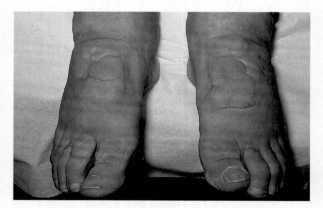

Fig. 39-3 **Pretibial myxoedema.** The patient had been thyrotoxic.

Hyperlipidaemia

Both primary (genetic metabolic defects) and secondary (associated with diabetes, hypothyroidism or the nephrotic syndrome) lipid abnormalities may produce a variety of xanthomatous deposits. These may be:

- ▪ *eruptive*: red-yellow papules on shoulders and buttocks (Fig. 39-4).

- ▪ *tendinous*: subcutaneous nodules; hand, foot or Achilles tendons.
- ▪ *plane*: yellow-orange macules in palmar creases.
- ▪ *tuberous*: yellow-orange nodules on knees and elbows.

Xanthelasma, seen as yellowish plaques on the eyelids, are not always due to a lipid abnormality. Treatment of xanthomas is usually aimed at underlying hyperlipidaemia.

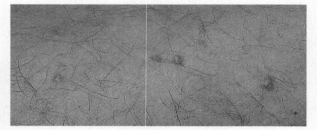

Fig. 39-4 **Eruptive xanthomas.** The patient had recently presented with diabetes mellitus.

Skin signs of nutritional and other internal disorders

Skin changes are common with nutritional deficiency and are not infrequent with gastrointestinal, hepatic and renal disease.

Nutritional deficiency

Protein malnutrition results in retarded growth, wasted muscles, oedema and skin changes of altered pigmentation, desquamation and ulcers with, in black Africans, dry and pale-brown/red hair. *Vitamin C deficiency* (scurvy) and *niacin deficiency* (pellagra) produce distinct lesions. In Europe, scurvy is mainly seen in elderly men who do not eat fresh fruit or vegetables. Deficiencies of other B vitamins and of iron also produce cutaneous changes (Table 39-2). *Acrodermatitis enteropathica* is a rare inherited defect of zinc absorption seen in weaned infants and cured by zinc supplements.

Gastrointestinal disease

Malabsorption and its deficiency states have accompanying skin problems that include dryness, eczema, ichthyosis, pigmentation and defects of the hair and

Table 39-2	**Skin signs of nutritional and internal disorders**
Disorder	**Skin signs**
Protein malnutrition	Pigmentation, dry skin, oedema, pale-brown/orange hair
Iron deficiency	Alopecia, koilonychia, itching, angular cheilitis
Scurvy	Perifollicular purpura, bleeding gums, woody oedema
Pellagra	Light-exposed dermatitis and pigmentation
Acrodermatitis enteropathica	Perianal/perioral red scaly pustular eruption in infants, failure to thrive, diarrhoea, poor wound healing
Malabsorption	Dry itchy skin, ichthyosis, eczema, oedema
Liver disease	Pruritus, jaundice, spider naevi, palmar erythema, white nails, pigmentation, xanthomas, porphyria cutanea tarda, zinc deficiency, striae, gynaecomastia, lichen planus
Renal failure	Pruritus, pigmentation, white/red nails, dry skin with fine scaling
Pancreatic disease	Panniculitis, thrombophlebitis, glucagonoma syndrome
Crohn's disease	Perianal abscesses, sinuses, fistulae, erythema nodosum, Sweet's disease, necrotizing vasculitis, aphthous stomatitis, glossitis
Ulcerative colitis	Pyoderma gangrenosum, erythema nodosum, Sweet's disease
Sarcoidosis	Nodules, plaques, erythema nodosum, dactylitis, lupus pernio, scar granulomas, small papules, nail involvement

nails. Some gut disorders show specific skin changes (Table 39-2). *Coeliac disease* is associated with an eczema (in addition to the link of dermatitis herpetiformis with gluten enteropathy). and both *Crohn's disease* and *ulcerative colitis* induce various eruptions. *Peutz-Jeghers syndrome* and *pseudoxanthoma elasticum* affect both the skin and the gut. *Bowel bypass surgery* induces a vesiculopustular eruption.

Other internal disorders

Hepatic and *renal diseases* often produce troublesome itching and pigmentation. Lesions may also be related to the underlying disease process, e.g. primary biliary cirrhosis (associated with systemic sclerosis) or vasculitis.

Sarcoidosis, a disorder of unknown aetiology in which granulomas commonly develop in the lung, lymph nodes, bone and nervous tissue, affects the skin in a third of cases. Cutaneous changes are variable and include brownish-red papules (typically on the face), nodules, plaques (on the limbs and shoulders, Fig. 39-5) and scar involvement. *Lupus pernio* is a particular pattern of sarcoidosis that appears as dusky-red infiltrated plaques on the nose or, occasionally, the fingers. *Erythema nodosum* may also result. Topical steroids have little effect. Resistant lesions may improve with intralesional steroid injection, but oral prednisolone or methotrexate is sometimes prescribed, particularly when there is progressive internal disease.

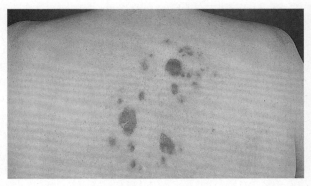

Fig. 39-5 **Sarcoidosis.** Plum-coloured plaques are seen on the upper back

Skin changes in pregnancy

Skin changes are common in pregnancy. Pigmentation generally increases, melanocytic naevi become more prominent, and spider naevi and abdominal striae develop. Telogen effluvium may occur in the postpartum period. Pruritus and an urticated papular eruption are not uncommon, although pemphigoid gestationis is rare. The effect on common dermatoses is variable and unpredictable: psoriasis tends to improve, but eczema may get worse.

Skin changes in internal conditions

■ Endocrine and metabolic disorders, nutritional deficiencies and malabsorption are frequently associated with skin changes.

■ Flushing may be physiological or induced by food, drugs or conditions such as thyrotoxicosis and carcinoid syndrome.

■ Hyperlipidaemias are associated with a variety of xanthomata and xanthelasma, although the latter can occur with normal lipid levels.

■ Liver and kidney failure, in particular, are complicated by pruritus and pigmentation. Treatment is often difficult.

■ Inflammatory bowel disease and sarcoidosis have specific skin manifestations, often granulomatous or with cellular infiltration.

■ Pregnancy can be associated with increased pigmentation (e.g. melasma), an urticated papular eruption and, rarely, with the blistering eruption pemphigoid gestationis.

Web resource

http://www.medderm.org.uk

Key words

diabetic dermopathy　糖尿病性皮肤病变

necrobiosis lipoidica　类脂质渐进性坏死

granuloma annulare　环状肉芽肿

pretibial myxedema　胫前黏液水肿

flushing　面部潮红

xanthoma　黄瘤

xanthelasma　睑黄瘤

acrodermatitis enteropathica　肠病性肢端皮炎

sarcoidosis　结节病

lupus pernio　冻疮样狼疮

erythema nodosum　结节性红斑

telogen effluvium　休止期脱发

Review questions

1. What are the most common skin disorders observed in poorly control diabetes?

2. What is the internal disease pretibial myxedema associated with? How is it formed?

3. What is the common skin signs related to hyperlipidaemias?

4. What are the specific skin changes highly related to gastrointestinal disease?

5. What are the skin disorders commonly presented in pregnancy?

(Liangchun Wang)

Chapter 40   Drug eruptions

Reactions to drugs are common and often produce an eruption. Almost any drug can result in any reaction, although some patterns are more common with certain drugs. Not all reactions are 'allergic' in nature.

Aetiopathogenesis

Drug-induced skin reactions have several possible pharmacological or idiosyncratic, as well as immune mediated mechanisms. Pharmacological mechanisms include:

- *Deposition* of the drug (or metabolites) in the skin, e.g. gold.
- *Excessive therapeutic effect*, e.g. purpura from overdosage with anticoagulants.
- *Pharmacological side-effects*, e.g. bone marrow suppression by cytotoxics.
- *Unknown*, e.g. when drugs exacerbate psoriasis.

Idiosyncratic: Some people are more susceptible than others to a reaction, for example, patients with the histocompatibility allele HLA-B*5701 are at high risk of Stevens-Johnson syndrome (SJS) from the anti-human immunodeficiency drug abacavir.

Immunological (type I ~ IV reactions):

Type I: mediated by IgE, e.g. urticaria or anaphylactic shock.

Type II: antibody-dependent cytotoxicity, e.g. thrombocytolytic purpura.

Type III: immune complex, e.g. vasculitis, serum sickness.

Type IV: cell mediated, e.g. exanthema.

Clinical presentation

Drug eruptions present in many guises and come into the differential diagnosis of several rashes. It is vital to obtain a detailed drug ingestion history. This must include 'over-the-counter' preparations (e.g. for headaches or constipation) not normally regarded as 'drugs' by the patient. A drug introduced during a 2-week period before the eruption starts must be viewed as the most likely culprit, although a reaction may occur to a drug taken safely for years. The majority of drug eruptions fit into a defined category (Table 40-1). The most severe and characteristic ones are outlined below. Other patterns are discussed in the relevant chapters. Drugs including non-steroidals or angiotensin-converting enzyme (ACE) inhibitors, but especially lithium and chloroquine, can exacerbate existing psoriasis. Other agents, e.g. beta-blockers and gold, may provoke a psoriasis-like eruption.

Drug-induced exanthem

Drug-induced exanthem, the commonest type of drug eruption, may be *morbilliform* (measles-like) or *maculopapular*, or may resemble *scarlatiniform*. It usually affects the trunk more than the extremities (Fig. 40-1), and may be accompanied by mild fever or followed by peeling of the skin. Haematological or biochemical disturbance does not arise. The eruption clears 1~2 weeks after stopping the offending drug.

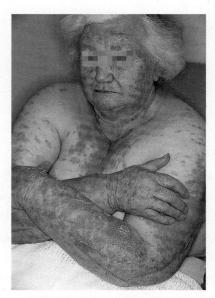

Fig. 40-1 **Drug-induced exanthem.** This morbilliform variant was due to chlorpropamide.

Table 40-1 **Patterns of drug-induced skin disease**

Drug eruption	Description	Drugs commonly responsible
Acneiform	Like acne: papulopustules, no comedones	Androgens, bromides, dantrolene, isoniazid, lithium, phenobarbital, quinidine, steroids
Bullous	Various types; some phototoxic, some 'fixed'	Barbiturates (overdose), furosemide, nalidixic acid (phototoxic), penicillamine (pemphigus-like)
Drug-induced exanthem	Commonest pattern (see text)	Antibiotics (e.g. amoxicillin), proton pump inhibitors, gold, thiazides, allopurinol, carbamazepine
Eczematous	Not common; seen when topical sensitization is followed by systemic treatment	Neomycin, penicillin, sulphonamide, ethylenediamine (cross-reacts with aminophylline), benzocaine (cross-reacts with chlorpropamide), parabens, allopurinol
Erythema multiforme	Target lesions	Antibiotics, anticonvulsants, ACE inhibitors, calcium channel blockers, non-steroidals
Erythroderma	Exfoliative dermatitis	Allopurinol, captopril, carbamazepine, diltiazem, gold, isoniazid, omeprazole, phenytoin
Fixed drug eruption	Round red-purple plaques recur at same site	Antibiotics, tranquillizers, non-steroidals, phenolphthalein, paracetamol, quinine
Hair loss	Telogen effluvium Anagen effluvium	Anticoagulants, bezafibrate, carbimazole, oral contraceptive pill, propranolol, albendazole, cytotoxic drugs, acitretin
Hypertrichosis	Excess vellus hair growth	Minoxidil, cyclosporin, phenytoin, penicillamine, corticosteroids, androgens
Lupus erythematosus (LE)	LE-like syndrome	Hydralazine, isoniazid, penicillamine, anticonvulsants, beta-blockers, etanercept
Lichenoid	Like lichen planus	Chloroquine, beta-blockers, anti-TB drugs, penicillamine, diuretics, gold, captopril
Photosensitive	Sun-exposed sites, may blister or pigment (Fig. 40-4)	Non-steroidals, ACE inhibitors, amiodarone, thiazides, tetracyclines, phenothiazines
Pigmentation	Melanin or drug deposition (Fig.40-5)	Amiodarone, bleomycin, psoralens, chlorpromazine, minocycline, antimalarials
Psoriasiform	Psoriasis-like appearance (see text)	Beta-blockers, gold, methyldopa; lithium and antimalarials exacerbate psoriasis
Toxic epidermal necrolysis	Blistering skin with mucosal involvement (see text)	Antibiotics, anticonvulsants, non-steroidals, omeprazole, allopurinol, barbiturates
Urticaria	Many mechanisms	ACE inhibitors, penicillins, opiates, non-steroidals, X-ray contrast media, vaccines
Vasculitis	Immune complex reaction	Allopurinol, captopril, penicillins, phenytoin, sulphonamides, thiazides

Urticarial eruptions

Urticarial eruptions characterized by transient wheals of the skin and mucous membranes with pruritus. Individual lesions characteristically last for less than 24h. Angioedema occurs if the deep dermal and subcutaneous tissues are involved. It occurs most commonly on the lips, eyes, and mucous membranes and may last for several days with or without urticarial lesions.

Stevens-Johnson syndrome, toxic epidermal necrolysis

Stevens-Johnson syndrome (SJS) and toxic epidermal necrolysis (TEN) represent a spectrum of disease, characterized by severe mucosal ulceration and blistering of the skin with different body surface area detachment (SJS 1%~10%; SJS/TEN overlap 10%~30%; TEN>30%). Both show significant systemic disturbance. Mucosal lesions may lead to scarring with a significant morbidity if the patient survives. The extensive skin loss results in problems of fluid and electrolyte balance, as seen with extensive burns, and TEN is usually managed in a burns or intensive care unit (Fig. 40-2). Overall mortality is up to 20%~30%.

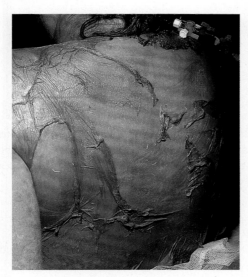

Fig. 40-2　**Toxic epidermal necrolysis.** The damaged epidermis has sheared off to leave extensive areas of eroded skin.

Drug reaction with eosinophilia and systemic symptoms (DRESS)

DRESS commonly has a delayed onset of 3~4 weeks. The rash initially starts similarly to a drug-induced exanthem, but quickly it becomes apparent that the individual is systemically unwell. There is significant amount of tissue oedema, often on the head and neck, and widespread lymphadenopathy. Small pinpoint pustules and superficial blisters may be evident. Systemic upset is characterized by fever and eosinophilia. Liver dysfunction is common but any organ system can become involved and may fail. On cessation of the offending drug, the rash may improve only to worsen again days later leading to confusion regarding the diagnosis. Reactivation of childhood viruses such as HHV6 and HHV7 have been demonstrated. Oral prednisolone is usually effective.

Acute generalized exanthematous pustulosis (AGEP)

AGEP often arises rapidly after a new medication (<5 days). The condition is characterized by the presence of large sterile pustules which may form sheets. The patient may have a mild systemic upset with a fever and usually has a neutrophilia. Pustular psoriasis can be difficult to distinguish.

Fixed drug eruption

This specific but uncommon eruption is characterized by round red or purplish plaques (Fig. 40-3) that recur at the same site each time the causative agent is taken. The lesions may blister and leave pigmentation on clearing.

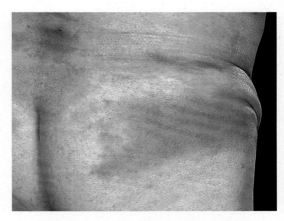

Fig. 40-3　**Fixed drug eruption.** The typical dusky erythematous lesion followed the ingestion of penicillin.

Fixed drug eruption, phototoxic reaction, drug-induced pemphigus and barbiturate overdosage (at pressure sites) may all blister (Table 40-1).

Differential diagnosis

The exact differential diagnosis depends on the type of drug eruption. The determination of which drug is responsible depends on a detailed prescribing timeline and a knowledge of the potential of each drug to cause a reaction (Table 40-2). In severe or extensive cases, photography and histology should be obtained. Allergen-specific immunoglobulin (Ig) E tests are not helpful, but patch tests may be of use in diagnosing a drug eruption. Assays of drug-induced T cell activation show promise but remain largely research based.

Table 40-2 **Eruptions seen with some commonly prescribed drugs**

Drug	Eruption
ACE inhibitors	Pruritus, urticaria, toxic erythema
Antibiotics	Toxic erythema, urticaria, fixed drug eruption, erythema multiforme
Beta-blockers	Psoriasiform, Raynaud's phenomenon, lichenoid eruption
Non-steroidal anti-inflammatories	Toxic erythema, erythroderma, toxic epidermal necrolysis
Oral contraceptives	Melasma, alopecia, acne, candidiasis
Phenothiazines	Photosensitivity, (Fig.40- 4) pigmentation (Fig.40- 5)
Thiazides	Toxic erythema, photosensitivity, lichenoid eruption, vasculitis

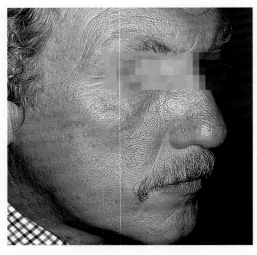

Fig. 40-5 **Pigmentation.** This was due to treatment with amiodarone for a cardiac arrhythmia. An erythematous eruption occurring within 2h of sun exposure is more common.

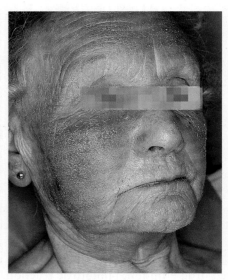

Fig. 40-4 **Photosensitivity.** This was caused by taking a thiazide diuretic, associated with being out of doors on a sunny day.

> *Drug eruptions*
> - Drug reactions may be pharmacological or idiosyncratic, as well as immune mediated.
> - Drugs that commonly cause drug eruptions are antibiotics, e.g.amoxicillin, *ACE inhibitors*, *anticonvulsants*, allopurinol and *non-steroidal anti-inflammatory drugs*.
> - The commonest pattern is a *drug-induced exanthem*, often morbilliform.
> - The most severe involvement is *toxic epidermal necrolysis*, which may be fatal.
> - A drug eruption typically begins within 3 days of starting a drug (if it has been taken before) and clears about 2 weeks after stopping it.
> - Withdrawal of the drug and avoidance of related compounds are necessary.
> - Provocation tests are not recommended because of the possibility of a severe reaction.

Management

Withdrawal of the offending drug usually leads to clearance of the eruption within 2 weeks or so. Simple emollients or topical steroids can help to ease the eruption until it resolves. Antihistamines can be applied to treat mild eruptions while systematic use of steroids may be taken into consideration to treat severe drug eruptions. Patients should be given advice about which drugs they must avoid. Oral challenge testing is not recommended because of the possibility of inducing a severe reaction.

Key words

drug-induced exanthema　发疹型药疹

toxic epidermal necrolysis　中毒性表皮坏死松解症

drug reaction with eosinophilia and systemic symptoms　药物超敏综合征

acute generalized exanthematous pustulosis　急性泛发性发疹性脓疱病

fixed drug eruption　固定型药疹

urticarial eruptions　荨麻疹型药疹

Idiosyncratic　特异体质的

phototoxic reaction　光毒性反应

allergen-specific immunoglobulin (Ig) E tests   抗原
特异性 IgE 试验

patch test   斑贴试验

oral challenge testing   口服激发试验

Review questions

1. What is the commonest type of drug eruption?

2. What is the most severe type of drug eruption?

3. Please give a brief description of management of drug eruption.

(Jinhua Xu)

Chapter 41   Associations with malignancy

Internal malignancy causes a variety of skin changes (Table 41-1). Apart from direct infiltration, the mechanisms of these effects are often poorly understood. Some genetic conditions associated with malignancy include characteristic skin lesions that may arise before or after the cancer (e.g. mucosal lentigines in Peutz-Jeghers syndrome associated with bowel malignancy).

Table 41-1	Cutaneous manifestations of malignancy
Condition associated	**Commonest malignancies**
Almost always	
Acanthosis nigricans	Gastrointestinal tract
Erythema gyratum repens	Lung, breast
Extramammary Paget's disease	Apocrine glands
Necrolytic migratory erythema	Pancreas (alpha cells)
Paget's disease of the nipple	Breast
Skin secondaries	Breast, gastrointestinal, ovary, lung, kidney
Occasionally	
Acquired ichthyosis	Lymphoma (Hodgkin's disease)
Dermatomyositis	Lung, breast, stomach
Erythroderma	T cell lymphoma
Flushing	Carcinoid syndrome
Generalized pruritus	Hodgkin's disease, polycythaemia rubra vera
Hyperpigmentation	Cachectic malignancy
Hypertrichosis	Various tumours
Migratory thrombophlebitis	Pancreas, lung, stomach
Paraneoplastic pemphigus	B cell lymphoma, thymoma
Pyoderma gangrenosum	Leukaemia, myeloma
Tylosis	Oesophagus

Conditions associated with malignancy

The following rare skin eruptions are characteristic and strongly indicate an underlying malignancy:

- acanthosis nigricans
- erythema gyratum repens
- necrolytic migratory erythema
- Paget's disease of the nipple
- extramammary Paget's disease
- skin secondaries.

Acanthosis nigricans

True acanthosis nigricans is uncommon. The flexures and neck typically show epidermal thickening and pigmentation (Fig. 41-1), and the skin is velvety or papillomatous. Warty lesions are seen around the mouth and on the palms and soles. *Benign acquired acanthosis nigricans* is more frequent and describes similar milder changes, seen with obesity or endocrine disorders such as insulin-resistant diabetes or acromegaly. Very rarely, acanthosis nigricans is *inherited* and appears in childhood or at puberty. In the malignancy-associated type, usually found in a middle-aged or elderly patient, the cancer is most commonly of the gastrointestinal tract. Growth factors, released from the tumour or associated with the endocrine disorder, cause the skin changes. The underlying disease must be identified and treated.

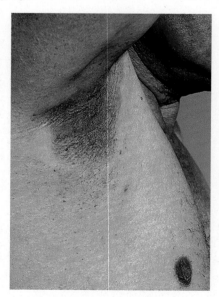

Fig. 41-1   **Acanthosis nigricans.** Pigmented velvety papillomatosis at the axilla and nipples is shown.

Erythema gyratum repens

Erythema gyratum repens is an exceptionally rare pattern of concentric scaly rings of erythema that shift visibly from day to day (Fig. 41-2). The appearance resembles wood grain. An underlying neoplasm, frequently a carcinoma of the lung, is almost invariably detected.

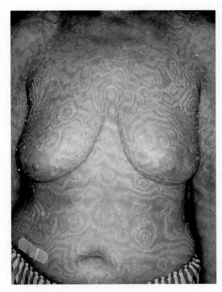

Fig. 41-2   **Erythema gyratum repens.** Note the 'wood grain' pattern.

Necrolytic migratory erythema

Necrolytic migratory erythema is a rare paraneoplastic eruption of serpiginous erythematous plaques, with a migratory eroded edge. It typically starts in the perineum. The eruption indicates a tumour, or occasionally a hyperplasia, of the glucagon-secreting alpha cells of the pancreas (a *glucagonoma*). Weight loss, anaemia, mild diabetes, diarrhoea and glossitis are associated. Liver metastases are often present at diagnosis.

Paget's disease and extramammary Paget's disease

Paget's disease presents as a unilateral eczema-like plaque of the nipple areola and represents the intraepidermal spread of an intraductal breast carcinoma. Extramammary Paget's disease is seen as an eczema-like eruption around the perineum or axilla. It usually results from intraepidermal spread of a ductal apocrine carcinoma. A skin biopsy confirms the diagnosis prior to surgical excision.

Secondary deposits

Cutaneous metastases are not uncommon. They occur late, indicate a poor prognosis and may be the presenting sign of an internal tumour. Skin secondaries are multiple or solitary and appear as firm asymptomatic pink nodules (Fig. 41-3). The scalp, umbilicus and upper trunk are favoured sites. They occur most commonly with tumours of the breast, gastrointestinal tract, ovary and lung, and with malignant melanoma. Leukaemias and lymphomas often show skin involvement. Direct infiltration of the skin causing sclerosis - carcinoma en cuirasse - is sometimes found with carcinoma of the breast (Fig. 41-4). Peau d'orange appearance and carcinoma erysipeloides (well demarcated red patch) and telangiectatic cutaneous metastases patterns are also recognized.

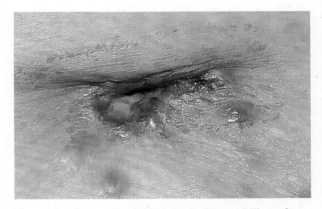

Fig. 41-3   **Secondary deposit at the umbilicus from a carcinoma of the breast.**

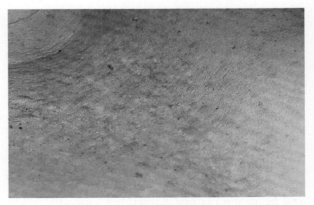

Fig. 41-4   **Carcinoma en cuirasse.** Direct pebbly infiltration of the skin of the chest wall from a carcinoma of the breast.

Conditions occasionally associated with malignancy

Conditions occasionally associated with underlying neoplasia but also seen with benign disease include:

- acquired ichthyosis
- dermatomyositis
- erythroderma
- flushing
- generalized pruritus
- hyperpigmentation
- hypertrichosis
- pyoderma gangrenosum
- superficial thrombophlebitis
- tylosis (keratoderma).

Acquired ichthyosis

Ichthyosis is usually inherited and starts in infancy, but it may be acquired in adult life due to an underlying malignancy (e.g. Hodgkin's disease), essential fatty acid deficiency (e.g. caused by intestinal bypass malabsorption) or drug therapy with nicotinic acid, allopurinol and clofazimine.

Generalized pruritus

Generalized pruritus not associated with an eruption has several causes:

- idiopathic ('senile')
- iron deficiency
- liver disease (cholestasis)
- malignancy, e.g. Hodgkin's disease
- neurological disorders
- polycythaemia
- renal failure (chronic)
- thyroid dysfunction.

Patients with generalized pruritus need careful examination and investigation to exclude liver disease (e.g. biliary obstruction), iron deficiency, polycythaemia, hypothyroidism, hyperthyroidism and renal failure. Pruritus may occur with multiple sclerosis and neurofibromatosis. Sometimes, especially in the elderly, no cause is found, and the itching is labelled *idiopathic*. The commonest malignant causes of pruritus are Hodgkin's disease (one-third of patients with this disease itch) and polycythaemia rubra vera. The aetiology of the itching is poorly understood. Treatment, once any underlying disorder has been dealt with, is symptomatic. Sedative antihistamines, calamine lotion and topical antipruritics (e.g. 0.5% menthol in aqueous cream) are used.

Hyperpigmentation

Malignancy-associated pigmentation may result from ectopic adrenocorticotrophic hormone (ACTH) or melanocyte-stimulating hormone (MSH)-like hormone production by the tumour. It is also seen in patients with malignant cachexia. The axillae, groins and nipples are involved.

Pyoderma gangrenosum

Pyoderma gangrenosum starts as a pustule or inflamed nodule, which breaks down to produce an ulcer with an undermined purplish margin and a surrounding erythema (Fig. 41-5). The ulcer may extend rapidly. Lesions may be multiple. A bacterial gangrene (e.g. necrotizing fasciitis) is sometimes misdiagnosed. Pyoderma gangrenosum often occurs on the trunk or lower limbs. An immune-mediated process is suggested. The following diseases are associated:

- ulcerative colitis, Crohn's disease
- chronic autoimmune liver disease
- rheumatoid arthritis
- Behçet's syndrome

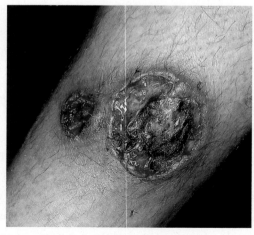

Fig. 41-5 **Pyoderma gangrenosum.** Necrotic ulcers shown on the lower leg.

■ multiple myeloma and monoclonal gammopathy
■ leukaemia (a bullous form is seen).

Treatment is with systemic steroids, ciclosporin or anti-tumour necrosis factor (TNF) monoclonal antibodies. Minocycline helps mild disease. Cases associated with bowel disease can improve as this is controlled.

Superficial thrombophlebitis

Migratory superficial thrombophlebitis, mainly associated with carcinoma of the pancreas or lung, also occurs with Behçet's syndrome.

Associations with malignancy

■ **Acanthosis nigricans**, characterized by pigmentation and epidermal thickening of the flexures, neck, palms and soles, is seen with gastrointestinal cancers.

■ **Benign acanthosis nigricans** is more common and occurs with obesity or endocrine disorders.

■ **Erythema gyratum repens** is a migratory erythema almost invariably associated with a neoplasm.

■ **Paget's disease**, an eczema-like plaque at the nipple, is due to epidermal spread of an intraductal carcinoma. The *extramammary* form comes from an apocrine carcinoma.

■ **Secondary deposits** are not uncommon and may present as single or multiple pink firm nodules, often on the scalp or upper trunk. They occur with tumours of the breast, gastrointestinal tract, ovary and lung and with malignant melanoma.

■ **Acquired ichthyosis** is associated with Hodgkin's disease, fatty acid deficiency (e.g. intestinal bypass malabsorption) and as a side-effect of some drugs.

■ **Generalized pruritus** may occur with malignancy (e.g. Hodgkin's disease), liver disease, renal failure, iron deficiency and thyroid dysfunction.

■ **Pyoderma gangrenosum** is a necrotic ulceration seen with ulcerative colitis, Crohn's disease, rheumatoid arthritis, multiple myeloma or leukaemia.

Web resource

http://emedicine.medscape.com/article/1095113-overview

Key words

acanthosis nigricans　黑棘皮病

erythema gyratum repens　匐行性回状红斑

necrolytic migratory erythema　坏死松解性游走性红斑

Paget's disease of the nipple　乳头湿疹样癌

extramammary Paget's disease　乳房外湿疹样癌

skin secondaries　皮肤转移瘤

malignant melanoma　恶性黑色素瘤

carcinoma erysipeloides　丹毒样癌

acquired ichthyosis　获得性鱼鳞病

dermatomyositis　皮肌炎

erythroderma　红皮病

generalized pruritus　泛发性瘙痒症

pyoderma gangrenosum　坏疽性脓皮病

Review questions

1. What are the six skin eruptions that strongly indicate an underlying malignancy?

2. What are the malignancies often associated to Paget's disease and extramammary Paget's disease?

3. What are the common features of skin sencondaries?

4. What are the causes of generalized pruritus with regard to extracutaneous disorders?

(Liangchun Wang)

Chapter 42   Keratinization and blistering syndromes

Common skin disorders, e.g. atopic eczema or psoriasis, have a genetic component that is often subject to environmental influences. The *genodermatoses* differ in being single gene defects and include keratinization, blistering and neurocutaneous syndromes.

Ichthyoses

The ichthyoses are inherited disorders of keratinization and epidermal differentiation. They are characterized by dry scaly skin and vary from mild and asymptomatic to severe and incompatible with life (Table 42-1). Keratinization is abnormal. Some of the biochemical defects have been identified, e.g. steroid sulphatase is deficient in X-linked ichthyosis.

Clinical presentation

Ichthyosis vulgaris is common and unrecognized if mild. Small branny scales are seen on the extensor aspects of the limbs and the back (Fig. 42-1). The flexures are often spared.

The other types of ichthyosis are uncommon or rare and can usually be identified by their clinical features, onset and inheritance. Autosomal dominant conditions tend to improve with age, whereas recessive ichthyoses may worsen. *Collodion baby* describes a newborn infant with a tight shiny skin that causes feeding problems and ectropion. It is mainly due to non-bullous ichthyosiform erythroderma. *Acquired ichthyosis* usually starts in adulthood.

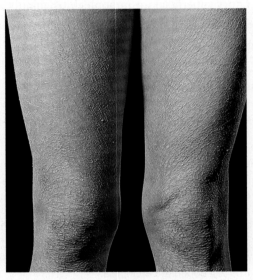

Fig. 42-1   **Ichthyosis vulgaris showing bran-like scaling.**

Management

Emollient ointments, creams and bath additives are essential and adequate for mild ichthyosis. Urea-containing creams (e.g. Aquadrate or Calmurid) and topical retinoids (e.g. tretinoin cream) help, but severe forms may need oral acitretin.

Table 42-1	**A classification of the ichthyoses**	
Disorder	**Inheritance**	**Clinical features**
Ichthyosis vulgaris	Autosomal dominant	Common (1 in 250). Onset 1~4 years. It occurs with atopic eczema. Often mild. Small bran-like scale seen. Flexures spared. Defect in filaggrin, needed for keratin assembly
X-linked ichthyosis	X-linked recessive	1 in 2 000 males. Generalized involvement with large brown scale. Onset in first week of life. Improves in summer. Due to a deficiency of steroid sulphatase
Non-bullous ichthyosiform erythroderma*	Autosomal recessive	Rare (1 in 300 000). At birth may present as collodion baby. Red scaly skin and ectropion may follow. Erythema improves with age
Bullous ichthyosiform erythroderma†	Autosomal dominant	Rare (<1 in 100 000). Redness and blisters occur after birth but fade. Warty rippled hyperkeratosis appears in childhood

*Lamellar ichthyosis is similar but rarer.
†Also called epidermolytic hyperkeratosis.

Keratosis pilaris

Keratosis pilaris is a common, sometimes inherited condition in which multiple small horny follicular plugs affect the upper thigh, upper arm and face (Fig. 42-2). It is occasionally associated with ichthyosis vulgaris. Application of 5% salicylic acid ointment or 10% urea cream lessens, but does not cure, the problem.

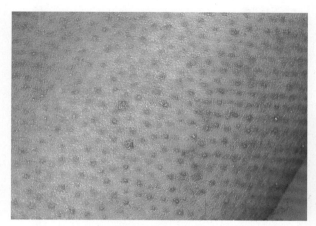

Fig. 42-2   **Keratosis pilaris on the upper arm.**

Epidermolysis bullosa

Epidermolysis bullosa (EB) defines a group of genetically inherited diseases characterized by skin fragility and blistering on minimal trauma. They range from being mild and trivial to being incompatible with life (Table 42-2).

Aetiopathogenesis

Keratin synthesis is defective in simple EB (genes mapped to chromosomes 12 and 17). Collagen VII is abnormal in dystrophic EB (gene sited on chromosome 3). Anchoring fibrils are defective in certain types of EB.

Clinical presentation and management

Simple EB is fairly common and requires avoidance of trauma. The more severe forms (Table 42-2; Fig. 42-3) need to be managed in specialized centres. Avoidance of trauma, supportive measures and the control of infection are important. Treatment with various drugs has given disappointing results. *Acquired EB*, with an onset in adult life, shows trauma-induced blistering and resembles pemphigoid on immunofluorescent studies.

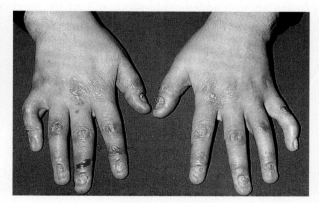

Fig. 42-3   **Epidermolysis bullosa.** The dystrophic dominant type is shown.

Prenatal diagnosis of inherited disorders

DNA-based prenatal diagnosis is now possible for junctional and recessive dystrophic EB, bullous ichthyosiform erythroderma and oculocutaneous albinism. DNA is obtained in the first trimester from chorionic villus samples or amniotic cells. Mid-second trimester fetal skin biopsy is still used for dis-

Table 42-2 **The main types of epidermolysis bullosa (EB)**		
Disease	**Inheritance**	**Clinical features**
Simple EB	Autosomal dominant	Commonest type. Often mild and limited to hands and feet. Blisters caused by friction. Nails and mouth unaffected
Junctional EB	Autosomal recessive	Rare and often lethal. At birth, large erosions seen around mouth and anus. Slow to heal. No effective treatment
Dystrophic EB	Autosomal dominant	Hands, knees and elbows are affected. Scarring with milia is found. Deformity of the nails may occur
Dystrophic EB	Autosomal recessive	Starts in infancy. Severe blistering results in fusion of fingers and toes, with mucosal lesions and oesophageal stricture

eases where the gene is unknown but biopsy changes are specific.

Hailey-Hailey disease

Hailey-Hailey disease, also known as familial benign chronic pemphigus, is a rare autosomal dominant cutaneous disorder characterized by erythema, vesicles, and erosions involving the body folds, particularly the groin and axillary regions. Other sites of the body, such as the neck, perianal, and submammary regions, may likewise be affected. Hailey-Hailey disease is caused by heterozygous mutation in the *ATP2C1* gene on chromosome 3q22. Topical corticosteroids with added antibiotics could get the good treatment. Carbon dioxide laser vaporization is also effective.

> *Inherited keratinization and blistering disorders*
> - **The ichthyoses** are inherited disorders of keratinization. The skin is dry and scaly. Emollient therapy is helpful. Certain ichthyoses may present at birth as a collodion baby.
> - **Keratosis pilaris** is a common condition in which horny follicular plugs are seen on the limbs and face. Treatment is difficult; emollients may help.
> - **Epidermolysis bullosa** describes inherited bullous diseases ranging from mild blistering induced by ill-fitting shoes to severe and lethal blistering present at birth.
> - **Hailey-Hailey disease** is a autosomal dominant skin disease characterized by erythema, vesicles, and erosions main involving the axillary regions

Web resource

http://www.ncbi.nlm.nih.gov/sites/entrez?db=omim&TabCmd=Limits

Key words

ichthyosis　鱼鳞病

keratosis pilaris　毛发角化病

epidermolysis bullosa　大疱性表皮松解症

familial benign chronic pemphigus　家族性慢性良性天疱疮

Review questions

1. Please describe the clinical features of ichthyosis vulgaris.
2. What are reasons for the different types of inherited epidermolysis bullosa?

(Min Gao)

Chapter 43   Neurocutaneous disorders and other syndromes

Certain inherited skin disorders also have significant involvement of internal organs. The neurocutaneous disorders, the inherited diseases of connective tissue and the premature ageing syndromes are included.

Neurofibromatosis

von Recklinghausen's neurofibromatosis (NF1) is relatively common, affecting about 1 in 3000 births. Café-au-lait spots, cutaneous neurofibromas and other bony or neurological abnormalities characterize NF1. The disease shows autosomal dominant inheritance, although 50% of cases are new mutations.

Aetiopathogenesis

The *NF1* gene is a tumour suppressor gene, mapped to chromosome 17. This finding offers the prospect of devising a prenatal DNA screening test.

Clinical presentation

The two main cutaneous features are:
- *Café-au-lait spots*: round or oval coffee-coloured macules, due to increased melanin pigment. They often appear in the first year of life. One or two café-au-lait spots are seen in 10% of normal people but, in neurofibromatosis, six or more are usually present. Freckling of the axilla is also found (Fig. 43-1).
- *Dermal neurofibromas*: small nodules that appear during childhood and increase in number at the time of puberty (Fig. 43-2). Their number varies from a few to several hundred.

A proportion of patients with NF1 have short stature and macrocephaly. Rare variants of the disease are occasionally seen. The commonest is NF2 (*central neurofibromatosis*) in which patients have bilateral acoustic neuromas but few, if any, café-au-lait spots

or dermal nodules. NF2 also shows autosomal dominant inheritance. The *NF2* gene is on chromosome 22.

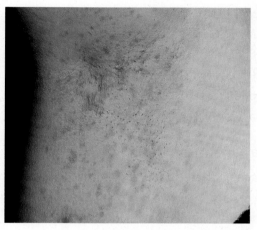

Fig. 43-1   **Neurofibromatosis showing axillary freckling.**

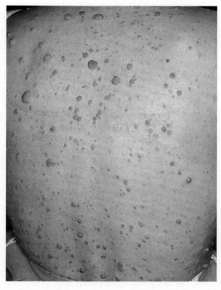

Fig. 43-2   **Neurofibromatosis.** Multiple neurofibromas are present on the back.

Complications

Complications develop in many cases and include the following:
- *Plexiform neurofibromas* are larger than their dermal

counterparts and measure up to several centimetres in size. They are associated with pigmentation and hypertrophy of the overlying skin or underlying bone, and present a cosmetic problem.

- *Benign tumours of the nervous system* may develop. These include optic gliomas, acoustic neuromas and spinal neurofibromas that arise from nerve roots of the spinal cord.
- *Sarcomatous change* in a neurofibroma, typically non-cutaneous, occurs in 1.5%~15% of cases.
- *Kyphoscoliosis* (in 2%) or bowing of the tibia and fibula may occur.
- *Other problems* include iris hamartomas (Lisch nodules), hypertension, epilepsy and learning difficulties.

Management

Once the diagnosis has been made, genetic counselling and the exclusion of any complicating factors are important. Troublesome nodules can be excised, and larger disfiguring neurofibromas removed by plastic surgery. Patients are often helped by contact with a patient support group.

Tuberous sclerosis complex

Tuberous sclerosis complex is an autosomal dominant condition of variable expression with an incidence of 1 in 10 000. About 60%~70% of patients have new mutations. Hamartomas occur in several organs. The abnormal genes have been mapped to chromosomes 9 and 16.

Clinical manifestations

The features may not appear until puberty. Patients typically show the following:

- *Adenoma sebaceum*: red-brown angiofibromatous papules that are usually found around the nose (Fig. 43-3). They appear in childhood.
- *Periungual fibromas*: pink fibrous projections are seen under the nail folds (Fig. 43-4).
- *Shagreen patches*: connective tissue naevi, soft, yellowish with a cobblestone surface, are found on the lumbosacral region.

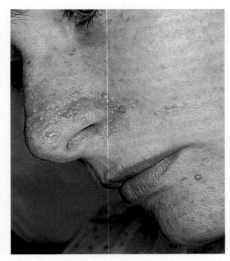

Fig. 43-3 **Tuberous sclerosis.** Angiofibromas are seen at the sides of the nose.

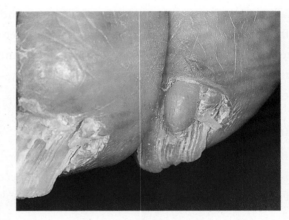

Fig. 43-4 **Tuberous sclerosis showing periungual fibromas.**

- *Ash-leaf macules*: small (1~3cm long) white oval macules, sometimes present at birth, and best seen with a Wood's light.
- *Neurological involvement*: learning difficulties and epilepsy affect 60%~70% of cases. Intracranial calcification is seen.
- *Other features*: retinal phacomas, cardiac rhabdomyomas and renal tumours are found.

Management

An affected individual should have a full clinical examination, often with radiographs and magnetic resonance imaging (MRI) of the head. Children are screened for ash-leaf macules using a Wood's light. The angiofibromas may be improved by hyfrecation or laser, but tend to recur. Genetic counselling is given once the diagnosis is made. The support group is helpful.

Neurocutaneous disorders and other syndromes
- **NF1 neurofibromatosis** is a relatively common autosomal dominant condition characterized by café-au-lait spots, dermal neurofibromas and often skeletal or neurological anomalies. The abnormal gene is on chromosome 17.
- **Tuberous sclerosis complex** is a not infrequent autosomal dominant disorder with prominent skin signs (e.g. facial angiofibromas and periungual fibromas), neurological problems (mental retardation and epilepsy) and ocular, cardiac and renal tumours.

Web resource

http://www.pxe.org.uk/
http://www.nhs.uk/conditions/neurofibromatosis/Pages/Introduction.aspx

Key words

neurofibromatosis　神经纤维瘤病
Café-au-lait spot　咖啡牛奶色(素)斑
hamartoma　错构瘤
kyphoscoliosis　脊柱后凸侧弯
tuberous sclerosis complex　结节性硬化症
adenoma sebaceum　皮脂腺腺瘤
periungual fibroma　甲周纤维瘤

Review questions

1. Please describe the clinical features of NF1.
2. Please describe the clinical features of tuberous sclerosis complex.

(Min Gao)

Chapter 44   Benign tumours

Skin tumours are common, and their incidence is rising in western countries. The treatment of skin tumours makes up a large part of current dermatological practice. Many skin tumours are benign, and these are described in this section. Viral warts, actinic keratoses and naevi are mentioned elsewhere.

Benign epidermal tumours

Seborrhoeic wart (basal cell papilloma)

A seborrhoeic wart (seborrhoeic keratosis) is a common, usually pigmented, benign tumour consisting of a proliferation of basal keratinocytes (Fig. 44-1). The cause is unknown, although they may be 'naevoid'. Seborrhoea is not a feature.

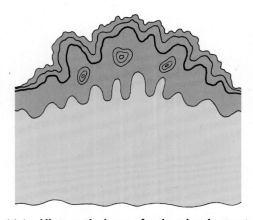

Fig. 44-1 **Histopathology of seborrhoeic wart.** The illustration shows a hyperkeratotic epidermis, thickened by basal cell proliferation, with keratin cysts.

Clinical presentation

Seborrhoeic warts have the following features:
- often multiple (Fig. 44-2), sometimes solitary
- affect the elderly or middle-aged
- mostly found on the trunk and face
- generally round or oval in shape
- start as small papules or plaques, often lightly pigmented or brown

- become darkly pigmented warty nodules, 1~6cm in diameter
- have a 'stuck-on' appearance, with keratin plugs and well-defined edges.

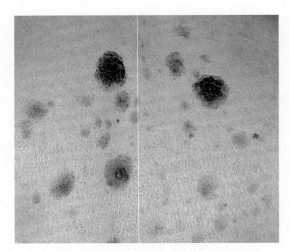

Fig. 44-2 **Seborrhoeic warts on the trunk, with a few small Campbell-de-Morgan spots.**

Differential diagnosis

The diagnosis is usually obvious from the physical findings and multiplicity of the lesions. Occasionally, a seborrhoeic wart can resemble an actinic keratosis, melanocytic naevus, pigmented basal cell carcinoma or malignant melanoma. Dermatoscopy is helpful in diagnosis.

Management

Multiple lesions can be adequately dealt with using liquid nitrogen cryotherapy. Thicker seborrhoeic warts are best treated by curettage or shave biopsy, with cautery or hyfrecation. If there is diagnostic doubt they can be excised. Histological examination is advised in all cases.

Skin tags (soft fibroma)

Skin tags are pedunculated benign fibroepithelial polyps, a few millimetres in length. They are common, mainly seen in the elderly or middle-aged, and show a predilection for the neck, axillae, groin and eyelids (Fig. 44-3). The cause is unknown, but they are often found in obese individuals. Occasionally, skin tags are confused with small melanocytic naevi or seborrhoeic warts. The treatment, usually for cosmetic reasons, is by snipping the stalk with scissors or cutting through it with a hyfrecator (under local anaesthesia if necessary).

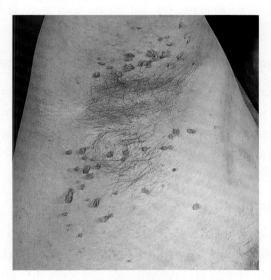

Fig. 44-3   **Skin tags in the axilla.**

Epidermal (epidermoid) cyst

Epidermal cysts, usually seen on the scalp, face or trunk, are sometimes incorrectly called sebaceous cysts. They are keratin filled and derived from the epidermis or, in the case of the related pilar cyst, the outer root sheath of the hair follicle. The cysts are firm, skin coloured, mobile and normally 1~3cm in diameter. Bacterial infection is a complication. Excision is curative.

Milium

Milia are mostly seen on the face, where they typically appear as small white keratin cysts (1~2mm in size) around the eyelids and on the upper cheeks. They are often seen in children, but may appear at any age. Occasionally, milia may develop as part of healing after a subepidermal blister, e.g. with porphyria cutanea tarda. Milial cysts can normally be extracted using a sterile needle.

Benign dermal tumours

Dermatofibroma (fibrous histiocytoma)

Dermatofibromas are common dermal nodules, and are usually asymptomatic. Histologically, they show a proliferation of histiocytes and fibroblasts, with dermal fibrosis and sometimes epidermal hyperplasia. They possibly represent a reaction pattern to an insect bite or other trauma, although often no such history is obtained.

Clinical presentation

Dermatofibromas are usually seen in young adults, most commonly women, and mainly occur on the lower legs. They are firm, dermal nodules 5~10mm in diameter and may be pigmented (Fig. 44-4). They enlarge slowly, if at all.

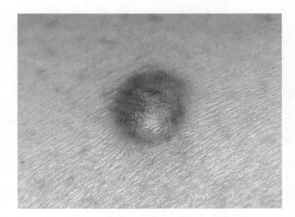

Fig. 44-4   **Dermatofibroma on the lower leg.**

Management

A pigmented dermatofibroma may be confused with a melanocytic naevus or a malignant melanoma. Excision of symptomatic or diagnostically doubtful lesions is recommended.

Pyogenic granuloma

A pyogenic granuloma is a rapidly developing bright red or blood-crusted nodule. It is neither pyogenic nor granulomatous, but is an acquired haemangioma.

Clinical presentation

A pyogenic granuloma typically:

■ develops at a site of trauma, e.g. a prick from a thorn

■ presents as a bright red, sometimes pedunculated, nodule 5-10mm in diameter that bleeds easily (Fig. 44-5)

■ enlarges rapidly over 2~3 weeks

■ is seen on a finger (also on lip, face and foot)

■ occurs in young adults or children.

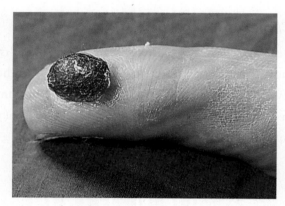

Fig. 44-5   **Pyogenic granuloma on the finger.**

Management

Curettage or cautery, or excision, is needed. Not infrequently, a pyogenic granuloma may recur after incomplete curettage.

Keloid

A keloid is an excessive proliferation of connective tissue in response to skin trauma and differs from a hypertrophic scar because it extends beyond the limit of the original injury. Keloids show the following characteristics:

■ Present as protuberant and firm smooth nodules or plaques (Fig. 44-6).

■ Occur mainly over the upper back, neck, chest and ear lobes.

■ Develop more commonly in black Africans.

■ Have their highest incidence in the second to fourth decades.

Treatment is with a topical silicone sheet or gel, or steroid injection.

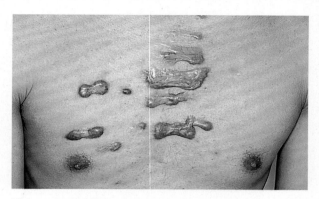

Fig. 44-6   **Keloids.** The nodules are seen on the chest of a patient with a history of acne.

Campbell-de-Morgan spot (cherry angioma)

Campbell-de-Morgan spots are benign capillary proliferations, commonly seen as small bright-red papules on the trunk in elderly or middle-aged patients (Fig. 44-2). If necessary, they can be removed by hyfrecation or cautery.

Tumours of the skin appendages

Tumours of the skin appendages, i.e. of the eccrine and apocrine sweat ducts, hair follicles and sebaceous glands, are relatively rare. Clinically, they often present as rather non-specific cutaneous nodules, and they are difficult to diagnose without histology following excision. Occasionally, these tumours are malignant.

Lipoma

Lipomas are benign tumours of fat, and present as soft masses in the subcutaneous tissue. They are often multiple and are mostly found on the trunk, neck and upper extremities. Sometimes they are painful. Removal is rarely needed.

Chondrodermatitis nodularis

Chondrodermatitis nodularis is not a neoplasm, but presents as a painful small nodule on the upper rim of the helix of the pinna, usually in elderly men. It is due to inflammation in the cartilage that may be a response to degenerate dermal collagen induced by pressure or chronic sun exposure. They are often confused with basal cell carcinomas. Excision is curative.

Benign tumours

Lesion	Age at onset	Main features
Epidermal		
Viral wart	Childhood mainly	Usually on hands or feet
Actinic keratosis	Old age	Sun-exposed areas
Seborrhoeic wart	Old/middle age	Keratosis, often on trunk or face
Milia	Childhood	White cysts, often on face
Epidermal cyst	After childhood	Mostly on face or scalp
Skin tags	Middle/old age	Seen on neck, axillae and groin
Dermal		
Dermatofibroma	Young adult, F > M	Nodule, often on leg
Melanocytic naevus	Teens/young adult	Brown macule or papule
Cherry angioma	Old/middle age	Small red papule on trunk
Pyogenic granuloma	Child/young adult	Red nodule, often on finger
Keloid	Second-fourth decades	Chest/neck, affects black Africans
Lipoma	Any age	Soft tumour on trunk or limbs
Chondrodermatitis nodularis	Old/middle age	Nodule on upper pinna, M > F

Web resource

http://www.aafp.org/afp/2003/0215/p729.html

Key words

wart   疣

seborrhoeic wart/seborrhoeic keratosis   老年疣 /
    脂溢性角化病

granuloma   肉芽肿

skin tag   皮赘

dermatofibroma   皮肤纤维瘤

keloid   瘢痕疙瘩

angioma   血管瘤

lipoma   脂肪瘤

skin appendages   皮肤附属器

cautery/hyfrecation   烧灼治疗

cryotherapy   冷冻治疗

Review questions

1. What is the difference between viral warts and seborrheic warts?
2. How to distinguish keloid from common scar?
3. Is there any relationship between keloid and dermatofibroma?

(Zhiqi Song)

Chapter 45   Naevi

A naevus is a benign proliferation of one or more of the normal constituent cells of the skin. Naevi may be present at birth or may develop later. The commonest naevi are those containing benign collections of melanocytic naevus cells, but other types of naevi are found (Table 45-1).

Table 45-1	A classification of naevi
Group	**Example**
Melanocytic	Congenital
	Junctional
	Intradermal
	Compound
	Spitz
	Blue
	Halo
	Becker's
	Dysplastic
Vascular	Salmon patch
	Port wine stain
	Strawberry
	Cavernous haemangioma
Epidermal	Warty naevus
Connective tissue	Tuberous sclerosis

Melanocytic naevi

Melanocytic naevi ('moles') are common. They are present in most Caucasoids but are less prevalent in mongoloids and black Africans.

Aetiopathogenesis and pathology

The naevus cells in melanocytic naevi are thought to be derived from melanocytes that migrate to the epidermis from the neural crest during embryonic development. The reason for the development of naevi is unknown, but there seems to be an inherited trait in many families.

The position of the naevus cells within the dermis determines the type of naevus (Fig. 45-1). The junctional type has clusters of naevus cells at the dermo-epidermal junction, the intradermal type has nests of naevus cells in the dermis and the compound naevus shows both components.

Naevus cells produce melanin and, if the pigment is deep in the dermis, an optical effect can give the lesion a blue colour, as in a blue naevus.

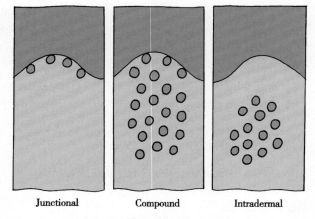

Junctional   Compound   Intradermal

Fig. 45-1 **Types of melanocytic naevus.** The site of the naevus cells, either at the dermoepidermal junction or in the dermis, or at both places, determines the type of melanocytic naevus.

Clinical presentation

A congenital naevus, that is one present at or soon after birth, is seen in about 1%~3% of infants, but most naevi develop during childhood or adolescence. Their number reaches a peak in the third decade, and they tend to become less numerous thereafter. However, it is not unusual to see a few new naevi appear after the third decade, especially if provoked by excessive sun exposure or pregnancy. The average young white adult has between 20 and 50 melanocytic naevi. Dermoscopy is helpful in assessment. The clinical features of different types of naevus are as follows:

- *Congenital naevi.* Present at or shortly after birth, they are usually more than 1cm in size, vary in colour from light brown to black and often become protuberant and hairy. They can be disfiguring, as in the rare bathing trunk naevus, and carry a lifetime risk of up to 5% for the development of malignant melanoma.

- *Junctional naevi.* These are flat macules, varying in size from 2 to 10mm and in colour from light to dark brown (Fig. 45-2). They are usually round or oval in shape and have a predilection for the palms, soles and genitalia.

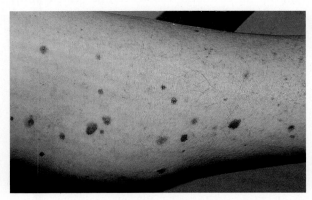

Fig. 45-2   **Multiple junctional (and compound) naevi on the lower leg.**

- *Intradermal naevi.* The intradermal naevus is a dome-shaped papule or nodule that may be skin coloured or pigmented, and is most often seen on the face or neck.
- *Compound naevi.* Compound naevi are usually less than 10mm in diameter, have a smooth surface and vary in their degree of pigmentation (Fig. 45-3). Larger lesions may develop a warty or cerebriform appearance. They may occur anywhere on the skin surface.

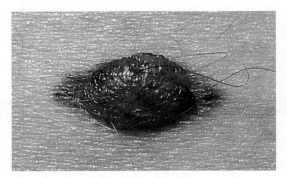

Fig. 45-3   **A compound melanocytic naevus.**

- *Spitz naevi.* A Spitz naevus is a firm, reddish-brown, rounded nodule seen typically on the face or leg of a child. The initial growth may be rapid. Histologically, the naevus cells are proliferative, and the dermal blood vessels are dilated. Differentiation from malignant melanoma is important.
- *Blue naevi.* This variant, so-called because of its steely-blue colour, is usually solitary and is most common on the extremities, particularly the hands and feet.
- *Halo naevi.* Halo (or Sutton's) naevi are mainly seen on the trunk in children or adolescents and represent the destruction, by the body's immune system, of naevus cells in a naevus. A white halo of depigmentation surrounds the pre-existing naevus that subsequently involutes (Fig. 45-4). This may be due to antimelanocyte autoimmune attack. There is an association with vitiligo. Multiple halo naevi often appear simultaneously.

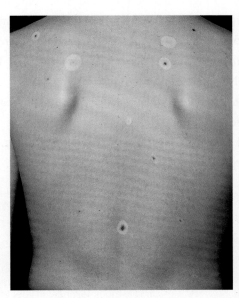

Fig. 45-4   **Multiple halo naevi on the back of an adolescent.**

- *Becker's naevi.* This rare variant usually develops in adolescent males as a unilateral lesion on the upper back or chest (Fig. 45-5). Hyperpigmented at first, it later becomes hairy and is prone to acne. It may represent mosaicism.
- *Dysplastic naevi.* Dysplastic (atypical) naevi show some irregularity in outline and in pigmentation.

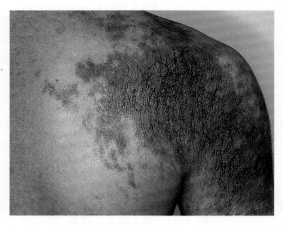

Fig. 45-5 **A Becker's naevus on the shoulder of a young man.**

Management

Over recent years, publicity in the media and in public health campaigns has promoted the early diagnosis of malignant melanoma. This has led to a greater public awareness about the significance of change in pigmented lesions, and many patients are now referred because of concern about their 'moles'. Any change merits serious attention. The differential diagnosis of melanocytic naevi is shown in Table 45-2. Naevi are excised because of:

- *concern about malignancy*, e.g. recent increase in size or itching
- *an increased risk of malignant change*, e.g. in a large congenital naevus

Table 45-2 **Differential diagnosis of melanocytic naevi**	
Lesion	**Distinguishing features**
Freckle	Tan-coloured macules on sun-exposed sites
Lentigine	Usually multiple, onset in later life
Seborrhoeic wart	Stuck-on appearance, warty lesions, may show keratin plugs, but easily confused
Haemangioma	Vascular but may show pigmentation
Dermatofibroma	On legs, elevated nodule, firm and pigmented
Pigmented basal cell carcinoma	Often on face, pearly edge, increase in size, can ulcerate, other photo-damage may coexist
Malignant mela-noma	Variable colour and outline, may have increased in size, be inflamed, bleed or be itchy

- *cosmetic reasons*, e.g. ugly naevi, usually on the face or neck
- *repeated inflammation*, e.g. bacterial folliculitis, often in hairy facial naevi
- *recurrent trauma*, e.g. naevi on the back that catch on bra straps.

All excised naevi should be sent for histology. Some clearly benign protuberant naevi that require removal for cosmetic reasons can be dealt with by shave biopsy.

Epidermal naevi

Epidermal naevi are usually present at birth or develop in early childhood. They are warty, often pigmented and frequently linear (Fig. 45-6). Most are a few centimetres long, but they can be much larger and involve the length of a limb or the side of the trunk. They can be excised, but recurrence is common. A variant on the scalp, *naevus sebaceus*, carries a risk of malignant transformation and should be excised.

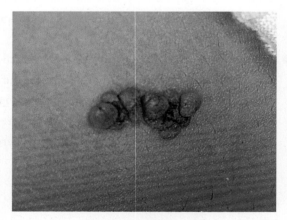

Fig. 45-6 **An epidermal naevus on the thigh.**

Connective tissue naevi

Connective tissue naevi are rare. They appear as smooth, skin-coloured papules or plaques and may be multiple. Coarse collagen bundles are seen in the dermis on histology. An example is the collagen-containing cobblestone naevus (shagreen patch) seen in tuberous sclerosis.

Naevi

- **Melanocytic naevi** are very common, usually multiple, pigmented and benign. They appear during childhood or adolescence. Young white adults have 20~50. Variants include:
  - *congenital naevi*: present at birth, may be protuberant or hairy and have a small risk of malignant change
  - *junctional naevi*: flat macules, often round or oval. Typically found on soles, palms or genitalia
  - *intradermal naevi*: dome-shaped, usually skin-coloured papules. Typically seen on the face
  - *compound naevi*: pigmented nodules or papules, sometimes warty or hairy. Histology shows junctional and dermal components
  - *Spitz naevi*: firm reddish-brown nodules typically seen on the face or legs in children
  - *blue naevi*: steely-blue in colour due to melanin in the deep dermis. They are mainly solitary and found on the extremities
  - *halo naevi*: show depigmentation where a naevus has involuted due to autoimmune attack. Mostly seen on the trunk
  - *Becker's naevi*: pigmented hairy lesions on the upper back or chest, usually in males and appearing in adolescence.
- **Epidermal naevi** are warty, pigmented and often linear. Usually small, they are sometimes extensive. A scalp variant, *naevus sebaceus*, should be excised as it has malignant potential.
- **Connective tissue naevi** are skin-coloured papules composed of coarse collagen in the dermis. They can occur as cobblestone naevi (shagreen patches) in tuberous sclerosis.

Web resource

http://emedicine.medscape.com/article/1058445-overview

Key words

naevus 痣
melanocytic naevus 黑素细胞痣
congenital naevus 先天痣
junctional naevus 交界痣
intradermal naevus 皮内痣
compound naevus 复合痣
blue naevus 蓝痣
halo naevus 晕痣
dysplastic naevus 发育不良痣
epidermal naevus 表皮痣
connective tissue naevus 结缔组织痣

Review questions

1. What's the classification of naevi?
2. What are the main types of melanocytic naevi?
3. Under what situation should the naevi be excised?

(Zhiqi Song)

Chapter 46   Skin cancer - Basal cell carcinoma

Malignant skin tumours are among the most common of all cancers. They are more frequent in light-skinned races, and ultraviolet (UV) radiation seems to be involved in their aetiology. The incidence of *non-melanoma skin cancer* in Caucasoids in the USA was recently estimated at 230 per 100 000 per year, compared with 3 per 100 000 for African Americans. The majority of malignant skin tumours (Table 46-1) are epidermal in origin and are either basal cell or squamous cell carcinomas or malignant melanomas. Premalignant epidermal conditions are common, but dermal malignancies are comparatively rare.

Table 46-1 **A classification of malignant skin tumours and premalignant conditions**		
Cell origin	Premalignant condition	Malignant tumour
Keratinocyte	Actinic keratosis, *in situ* squamous cell carcinoma	Basal cell carcinoma Squamous cell carcinoma
Melanocyte	Dysplastic naevus	Malignant melanoma
Fibroblast		Dermatofibrosarcoma
Lymphocyte		Lymphoma
Endothelium		Kaposi's sarcoma
Non-cutaneous		Secondary

Basal cell carcinoma

Basal cell carcinomas (BCCs, rodent ulcers) are the commonest form of skin cancer and are typically seen on the face in elderly or middle-aged subjects. Although there is strong epidemiological evidence for the role of UV radiation in the pathogenesis of BCCs, the tumours do not distribute to the most sun-exposed sites and BCCs of the dorsum of the hand, forearm and lip are uncommon. They arise from the basal keratinocytes of the epidermis, are locally invasive, but very rarely metastasize.

Aetiopathogenesis

Malignant transformation of basal cells may be induced by:
- prolonged UV exposure (and acute sunburn)
- immunosuppression (e.g. renal transplant recipients)
- arsenic ingestion, e.g. in 'tonics' or drinking water
- X-rays and other ionizing radiation
- chronic scarring, e.g. burns or vaccination scars
- genetic predisposition, e.g. basal cell naevus syndrome and xeroderma pigmentosum.

Basal cell carcinomas are most common in Caucasoids with a fair 'celtic' skin who live near the equator, and are seen more in males than in females. In the UK, they mainly occur in those over the age of 40 years, although, in Australia, they may be seen in the third decade.

Pathology

The tumour is classically composed of uniform basophilic cells, in well-defined islands, that invade the dermis from the epidermis as buds, lobules or strands (Fig. 46-1).

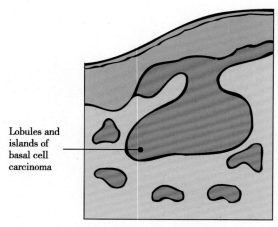

Lobules and islands of basal cell carcinoma

Fig. 46-1 **The histological structure of a basal cell carcinoma.**

Clinical presentation

Basal cell carcinomas occur mainly on light-exposed sites, commonly around the nose, the inner canthus of the eyelids and the temple. They grow slowly but relentlessly, are locally invasive and may destroy cartilage, bone and soft tissue structures. A lesion has often been present for 2 years or more before the patient seeks advice. Often more than one tumour is evident. There are four main types of basal cell carcinoma, all of which may occasionally be pigmented:

- *Nodular*. This is the commonest type of lesion and usually starts as a small, skin-coloured papule that shows fine telangiectasia and a glistening pearly edge (Fig. 46-2). Central necrosis often occurs and leaves a small ulcer with an adherent crust. The lesions are mostly less than 1cm in diameter, but grow larger if present for several years. Clinically, they usually present as a thickened plaque rather than a tumour and, although firm to palpation, this may be difficult to establish in smaller lesions. Nodular BCCs often have slightly raised margins with a central depression. Superficial branching telangiectasia are characteristic and are seen on dermoscopy as 'arborizing' (Fig. 46-3). Stretching the skin between two fingers will often accentuate the margins giving them a pale white 'pearly' colour.
- *Cystic*. These become tense and translucent and show cystic spaces on histology.
- *Multicentric*. Superficial tumours, often multiple, plaque-like and several centimetres in diameter, are sometimes seen especially on the trunk (Fig. 46-4). They have a rim-like edge and are frequently lightly pigmented.
- *Morphoeic*. This scarring (cicatricial) variant, most common on the face, often shows a white or yellow morphoea-like plaque that may be centrally depressed (Fig. 46-5).

Differential diagnosis

The differential diagnosis depends on the type, pigmentation and location of the basal cell carcinoma:

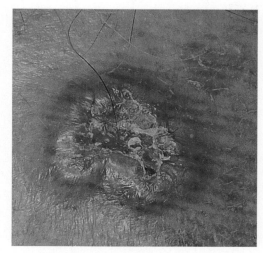

Fig. 46-2　**Basal cell carcinoma.** The lesion shows the typical pearly edge, telangiectasia and central crusting.

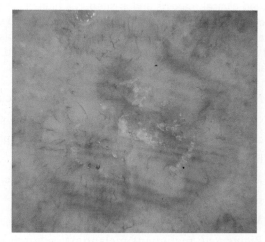

Fig. 46-3　**Dermsocopic view of basal cell carcinoma.** Note the arborizing telangiectasia.

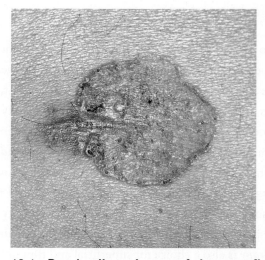

Fig. 46-4　**Basal cell carcinoma of the superficial multifocal type.** This was located on the trunk. A biopsy (scar visible) confirmed the diagnosis.

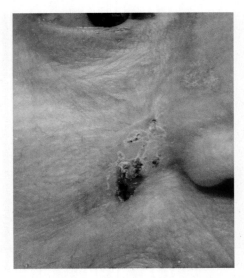

Fig. 46-5 **Basal cell carcinoma of the right cheek in an immunosuppressed patient**. This BCC has poorly defined clinical margins and is sited in a high-risk area. Discussion of planned management with a multidisciplinary team including a dermatological surgeon, plastic and maxillofacial surgeon and radiotherapist would be ideal.

- *Nodular/cystic*: intradermal naevus, molluscum contagiosum, keratoacanthoma, squamous cell carcinoma, sebaceous hyperplasia (a benign proliferation of sebaceous glands).
- *Multicentric*: discoid eczema, psoriatic plaque, *in situ* squamous cell carcinoma.
- *Morphoeic*: morphoea, scar.
- *Pigmented*: malignant melanoma, seborrhoeic wart, compound naevus.

Management

The most appropriate treatment for any one tumour depends on its size, site, type and the patient's age. If possible, complete *excision* is the best treatment, as this allows a histological check on the adequacy of removal. If excision is difficult or not possible, incisional biopsy (to confirm the diagnosis) and *radiotherapy* are suitable for those aged 60 years and over. Large tumours around the eye (Fig. 46-6) and the nasolabial fold, especially if of the morphoeic type, are best managed by surgical excision. *Photodynamic therapy* is also a choice for superficial and thin nodular BCC (thickness <2mm), especially for multiple or inoperable lesions. *Mohs' micrographic surgery* may

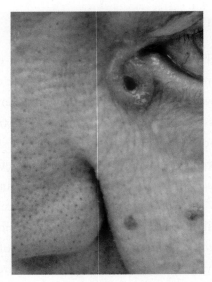

Fig. 46-6 **Basal cell carcinoma of the lower lid**. These lesions require careful surgical management to protect the lacrimal anatomy and prevent scar induced retraction of the eyelid margin.

be employed, as the margins of these tumours are often difficult to determine and may be extensive. *Curettage and cautery* is sometimes used for lesions on the trunk or upper extremities. *Cryosurgery* or topical *imiquimod* are acceptable modalities for multiple, superficial lesions, e.g. on the trunk.

The recurrence rate is about 5% at 5 years for most methods of treatment. Follow-up is particularly important if there is concern about the adequacy of treatment.

Basal cell carcinoma
- **Basal cell carcinoma** (rodent ulcer) is a common tumour often seen on the face of elderly or middle-aged patients who may have had excessive sun exposure. It:
  - is locally invasive but almost never metastasizes
  - is best removed by surgical excision with an adequate margin
  - can be treated by radiotherapy, by curettage and cautery, using cryosurgery or with topical imiquimod in certain biopsy-proven tumours.
- **Basal cell carcinomas with a worse prognosis** (high risk) include:
  - large size (>2cm)
  - central face location: eyes, nose, lips, ears
  - poorly defined clinical margins
  - histological features: morphoeic subtype, perineural or perivascular involvement
  - host immunosuppression
  - recurrence from previous failure of treatment.

Key words

basal cell carcinoma　基底细胞癌
radiotherapy　放射治疗
photodynamic therapy　光动力学治疗
Mohs' micrographic surgery　莫氏显微手术
cryosurgery　冷冻术

Review questions

1. Where is the most common area affected by BCC?
2. What are the common treatment methods for BCC?

(Xiuli Wang)

Chapter 47   Skin cancer - Squamous cell carcinoma

Squamous cell carcinoma (SCC) is a heterogeneous disease comprising clinically distinct but histologically similar entities with differing risk factors implicated in their aetiopathogenesis.

Aetiopathogenesis

Squamous cell carcinoma is derived from moderately well-differentiated keratinocytes. Ultraviolet (UV) radiation is clearly the strongest predisposing risk factor for this condition. The evidence for this is extensive and includes: a direct correlation between average annual UV radiation and risk of SCC; increased incidence with proximity to the equator; high incidence in albinos versus non-albinos in tropical climates; and an association with the development of features of photoageing such as wrinkles. The increased incidence of SCC in the last 25 years parallels an increased exposure to UVA due to both UVB protective sunscreens, which prevent sunburn but prolong exposure to UVA, and also the increased use of sunbeds.

Predisposing factors include:

- chronic actinic damage, accumulating over a lifetime of sun exposure ; psoralen with ultraviolet A (PUVA) treatment can predispose
- immunosuppression, e.g. in renal transplant patients
- X-rays or other ionizing radiation; radiant heat (e.g. from a fire; see erythema ab igne)
- chronic ulceration and scarring (e.g. a burn, lupus vulgaris or discoid lupus erythematosus, genetic blistering diseases)
- smoking pipes and cigars (relevant for lip lesions)
- industrial carcinogens (e.g. coal tars, oils)
- human papilloma (wart) virus
- genetic factors (e.g. albinos, xeroderma pigmentosum)

Pathology

The malignant keratinocytes, which retain the ability to produce keratin, destroy the dermoepidermal junction and invade the dermis in an irregular manner (Fig. 47-1).

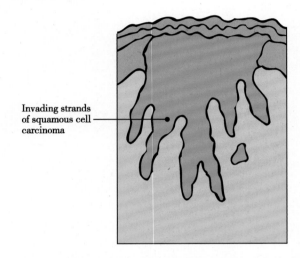

Invading strands of squamous cell carcinoma

Fig. 47-1 **The histological structure of a squamous cell carcinoma.**

Bowen's disease (*in situ* squamous cell carcinoma)

Bowen's disease is common and typically occurs on the lower leg in elderly women. The lesions are solitary or multiple. Previous exposure to arsenicals predisposes to the condition.

Pink or lightly pigmented scaly plaques, up to several centimetres in size, are found on the lower leg or trunk (Fig. 47-2). Transformation into invasive squamous cell carcinoma is infrequent. Bowen's disease may resemble discoid eczema, psoriasis or superficial basal cell carcinoma. Histologically, the epidermis is thickened and the keratinocytes are atypical, but not invasive. Small biopsy samples may not be representative of the entire lesion and if there is clinical doubt then larger or excisional biopsies should be undertaken.

Bowen's disease is treated by cryotherapy, curettage, excision, topical 5-fluorouracil or imiquimod, or photodynamic therapy.

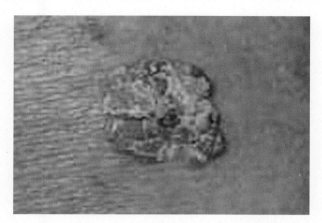

Fig. 47-2 **In situ squamous cell carcinoma on the lower leg.**

Keratoacanthoma

A keratoacanthoma is a rapidly growing tumour usually arising in the sun-exposed skin of the face or arms (Fig. 47-3). A keratoacanthoma is now generally considered a low-risk SCC, but was previously not regarded as malignant and may resolve spontaneously leaving a prominent scar. The tumour grows rapidly over a few weeks into a dome-shaped nodule up to 2cm in diameter. There is often a keratin plug, which may fall out to leave a crater.

Histologically, a keratoacanthoma resembles a SCC, although it shows more symmetry and shouldering. Excision is the preferred treatment, but thorough curettage and cautery will usually be satisfactory. If recurrence occurs after curettage, excision is recommended.

Squamous cell carcinoma

Squamous cell carcinoma is a malignant tumour arising from keratinocytes of the epidermis or hair follicle and is the second most common skin cancer. The incidence of SCC is thought to be approximately a quarter that of basal cell carcinoma (BCC), affecting 2 per 1000 population per annum. SCC mainly occurs in white-skinned people over 55 years of age, is three times more common in males than in females and may metastasize.

Clinical presentation

Squamous cell carcinomas usually develop in sun-exposed sites such as the face, neck, forearm or hand (Fig. 47-4). Commonly other signs of photodamage will be evident in adjacent skin: solar elastosis, hyperkeratosis, mottled pigmentation and telangiectasia. Premalignant changes such as actinic keratoses and Bowen's disease as well as other skin cancers may also be present. On mucous membranes, leukokeratosis and fissuring or actinic cheilitis are frequent. Lesions present in a variety of ways:

◼ A hyperkeratotic papule, plaque or cutaneous horn with an indurated base.

◼ A small ulcer that refuses to heal.

◼ A firm ulcerated or crusted nodule (Fig. 47-4).

◼ A friable, fungating tumour that bleeds and weeps.

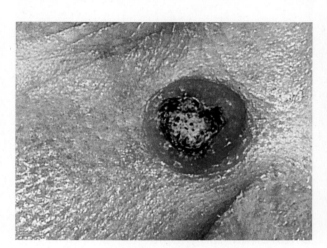

Fig. 47-3 **Keratoacanthoma on the face.**

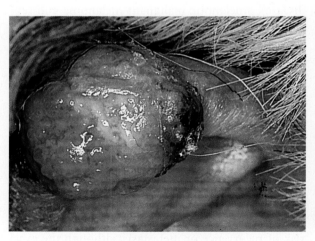

Fig. 47-4 **Squamous cell carcinoma.** The cancer is seen here on the upper pinna in a patient with actinically damaged skin.

The tumour may start within an actinic keratosis as a small papule that, if left, progresses to ulcerate and form a crust. This type of SCC does not commonly metastasize. Ulcerating forms of SCC which develop at the edge of ulcers (Fig. 47-5), in scars and at sites of radiation damage are frequently more aggressive. Metastasis is found in 10% or more of these cancers. An important clinical marker of SCC is its rapidity of growth. Most patients will report a lesion that grows over several months, in contrast to a BCC which would frequently develop slowly over 6 or more months. Tenderness is also an important symptom identified in SCCs and is thought to represent the extension of the SCC around nerves.

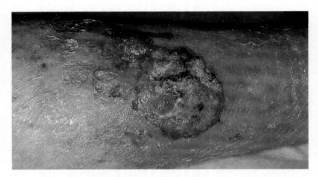

Fig. 47-5 **Squamous cell carcinoma on the lower leg.** The tumour occurred at the site of a longstanding ulcer.

Differential diagnosis

A SCC needs to be distinguished from keratoacanthoma, actinic keratosis, BCC, *in situ* SCC (Bowen's disease), amelanotic malignant melanoma and seborrhoeic keratosis. Excisional or incisional biopsy is needed in every case to confirm the diagnosis or adequacy of excision.

Management

Surgical excision is the treatment of choice. Large lesions may require a skin graft. In the elderly, SCCs of the face or scalp can be treated by *radiotherapy* (after an incisional biopsy for histological diagnosis). SCCs can be subdivided into high risk and low risk of recurrence or metastasis, although the exact boundaries are somewhat controversial. Generally agreed features of a high-risk SCC are given in the

Box. Patients are examined for lymph node metastasis at presentation: suspicious nodes are biopsied. Carefully agreed follow-up, especially for high-risk SCCs, is recommended.

Squamous cell carcinoma

- **Bowen's disease** is *in situ* squamous carcinoma, characterized with the sharply demarcated hyperkeratotic macule, papule or plaque, and it always follows a slowly aggressive course. Treatment is with cryotherapy, topical, surgical or photodynamic therapy.
- **Keratoacanthoma** is a spontaneously resolving lesion that bears clinical and histological resemblance to SCC. Excision is recommended.
- **Squamous cell carcinoma** is often seen in the sun-exposed skin of white people in association with signs of actinic damage. A more aggressive form of the tumour is found with chronic scarring. All types are treated by surgical excision.
- **Squamous cell carcinomas with a worse prognosis (high risk) include:**
  - body site involved: lip, ear, non-sun-exposed areas (perineum, sacrum, sole)
  - greater than 2cm in diameter
  - histological factors: >4mm in depth (histologically) or reaching the subcutis (Clark level V), poor differentiation, perineural involvement
  - host immunosuppression
  - recurrence from previous failure of treatment.

Web resources

http://dermnetnz.org/lesions/squamous-cell-carcinoma.html

Key words

squamous cell carcinoma (SCC)　鳞状细胞癌
actinic damage　光化损伤
Bowen's disease　鲍恩病
in situ　原位
cryotherapy　冷冻疗法
keratoacanthoma　角化棘皮瘤
solar elastosis　日光性弹力组织变性
actinic keratosis (AK)　光线性角化病

Review questions

1. Considering the already recognized pathogenic factors of SCC, what kind of people should be paid special attention to?

2. What are the main differences in clinical manifestation, among Bowen's disease, keratoacanthoma and SCC?

3. How to differentiate BCC from SCC?

4. How to make proper therapeutic decision for SCC?

5. How to roughly evaluate the prognosis of SCC?

(Juan Tao)

Chapter 48   Skin cancer - Malignant melanoma

Malignant melanoma is a malignant tumour of melanocytes, usually arising in the epidermis. In rare cases, it also appears in the dermis or the mucosal epithelial lining. It is the most lethal of the main skin tumours and has increased in incidence over the last three decades in the Caucasian races. The important pathogenic role of excessive ultraviolet (UV) radiation exposure has been the subject of public education campaigns. Friction is also regarded as the main predisposition in Asians. Genetics may be important, and up to 5% of patients have a family history of malignant melanoma.

Clinical presentation

Four main clinicopathological variants are recognized. These are described below.

Superficial spreading malignant melanoma

This type accounts for 50% of all British cases, shows a female preponderance and is commonest on the lower leg and trunk. The tumour is macular and shows variable pigmentation, often with regression (Fig. 48-1).

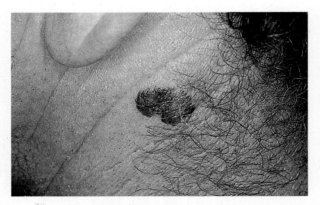

Fig. 48-1   **Superficial spreading malignant melanoma.**

Lentigo maligna melanoma

Malignant melanoma developing in a longstanding lentigo maligna (Fig. 48-2) constitutes 15% of UK cases, but a relatively smaller proportion in Asian cases. It always starts as the lentigo maligna (LM), which represents a macular intraepidermal neoplasm and is actually a melanoma *in situ*. A lentigo maligna arises in sun-damaged skin, often on the face of an elderly person who has spent many years in an outdoor occupation.

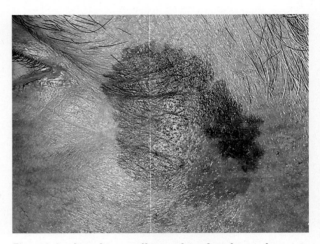

Fig. 48-2   **Lentigo maligna showing irregular outline and pigmentation.**

Acral lentiginous malignant melanoma

The acral lentiginous type makes up 1 in 10 of British cases, but is the most common form in brown- and black-skinned races. The tumour affects the palms, soles (Fig. 48-3) and nail beds, which may appear as a gradually enlarging "stain", is often diagnosed late and has poor survival figures.

Nodular malignant melanoma

The nodular variant is seen in 25% of British patients; it shows a male preponderance and is commonest on the trunk. The pigmented nodule (Fig. 48-4) may grow rapidly and ulcerate.

The *differential diagnosis* of malignant melanoma includes:

■ benign melanocytic naevus

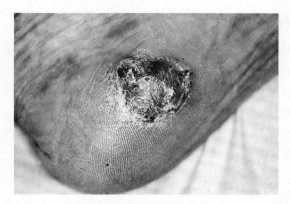

Fig. 48-3 **Acral lentiginous malignant melanoma.**

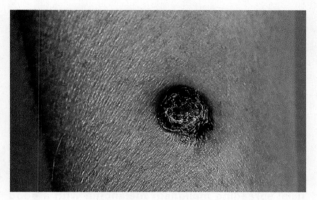

Fig. 48-4 **Nodular malignant melanoma.**

- seborrhoeic wart
- haemangioma
- dermatofibroma
- pigmented basal cell carcinoma
- benign lentigo

Epidemiology

Malignant melanoma has an incidence in the UK of 15~20 per 100 000 population per year. The incidence has been rising at 7% each year and has trebled in the last two decades in the UK. In the UK, women are affected twice as frequently as men. Superficial spreading and nodular melanomas tend to occur in those in the 20~60-year age group, whereas lentigo malignant melanomas mostly affect those over 60 years old. In males, the commonest site is the back; in females, it is the lower leg (about half occur here).

Staging

Malignant melanomas usually progress through two phases: *horizontal* growth in the epidermis then *vertical* invasion of the dermis (Fig. 48-5).

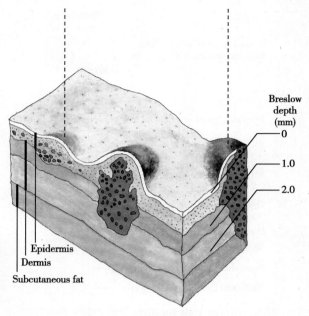

Fig. 48-5 **Staging.**

Local invasion by the tumour is assessed using the *Breslow method*, which is the measurement in millimetres of the distance between the granular cell layer to the deepest identifiable melanoma cell. Metastasis is uncommon in tumours restricted to the epidermis.

Aetiopathogenesis

The main risk factor that increases risk of melanoma is exposure to UV radiation. Some people are more at risk of melanoma than others (Fig. 48-6). Histological evidence of a pre-existing melanocytic naevus is found in 30% of malignant melanomas but, with the exception of dysplastic or congenital naevi (Fig. 48-7), the risk of change in a common melanocytic naevus is small. Besides, the genetic variances of different races also play an important role in the pathogenesis of the malignant melanoma.

Dermatopathology

Atypical melanocytes are found in the epidermis or dermis layers, or even deeper tissues. Special stains (such as S-100 and HMB-45) contribute to more efficient diagnosis.

Diagnosis

Any of the following changes in a naevus or pigmented lesion may suggest malignant melanoma:

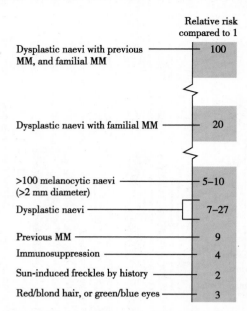

Relative risk compared to 1

Dysplastic naevi with previous MM, and familial MM	100
Dysplastic naevi with familial MM	20
>100 melanocytic naevi (>2 mm diameter)	5–10
Dysplastic naevi	7–27
Previous MM	9
Immunosuppression	4
Sun-induced freckles by history	2
Red/blond hair, or green/blue eyes	3

Fig. 48-6 **Major risk factors.** The major risk factors and their relative risk for the development of malignant melanoma (MM) are shown. Int J Dermatol. 2010; 49: 362-376.

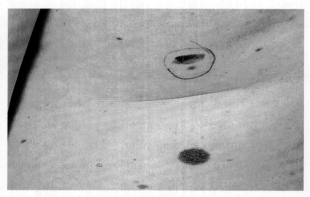

Fig. 48-7 **Dysplastic naevus syndrome.** This condition, which may be familial, is characterized by large numbers of atypical and 'dysplastic' naevi, which are often over 7mm in diameter with an irregular edge and variable pigmentation. Affected individuals have a greatly increased risk of developing malignant melanoma. They should avoid the sun and be closely observed. Changing or suspicious pigmented lesions should be excised for histological examination.

- *size*: usually a recent increase
- *shape*: irregular in outline
- *colour*: variation, darker or lighter
- *inflammation*: may be at the edge
- *crusting*: some ooze or bleed
- *itch*: a common symptom.

Prognosis

The prognosis relates to the tumour depth. The approximate 5-year survival rates are:

- <1mm 95%
- 1~2mm 90%
- 2.1~4mm 77%
- >4mm 65%

Examples of thin and thick tumours are given in Fig. 48-8 and Fig. 48-9.

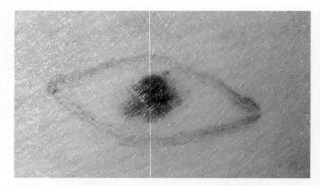

Fig. 48-8 **A thin (0.8-mm Breslow thickness) superficial spreading malignant melanoma with a good prognosis.**

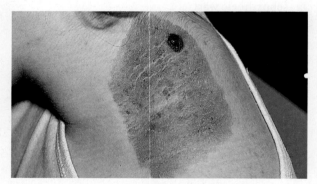

Fig. 48-9 **A thick (11-mm Breslow thickness) nodular malignant melanoma developing within a large congenital naevus.** Local lymph nodes were involved; the prognosis was poor.

Management

The primary treatment is narrow surgical excision followed by re-excision of the scar dependent upon Breslow thickness. *In situ* tumours require a 0.5-cm re-excision, those up to 1mm thick require a 1-cm margin, those of 1~2mm thickness need a 2-cm margin and thicker tumours require a 2~3-cm clearance. A skin graft may be necessary to close the defect.

Regular follow-up is needed to detect any recurrence, of which there are three main types:

1. *local* (Fig. 48-10)
2. *lymphatic* - either in the regional lymph nodes or in transit in the lymphatics draining from the tumour to the nodes
3. *blood-borne* to distant sites

Routine sentinel node biopsy or elective lymph node dissection is not recommended as a standard procedure at present. Radiotherapy is of limited use. Interferon-alpha may increase survival in patients with tumours more than 1.5mm thick. For metastatic disease, chemotherapy with dacarbazine is the current standard but has limited effectiveness and significant toxicity. New therapies including ipilimumab, a monoclonal antibody targeting the negative T cell regulator molecule, CTLA-4, has been shown to improve survival in advanced melanoma, and BRAF kinase inhibitors in BRAF-mutated melanomas have shown promise.

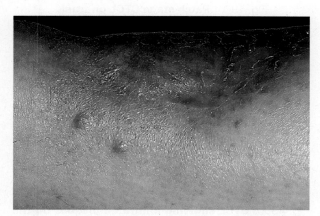

Fig. 48-10　**Hypomelanotic recurrent malignant melanoma.** Pink papules of recurrent tumour are evident at the edge of a previously excised and grafted site.

Prevention and public education

Early malignant melanoma is a curable disease, but thick lesions have a poor prognosis. Public health education should encourage early visits to the doctor for changing pigmented lesions and should discourage excessive sun exposure, especially in fair-skinned individuals or those with numerous melanocytic naevi. The best advice is:

- avoid burning in the sun
- report early any change in a mole.

> *Malignant melanoma*
> - Melanoma is the most lethal skin tumour with a rapid increasing incidence worldwide. White-skinned persons have a higher incidence than brown- and black-skinned ones.
> - The incidence is largely related to ultraviolet radiation and genetic heterogeneity.
> - Four principal clinicopathological variants of melanoma are recognized by now. The most common type in white persons is the superficial spreading one, while the acral lentiginous type occurs most often in brown- and black-ones.
> - Management to melanoma includes surgical excision, radiotherapy, chemotherapy, interferon-alpha and some immunomodulators.
> - The prognosis is related to tumour thickness.

Key words

malignant melanoma　恶性黑素瘤

melanocyte　黑素细胞

superficial spreading malignant melanoma (SSM)　浅表扩散性黑素瘤

lentigo maligna melanoma (LMM)　恶性雀斑样痣黑素瘤

acral lentiginous malignant melanoma (ALM)　肢端雀斑样痣黑素瘤

nodular malignant melanoma (NM)　结节性恶性黑素瘤

dysplastic naevi　发育不良痣

dysplastic naevus syndrome　发育不良痣综合征

Review questions

1. What is the well-recognized pathogenesis in melanoma development?
2. What are the characteristics of the four types of malignant melanoma?
3. What characteristics of a naevus or pigmented lesion should be paid special attention to?
4. How to distinguish a malignant melanoma from a benign melanocytic naevus based on the clinical and pathological features?
5. How to choose the proper treatment strategy to a 1.5mm-thick ALM on the face of a 65-year old man?

(Juan Tao)

Chapter 49   Cutaneous T cell lymphomas and malignant dermal tumours

Cutaneous T cell lymphoma (CTA) is the most common type of skin lymphoma, with an incidence of 0.6 per 100 000. B cell lymphoma of the skin is rare. Malignant tumours of the dermis are infrequent. The commonest are secondary deposits Kaposi's sarcoma and a malignancy of dermal fibroblasts (dermatofibrosarcoma).

Cutaneous T cell lymphoma (mycosis fungoides)

CTCL describes a lymphoma that evolves in the skin, although extracutaneous T cell tumours often produce secondary skin deposits. CTCL is a slowly progressive tumour of epidermotropic $CD3^+$, $CD4^+$ T lymphocytes that becomes systemic only in its terminal stage.

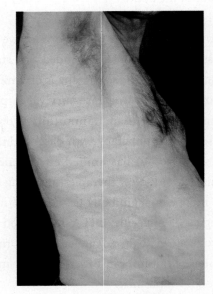

Fig. 49-1   **Patch stage CTCL on trunk.**

Clinical presentation

The course is usually protracted, although it is occasionally more rapidly progressive. The diagnosis is often delayed for some years as, in its initial stages, CTCL may resemble eczema or 'chronic superficial dermatitis' CTCL can be regarded as having four stages:

1. *Patch stage.* Describes small, scaly, slightly raised erythematous patches, typically on the trunk, that can resemble eczema (Fig. 49-1). It may persist for 10 years or more. Occasionally, the skin becomes atrophic, pigmented and telangiectatic (poikiloderma).

2. *Infiltrated plaques.* Fixed plaques develop, usually on the trunk but sometimes more widely distributed (Fig. 49-2). This stage may last for years.

3. *Tumour stage.* This later phase, characterized by tumorous nodules or ulcers within the plaques, has a 5-year survival of 40%~65% (Fig. 49-3).

4. *Systemic disease.* Involvement of lymph nodes or internal organs is a late finding. The Sézary syndrome is a variant.

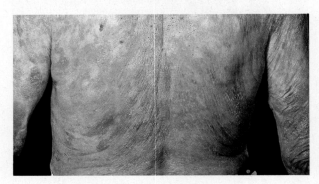

Fig. 49-2   **CTCL showing infiltrated plaques on the back and arms.**

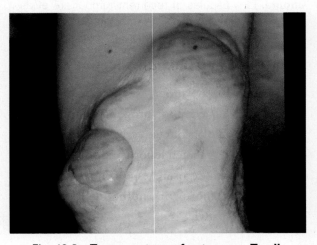

Fig. 49-3   **Tumour stage of cutaneous T cell.**

Dermatopathology

The typical histology of MF includes epidermotropism, the Pautrier's microabscess.

Differential diagnosis

Chronic superficial dermatitis, undifferentiated eczema and psoriasis are the main differential diagnoses. Those cases of chronic superficial dermatitis that show larger patches are said to be more likely to progress to CTCL. CD30+ lymphoproliferative disorders represent a subgroup of skin lymphomas. They present either as multiple nodules that heal with scarring and follow a protracted course (lymphomatoid papulosis) or as large cell lymphoma, in which ulcerated nodules appear on the trunk.

Management

Diagnosis relies on matching the clinical and pathological appearances T cell receptor gene analysis demonstrates clonality of the lymphocytic infiltrate. Current treatment is not curative but aimed at controlling the lymphoma. The patch-stage lesions often improve with moderately potent topical steroids and ultraviolet (UV) B therapy. More infiltrated plaques require PUVA or topical nitrogen mustard. Localized lesions respond to conventional radiotherapy. Advanced CTCL can be treated with extracorporal photopheresis, electron beam therapy, oral bexarotene, or combined chemotherapy.

Cutaneous T cell lymphomas and malignant dermal tumours

■ **Definition:** CTCL is an uncommon tumour resulting from infiltration of the skin by malignant clonal T lymphocytes.

■ **Stages:** CTCL progresses through patch stage to indurated plaques, and then to tumours and systemic involvement.

■ **Treatment:** therapy depends on the stage and extent of the disease. Localized patch stage CTCL responds to topical steroids and phototherapy. In more advanced disease, phototherapy, radiotherapy and oral bexarotene or chemotherapy may be prescribed.

■ **Malignant dermal tumors** are uncommon. Secondary deposits, Kaposi's sarcoma and other sarcomas can be found.

Key words

lymphoma   淋巴瘤

cutaneous T cell lymphoma (CTCL)   原发性皮肤 T 细胞淋巴瘤

Kaposi's sarcoma   卡波西肉瘤

secondary deposits   继发沉积

dermatofibrosarcoma   皮肤纤维肉瘤

mycosis fungoides (MF)   蕈样霉菌病 / 蕈样肉芽肿病

Sezary syndrome (SS)   塞扎里综合征

lymphoproliferative disorder   淋巴组织增生异常

lymphomatoid papulosis   淋巴瘤样丘疹病

extracorporal photopheresis   体外光化学疗法

electron beam therapy   电子束疗法

Review questions

1. Apart from the CTCL, what are the other kinds of malignant dermal tumors?
2. What are the four stages and what are their respect clinical characteristics in the successive progression of the CTCL?
3. What are the main differential diagnoses of the CTCL?
4. What is the theraputic principle to the CTCL in different stages?

(Juan Tao)

Special topics in dermatology

Chapter 50   Ultraviolet radiation and the skin

An interaction between skin and sunlight is inescapable. The potential for harm depends on the type and length of exposure. Photoageing is a growing problem, because of an increasingly aged population and a rise in the average individual exposure to ultraviolet (UV) radiation.

The electromagnetic radiation spectrum

The sun's emission of electromagnetic radiation ranges from low-wavelength ionizing cosmic, gamma and X-rays to the non-ionizing UV, visible and infrared higher wavelengths (Fig. 50-1). The ozone layer absorbs UVC, but UVA and smaller amounts of UVB reach ground level. UV radiation is maximal in the middle of the day (11.00~15.00h) and is increased by reflection from snow, water and sand. UVA penetrates the epidermis to reach the dermis. UVB is mostly absorbed by the stratum corneum - only 10% reaches the dermis. Most window glass absorbs UV less than 320 nm in wavelength. Artificial UV sources emit in the UVB or UVA spectrum. Sunbeds largely emit UVA.

Effects of light on normal skin

Physiological

UVB promotes the synthesis of vitamin D3 from its precursors in the skin, and UVA and UVB stimulate immediate pigmentation (due to photo-oxidation of melanin precursors), melanogenesis and epidermal thickening as a protective measure against UV damage.

Sunburn

If enough UVB is given, erythema always results. The threshold dose of UVB - the *minimal erythema dose* (MED) - is a guide to an individual's susceptibility. Excessive UVB exposure results in tingling of the skin, followed 2~12h later by erythema. The redness is maximal at 24h and fades over the next 2 or 3 days to leave desquamation and pigmentation. Severe sunburn causes oedema, pain, blistering and systemic upset. The early use of topical steroids may help sunburn; otherwise, a soothing shake lotion (e.g. calamine lotion) is applied. Individuals may be skin typed by their likelihood of burning in the sun (Table

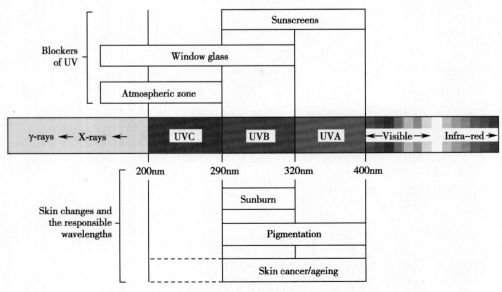

Fig. 50-1   **The sun's emission spectrum.**

50-1). Prevention is better than cure, and 'celts' with a fair 'type 1' skin should not sunbathe and must use a high protection factor sunblock cream on exposed sites. Some evidence suggests the sun avoidance message may have gone too far in that it could be causing white populations to become vitamin D deficient.

Table 50-1	**Skin type according to sunburn and suntan histories**
Skin type	**Reaction to sun exposure**
Type 1	Always burns, never tans
Type 2	Always burns, sometimes tans
Type 3	Sometimes burns, always tans
Type 4	Never burns, always tans
Type 5	Brown skin (e.g. Asian Caucasoid)
Type 6	Black skin (e.g. black African)

Sunbeds

Sunbeds emit UVA radiation and have been used by 10%~20% of adults in the UK. They will produce a tan in people with skin types 3 and over, but those with type 1 and 2 skin will not tan so well, if at all. Side-effects, particularly redness, itching and dry skin, are seen in half of all users. More serious effects can occur in patients taking drugs or applying preparations with a photosensitizing potential. An acute photosensitive eruption may develop, and intense pigmentation sometimes follows. Sunbeds can exacerbate polymorphic light eruption and systemic lupus erythematosus, and may induce porphyria-like skin fragility and blistering. They are a weak risk factor for malignant melanoma, and may cause premature skin ageing.

Dermatologists discourage sunbed use, particularly in the fair-skinned, in those with several melanocytic naevi and in anyone with a history of skin cancer. Patients who, despite these warnings, wish to use a sunbed should not do so more than twice a year and should limit each course to 10 sessions. Sunbeds are not recommended for the treatment of skin disease.

Phototherapy and photochemotherapy

Natural sunlight helps certain skin diseases, and both UVB and UVA are extensively used therapeutically. UVA alone has little effect and is combined with photosensitizing psoralens given systemically or topically.

Ultraviolet B

UVB (290~320nm) is given three times a week. The starting dose is decided from the patient's MED or skin type. The dosage is increased on each visit according to a schedule. A course of 10~30 treatments is usual. Narrow-band (311nm ± 2nm: TL01) UV lamps are superior to broadband and allow a lower dose of UV to be used.

UVB is used to treat psoriasis, pityriasis rosea and mycosis fungoides (cutaneous T cell lymphoma) and, occasionally, atopic eczema (atopic dermatitis) and vitiligo. It can be given to children and women during pregnancy. Its main side-effects are acute sunburn and an increased long-term risk of skin cancer.

When used to treat psoriasis, UVB may be combined with a topical preparation such as a vitamin D analogue, tar or dithranol, or with oral acitretin.

Photochemotherapy (PUVA)

In psoralen plus UVA (PUVA) therapy, 8-methoxypsoralen, taken orally 2h before UVA (320~400nm) exposure (Fig. 50-2), is photoactivated. This causes

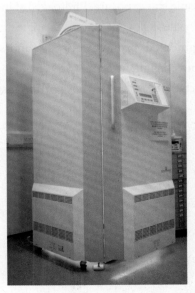

Fig. 50-2 **Photochemotherapy using UVA-emitting tubes.**

cross-linkage in DNA, inhibits cell division and suppresses cell-mediated immunity. PUVA is usually given for psoriasis or mycosis fungoides, and sometimes for atopic eczema, polymorphic light eruption or vitiligo. The initial dose of UVA is determined by the minimum toxic dose (the MED for PUVA) or skin type, and is increased according to a schedule. PUVA is given two or three times a week and leads to clearance of psoriasis (with tanning) in 15~25 treatments. Maintenance PUVA is not recommended. PUVA can be combined with acitretin ('Re-PUVA') but not methotrexate.

The immediate side-effects of pruritus, nausea and erythema are usually mild. The long-term risks of skin cancer and premature skin ageing are related to the number of treatments or total UVA dose. Careful records must be kept. Cataracts are theoretically possible, and UVA-opaque sunglasses must be worn for 24h after taking the psoralen.

Bath PUVA, in which the patient soaks in a bath containing a psoralen, is an alternative, especially if systemic side-effects make the oral route impractical. A lower dose of UVA is needed. *Local PUVA* using topical psoralen is useful for psoriasis or dermatitis of the hands or feet.

Photoageing

Photoageing describes the skin changes resulting from chronic sun exposure. Photoaged skin is coarse, wrinkled, pale-yellow in colour, telangiectatic, irregularly pigmented, prone to purpura and subject to benign and malignant neoplasms (Fig. 50-3). Some of these changes resemble those of intrinsic ageing,

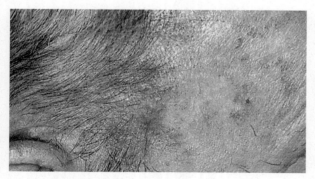

Fig. 50-3 Photoageing of the skin. Keratoses and pigmentation are evident.

but the two are not identical, as may be judged by comparing, in an elderly patient, the sun-exposed face with the sun-protected buttock. The features of photoageing are usually more striking, particularly the development of premalignant and malignant tumours. Some rare conditions, e.g. xeroderma pigmentosum, predispose to photoageing.

Management of photoageing

Prevention is the most effective treatment and is particularly important for those with a fair (type 1 or 2) skin. Avoidance of prolonged, direct sun exposure by wearing long-sleeved shirts and a wide-brimmed hat is useful, and sunscreens are applied to sites that are likely to receive some sun, such as the face or hands. The use of tretinoin or alpha hydroxy acids, in cream formulations, has been shown partially to reverse the clinical and histological changes of photoageing. Chemical peels and laser resurfacing are also used.

UV and the skin

- **UVB radiation** is mostly absorbed by the epidermis, but UVA can penetrate to the dermis. UVB promotes vitamin D synthesis. UVA and UVB stimulate melanogenesis and epidermal thickening.
- **Minimal erythema dose** is the threshold amount of UVB to cause erythema.
- **Sunburn** is maximal at 24h and fades at 2~3 days to leave desquamation and pigmentation of the skin.
- **Sunbeds** emit UVA and will induce a tan in those with type 3 or 4 skin. Side-effects are common.
- **Photoageing** describes coarse, wrinkled, yellowed skin, prone to tumours, resulting from excess sun exposure.
- **UVB therapy**, now mostly narrow-band TL01, is mainly used in psoriasis; a course of 10~30 treatments is usual.
- **PUVA** has been a common treatment for psoriasis; used less now. Skin cancer is one potential long-term sequela.
- **Treatment of photoageing**: prevention is best, but tretinoin cream can reverse some of the changes.

Web resource

http://www.skincarephysicians.com/psoriasisnet/phototherapy.html

Key words

photoageing 光老化

ultraviolet (UV) 紫外线

ultraviolet A (UVA) 紫外线 A 段

ultraviolet B (UVB) 紫外线 B 段

sunburn 日晒伤或日灼伤

minimal erythema dose (MED) 最小红斑量

photochemotherapy (PUVA) 光化学疗法

psoralen 补骨脂素

psoriasis 银屑病

sunscreen 防晒霜

Review questions

1. What kind of dermatoses can be treated using narrow-band UVB?

2. What are the side-effects of narrow-band UVB photo-therapy?

(Wei He)

Chapter 51   Cosmetics

A cosmetic may be defined as any substance that is applied to the body for cleansing, beautifying, promoting attractiveness or altering the appearance. Cosmetics in some form are used by almost everyone. The market for cosmetic sales is vast and far exceeds that of dermatological products. Over recent years, the fields of cosmetology and dermatology have converged so that patients often present having had a reaction to a cosmetic or asking for advice about cosmetic usage. Some cosmetics are now being marketed as 'cosmeceuticals' with the claim that they have an 'active' ingredient, for example one that can 'reverse ageing' or especially for Chinese that can 'lighten skin'.

The range of cosmetics and their usage

Cosmetics are normally used to enhance the appearance of the body, to clean it, to impart a pleasing smell or to mask an unpleasant one, or as a fashion accessory. Table 51-1 shows the range of common types of cosmetics.

Table 51-1	**The range of cosmetics**
Site	**Product**
Skin	Moisturizer, cleanser, soap, make-up remover, powder, rouge, foundation, toner, perfume, aftershave, bath additive, sunscreen
Hair	Shampoo, conditioner, bleach, colourant, permanent waving, straightening, lacquer, gel, hair-removing agents
Eyelids	Mascara, eyeshadow, eyeliner, pencil
Nails	Nail varnish, false nails
Lips	Lipstick, lipgloss, sunscreen

Constituents of cosmetics

The exact contents of a cosmetic depend on its proposed function. However, commonly used ingredients, some of which will be found in most cosmetics, are detailed in Table 51-2. Many cosmetics contain perfumes, preservatives and, quite often, a sunblock agent. Cosmetics are often emulsions (e.g. oil-in-water or water-in-oil) or gels. Full labelling of contents is usually required by governments, a measure strongly supported by dermatologists. This is a useful development for patients allergic to cosmetic ingredients because they are now able to avoid products that would be problematic. Certain preparations deserve special mention. They are discussed below.

Occlusives

Occlusives coat the stratum corneum to retard transepidermal water loss (TEWL). An Occlusive provides an emollient effect as well as decreases TWEL. The best occlusive ingredients currently available are petrolatum, mineral oil, plant oil and beeswax. Occlusives are usually combined with humectant ingredients.

Humectants

Humectants are water-soluble materials with high water absorption capabilities. They are able to attract water from the atmosphere and from the underlying epidermis. They are effective when combined with occlusives. Humectants are also popular additives to cosmetic moisturizers because they prevent product evaporation and thickening. The ingredients currently available are hyaluronic acid, glycerin, sorbitol.

Emollients

There are substances added to cosmetics to soften and smooth the skin. They function by filling the spaces between desquamating corneocytes to create a smooth surface. Many emollients such as hyaluronic acid, lanolin, mineral oil and petrolatum function as humectants and occlusive moisturizers as well.

Para-phenylenediamine (PPD) hair dye

Hair dyes, principally PPD, are widely used. Adverse reactions occur in 5%, usually as a scalp or facial

Table 51-2 **Some ingredients of cosmetics**

Ingredient	Action	Examples
Antioxidant	Prevent degradation	Butylhydroxyanisole, gallates, tocopherol
Colorant, dye	Colour	Cochineal, azo compounds, iron dioxides, para-phenylenediamine, titanium dioxide, metal salts, dihydroxyacetone in fake tan
Perfume	Smell or for masking smell	*Myroxylon pereirae*, limonene, geraniol, linalool
Preservative	Antimicrobial	Parabens, formaldehyde, iodo-propynyl butyl carbamate, methyl isothiazolin-one/chloro methyl isothiazolin-one, quaternium 15, bromo-nitropropane-diol, imidazolidinyl urea
Polyol	Humectant (retains water), emollient	Glycerol, propylene glycol, sorbitol, hyaluronic acid
Oil, fat, wax	Occlusive, Emollient, lustre	Vaseline, almond oil, lanolin
Sun filter	Absorb or reflect UV	Titanium dioxide, oxybenzone, avobenzone
Tensioactive agent	Emulsifier, surfactant, detergent	Soaps, stearic and oleic acids
Water	Hydration	Purified water

eczema. 'Henna' tattoos often contain 15-30% PPD and can induce allergy to PPD.

Nail preparations

Nail varnish is composed of a tosylamide-formaldehyde resin and colourants. Artificial nails are made of methacrylate acid esters and stuck on with acrylic glues.

Sunscreens

A sunscreen absorbs or reflects ultraviolet (UV) radiation. Absorbent agents are shown in Table 51-2. Titanium dioxide and zinc oxide are reflectant pigments. The sun protection factor (SPF) indicates the ratio of the reaction time to erythema when exposed to UV radiation for treated compared with untreated skin. Thus, using a factor 10 cream means that it should take 10 times longer for erythema to develop when in the sun. Some sunscreen creams are waterproof. Most need to be applied several times a day. Preparations available on prescription in China for patients with photodermatoses.

Camouflage cosmetics

These pigmented camouflage creams can be mixed to match the colour of the patient's skin and are useful for individuals who have vitiligo, disfiguring birthmarks or scars.

Skin-lightening creams

These may contain mercury or hydroquinone, both of which can cause contact allergy or, paradoxically, pigmentation.

Hypoallergenic formulations

These cosmetics are made of highly purified ingredients, selected with the knowledge of their allergenic and irritant potential. However, they still contain compounds that are potential irritants and allergens.

Reactions to cosmetics

Side-effects are comparatively rare when the vast usage of cosmetics is considered but, nonetheless, 12% or more of adults have had a reaction to a cosmetic. Some responses, e.g. stinging with aftershave due to the alcohol base, are expected and do not constitute a reaction. Some patients undoubtedly have a 'sensitive' skin and experience abreactions to a number of products. The preparations most likely to cause a problem are eye and facial cosmetics, antiperspirants and deodorants, hair colourants and soaps (Table 51-3). Reactions can be categorized as follows.

Irritant contact dermatitis

This is particularly seen in atopics and those with a 'sensitive' skin. Soaps, which are drying and alkaline (the normal pH of facial skin is about 5.5), and deodorants cause mostly irritant dermatitis (Fig. 51-1). Lanolins, detergents and preservatives may also be irritant.

Table 51-3	**Frequent adverse reactions to cosmetics**
Cosmetic	**Reaction**
Soap, detergent	Mostly irritant
Deodorant, antiperspirant	Irritant, sometimes allergic
Moisturizer	Irritant and allergic
Eye shadow	Mostly irritant
Mascara	Mostly irritant
Permanent wave agent	Irritant and allergic
Hair dye (mostly para-phenylenediamine)	Allergic
Shampoo	Mostly irritant

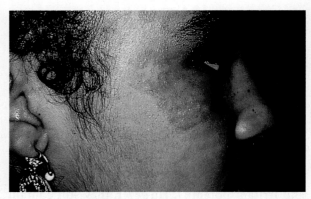

Fig. 51-1 **Irritant contact dermatitis to a component of a hair-removing cream.**

Allergic contact dermatitis

Allergic contact dermatitis most commonly develops to fragrances, preservatives, dyes (e.g. PPD), lanolins, metallic salts (in some eye cosmetics) and the permanent wave agent glyceryl mono-thioglycolate (Figs 51-2 and 51-3). The eruption usually develops at the place of application of the product (usually the face), but this is not always so, as substances can be transferred to another site where they cause symptoms. For example, contact allergy to tosylamide-formaldehyde resin (Fig. 51-4) in nail varnish most often manifests as an eruption around the eyelids or on the neck.

Contact urticaria and other adverse reactions

Contact urticaria presents as a wheal and flare response

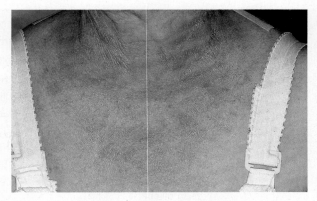

Fig. 51-2 **Allergic contact dermatitis on the neck due to fragrances.**

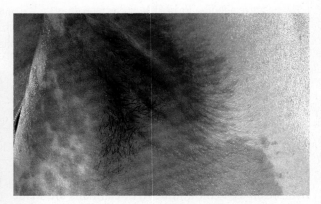

Fig. 51-3 **Allergic contact dermatitis at the axilla due to a component of a roll-on deodorant.**

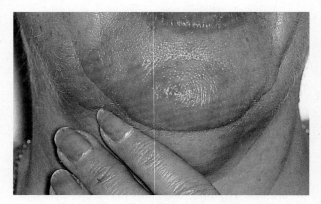

Fig. 51-4 **Contact sensitivity to tosylamide-formaldehyde resin in nail varnish, causing a facial dermatitis.**

within a few minutes of the application of a substance. It may occur with compounds in perfumes, shampoos and hair dyes. Other adverse reactions include nail dystrophies caused by nail cosmetic or artificial nail use, hair breakage and weathering due to improper use of permanent waving, hair straighteners or dyes, pigmentation and acne.

Management of cosmetic reactions

A patient intolerant of a cosmetic should stop the use of all cosmetics. If necessary, a topical steroid is prescribed until the reaction subsides. All the cosmetics and preparations that have been used must be examined for ingredients, and patch testing performed if appropriate. Alternative cosmetics can then be introduced, but kept to a minimum.

Cosmetics

- *A cosmetic is a* substance applied to the body for cleansing, to promote attractiveness or to alter the appearance. Now used by both sexes.
- *A cosmetic cream* typically contains emollients, emulsifiers, colourants, perfumes and preservatives to prevent oxidation and the growth of micro-organisms. Sun filters may also be included to prolong shelf-life and for their 'anti-photoageing' effect.
- *Reactions to cosmetics* may take the form of irritant or allergic contact dermatitis, contact urticaria or pigmentary change.
- The commonest causes of *irritant reactions* are soaps, shampoos and deodorants, often because of detergents or preservatives.
- The substances that most frequently cause *allergic contact dermatitis* are fragrances or preservatives (found in most cosmetics, e.g. moisturizers) and dyes (e.g. PPD found in hair colourants).

Web resource

http://www.medicinenet.com/cosmetic_allergies/article.htm

Key words

cosmetics　化妆品
hairdressing　美发

shampoo　洗发香波
lighten skin　皮肤美白
reverse ageing　逆龄
emulsion　乳剂
gel　凝胶
occlusives　锁水剂
humectant　保湿剂
emollient　柔肤剂 / 润肤剂
mascara　睫毛膏
eye shadow　眼影
eyeliner　眼线笔
pencil　眉笔
soap　肥皂
detergent　洗涤剂 / 清洁剂
deodorant antiperspirant　香体止汗剂
hair dye　染发剂
camouflage cosmetics　遮瑕膏
skin-lightening cream　美白乳膏
formulation　配方
colourant　着色剂
permanent wave agent　定型剂
tensioactive agent　表面活性剂
perfume　香水
preservative　防腐剂
antioxidant　抗氧化剂
nail varnish　指甲油
artificial nail　人工指甲

Review questions

1. What's the range of cosmetics?
2. What are the main ingredients of cosmetics?
3. Please comment on the frequent adverse reactions to cosmetics.

(Jianyun Lu)

Chapter 52 Basic dermatological surgery

The demand for the removal of benign and malignant skin lesions has increased considerably, such that skin surgery is now practised by many general practitioners as well as by dermatologists. Knowledge of basic surgical techniques is mandatory for all those who treat skin disease.

Instruments and methods

No-one should attempt a procedure if unsure about it. Those with limited experience should remove only benign lesions. All procedures are ideally performed in an *operating theatre* with trained nurses and adequate lighting. Sterile instruments, an aseptic technique and sterile gloves are essential. The operator plans the procedure, explains it to the patient, discusses the scar and obtains written consent. The direction of crease marks is assessed: any excision is usually made parallel to these lines.

The *basic instruments* (Fig. 52-1) include a #3 scalpel handle and #15 blade, a toothed Adson's forceps, a small smooth-jawed needle holder, a pair of fine scissors, artery forceps and a Gillies skin hook. Curettes and skin punches come in various sizes. A solution of 1% lidocaine (Xylocaine) with 1/200 000 adrenaline (epinephrine) is usually satisfactory as the *local anaesthetic*, but plain lidocaine must be used on

the fingers, toes and penis. The maximum safe dose for an 80kg person using 1% lidocaine and adrenaline (1/200 000) is 40~50ml. This volume is significantly reduced if higher concentrations of lidocaine or no adrenaline are used. The skin is prepared (but not sterilized) using, for example, 0.05% aqueous chlorhexidine (Unisept). Alcohol-based preparations are avoided as, if cautery is used, the solution may ignite. Sterile towels, placed around the operation site, reduce the chance of infection.

Absorbable subcutaneous sutures (e.g. polyglactin; Vicryl) are used for excisions where the wound may be deep or under tension. For cuticular stitches, monofilament nylon (e.g. Ethilon) and polypropylene (e.g. Prolene) are recommended. Use 5/0 or 6/0 sutures on the face, 3/0 on the back and legs, and 4/0 elsewhere. Stitches are preferably removed at 5~7 days on the face, 10~14 days on the legs or trunk and 7~8 days at other sites. Steristrips give extra support to a wound either in addition to sutures or when applied after their removal. An adherent tape or dressing (e.g. Micropore or Mepore) is used in most cases. For scalp biopsies, spray adhesive (e.g. Opsite spray) is useful.

Every biopsied lesion is sent for histology. If more than one specimen is taken from a patient, separate pots are used and each labelled before the biopsy is placed in it. The usual fixative is 10% formalin.

Safety aspects

Safety measures and protocols are essential within a dermatological surgery unit in order to minimize the risks of infection and accidental injury to both patients and staff. Control of blood-borne infections, especially human immunodeficiency virus (HIV) and hepatitis viruses, has two main components: prevention of transmission from patient to patient, and protection of the medical staff. It is now manda-

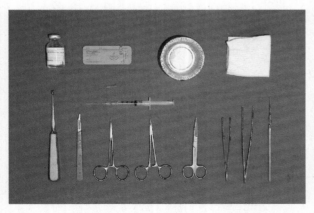

Fig. 52-1 **A typical surgical set for skin surgery.** A curette is included.

tory for all British medical and nursing staff to be adequately vaccinated against hepatitis B, and for hospitals to have both dedicated infection control staff and protocols to ensure instrument sterility. One approach suggested by the US Centers for Disease Control and Prevention (CDC) is to treat all patients as if they were infected with HIV, hepatitis B or other blood-borne pathogens and to adopt 'universal precautions'. Needle-stick injuries and other sharp instrument cuts are particularly important, and all members of the surgical team should take extreme care with the use and disposal of 'sharps'. It is extremely dangerous to either leave uncapped needles on the instrument tray or to attempt needle recapping by the two-handed method. Ideally, the surgeon should make a habit of both disposing of used needles and syringes immediately after use and removing all sharp disposable instruments (e.g. needles, scalpel blades) from the tray after the operation, placing these directly into 'sharps disposal' boxes. All relatives and those theatre personnel not directly concerned with the procedure should be excluded from the operating room. Clothing should be specific for surgery—apart from potentially introducing a variety of organisms to the procedure room, clothes may become contaminated. At the pre-operative consultation, a careful history may identify certain potential problems (e.g. diabetes, epilepsy) and the presence of cardiac pacemakers. A full drug history is important—aspirin and anticoagulants promote bleeding and non-selective β-blockers (e.g. propranolol) may rarely interact with epinephrine (adrenaline) in local anaesthetics, resulting in malignant hypertension. As there is always a risk of patient collapse in operating rooms, there must be adequate space available for an emergency resuscitation to be performed. Resuscitation drugs and equipment, together with both suction and an oxygen supply, should be readily available. All theatre personnel should be trained in advanced resuscitation techniques, including emergency electrocardiography and cardiac defibrillation.

Basic surgical techniques

Excisional biopsy

An excisional biopsy is planned after considering the local anatomy. The excision's axis depends on the skin creases (Fig. 52-2) and its margin on the nature of the lesion. The ellipse to be excised is drawn on the skin using a marker pen. An ellipse has an apical angle of about 30° and is usually three times as long as it is wide. If any shorter, 'dog-ears' appear at either end, although these can easily be corrected. After cleaning, local anaesthetic is infiltrated using a fine needle into the area of the lesion. Once numbed, the skin is incised vertically down to fat with the scalpel, in a smooth continuous manner to complete both arcs of the ellipse. The ellipse is freed from surrounding skin, secured at one end with a skin hook and removed from the underlying fat, usually using the scalpel blade (Fig. 52-3). In most cases, the wound can now be repaired, although any bleeding vessels will need to be stemmed with cautery, hyfrecation or suturing.

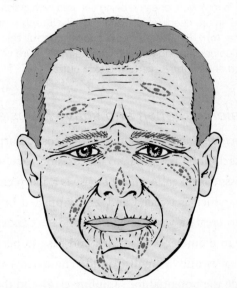

Fig. 52-2 **Facial crease lines, with some examples of excision ellipses.**

In a simple *interrupted skin suture*, the needle is inserted vertically through the skin surface down through the dermis and up the other side of the incision to trace a flaskshaped profile (see Fig. 52-3). The wound is apposed and slightly everted. Stitches should not be tied too tightly. Nylon or polypropylene sutures are tied with three knots in alternating directions to produce a square knot. Care is exercised at sites where keloids may form (e.g. the upper back, chest or jawline), where scars may be obvious (e.g. the face of a young woman) and when healing may be poor (e.g. the lower leg). In cosmetically sensitive sites, running subcuticular stitches are preferable.

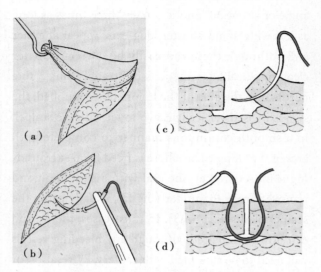

Fig. 52-3   **Ellipse removal and suture insertion. (a)** The ellipse is removed, one end being secured with a skin hook. **(b)** The suture needle is inserted vertically through the skin surface. **(c)** The suture needle pierces the full thickness of the epidermis and dermis. **(d)** The tied suture is 'flask' shaped and slightly everts the skin surface.

Incisional, punch and shave biopsies

An *incisional biopsy* is done for diagnostic purposes. The technique is similar to an excision except that less tissue is taken. A *punch biopsy* is a sharp circular blade, which is twisted and gently pushed into the skin to create a vertical cylindrical defect (normally 4mm in diameter). It is quick and easy to perform, and leaves only a small wound. The disadvantages include the potential for sampling error and the difficulty in stopping bleeding if a small arteriole is punctured at the base of the wound. Punch biopsy is used for removing small lesions or for diagnostic biopsies (Fig. 52-4).

Shave biopsy is employed for protuberant benign lesions, usually intradermal naevi or seborrhoeic warts. The lesion is shaved off parallel to, but slightly above, the skin surface. Haemostasis is achieved with cautery or hyfrecation. Not all the lesion is removed, and shaving is not used if malignancy is a possibility. Skin tags can be removed by simply snipping them off with scissors and cauterizing any bleeding points.

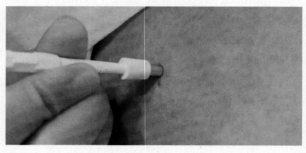

Fig. 52-4   **Punch biopsy.** After anaesthetizing, the skin is stretched at right angles to the tension lines, the punch blade is placed on the skin over the area to be biopsied and rotated under gentle pressure by rolling it between the thumb and the forefinger until it penetrates down to subcutaneous fat. The full-thickness cylinder of skin floats up and can be snipped off at the base. The defect is repaired with a single suture, cauterized or left to heal by secondary intention.

Curettage

Curettage is performed for seborrhoeic warts, pyogenic granulomas or single viral warts (e.g. on the face), but not for naevi or possibly malignant lesions. Basal cell carcinomas can be treated by repeated cycles of curettage and cautery but careful case selection is required. After being anaesthetized, the lesion is removed by a gentle scooping motion with the curette spoon or ring (Fig. 52-5), and then the base is cauterized. Curettings should be sent for histological analysis in 10% formalin.

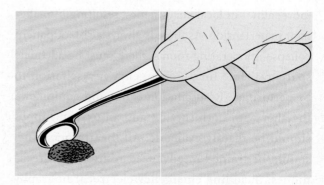

Fig. 52-5   **Curettage.** The lesion is removed using the curette spoon in a gentle scooping fashion. Most of the curettes now employed are disposable (use only once) ring curettes.

Other surgical techniques

Cautery

Cautery secures haemostasis and destroys tissue. The conventional cautery machine has an electrically heated wire and is self-sterilizing. The *Birtcher hyfrecator*, a unipolar diathermy, gives better controlled electrocautery. It is used to treat spider naevi and telangiectasia, and to give haemostasis, but should not routinely be employed in patients with cardiac pacemakers. Aluminium chloride 20% in an alcohol base (Driclor; Anhydrol Forte) or silver nitrate sticks provide chemical cautery.

Cryotherapy

Cryotherapy using liquid nitrogen is effective for viral warts, molluscum contagiosum, seborrhoeic warts, actinic keratoses, *in situ* squamous cell carcinoma and, in some instances, biopsy-proven basal cell carcinoma. The liquid nitrogen (at –196 ℃) is delivered by spray gun (e.g. Cry-Ac) or cotton wool bud and injures cells by ice formation.

Cryotherapy is believed to cause cell death in four ways. ① Ice crystals formed in the cell damage cellular components; ② Uneven intracellular ice formation during freezing leads to osmotic differences arising during thawing, which in turn causes cell disruption; ③ Cold injury to small blood vessels results in ischaemic damage; ④ Immunological stimulation produced by the release of antigenic components results in cell damage. The extent of injury is determined by the rate of freezing, the coldest temperature reached, the freeze time and the rate of thawing. Maximum damage is produced by rapid freezing and slow thawing. Repeating the freeze-thaw cycle produces much greater tissue damage than a single freeze because the greater conductivity of the previously frozen skin and the already impaired circulation both allow a greater and faster depth of cold penetration. It is suggested that a temperature of –30 ℃ is required to produce cell death. In practice tissue temperatures achieved during cryotherapy do not need to be measured because clinical studies have determined the duration of liquid nitrogen spray freeze times for common skin conditions.

After immersion in a flask containing liquid nitrogen, a cotton wool bud on a stick is applied to the lesion for about 10s until a thin frozen halo appears at the base. The spray gun is used from a distance of about 10mm for a similar length of freeze (Fig. 52-6). Longer freeze times are given for suitable malignant lesions. Blisters may develop within 24h. They are punctured and a dry dressing applied. Cryotherapy pain is significant but usually transient, and tissue swelling is common. Haemorrhagic blisters may occur but blister formation is not necessary for the cure of lesions such as viral warts. Skin necrosis is a desirable part of the treatment of neoplastic and many preneoplastic lesions, and several weeks may elapse before healing is complete. Hypopigmentation is common after liquid nitrogen cryosurgery, is particularly noticeable in dark-skinned patients and may be permanent. Temporary post-inflammatory hyperpigmentation is to be expected following less severe freezing. Nerve damage resulting in paraesthesiae, distal anaesthesia and motor paralysis occasionally occurs. Treatment is repeated after 4 weeks if necessary.

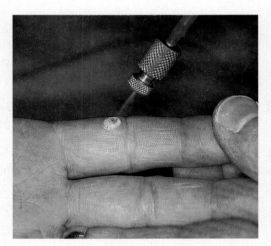

Fig. 52-6 **Liquid nitrogen treatment using a cryotherapy apparatus.**

Electrofulguration

These effects are produced using a monoterminal or unipolar electrode. Electrodesiccation occurs when the needle remains in contact with the skin and no spark occurs. Because the current concentration is greater at the point of contact, the tissue damage is deeper compared with electrofulguration. During the latter, the needle tip is not in contact with the skin and a spark jumps between the skin and the needle, but its energy is spread over a greater area. The resulting heat causes superficial damage to the tissues and is an effective way of stopping bleeding. Various needle tips have been developed for specific circumstances. Because of the risk of virus transmission, a different, clean needle must be used for each patient.

Basic dermatological surgery

- **Skin surgery** is best performed in an operating theatre with aseptic technique, adequate lighting and trained nurses.
- **Local anaesthetic**: 1% lidocaine with 1/200 000 adrenaline (epinephrine) is an adequate local anaesthetic for most sites.
- **Nylon or polypropylene sutures** should be used. Smallest diameter sutures are used on the face.
- **Histopathology** is performed on all biopsy material, which needs to be labelled carefully.
- **Excisions** are done as an ellipse, parallel to the crease marks, and are about three times as long as wide, with 30° angles at the ends.
- **Shave biopsy** is a technique suitable for the removal of benign naevi.
- **Punch biopsy** is a useful technique for removing small lesions or for full-thickness diagnostic biopsy.
- **Curettage** is a good treatment for seborrhoeic warts, single viral warts and pyogenic granulomas.
- **Cautery**, e.g. hyfrecation, secures haemostasis and destroys tissue.
- **Cryotherapy** is used for viral and seborrhoeic warts, premalignant conditions and some tumours.
- **Electrofulguration** causes superficial damage to the tissues and is an effective way of stopping bleeding.

Key words

local anaesthesia　局部麻醉
excision　切除术
shave biopsy　削切活检
punch biopsy　环钻活检
curettage　刮除术
cautery　电烙术
cryotherapy　冷冻疗法
liquid nitrogen　液氮
electrofulguration　电灼疗法

Review questions

1. What is the difference between skin tension lines and Langer's lines?
2. What is an ideal local anaesthetic agent?
3. What is the disadvantages of shave biopsy?
4. What types of basal cell carcinoma (BCC) should not be treated by curettage?
5. What is the buried suture?

(Weimin Shi)

Chapter 53 Advanced dermatological surgery

Some dermatologists specialize in the field of skin surgery. All registrars and residents in dermatology are trained in these techniques. An outline of the subject is given here, including the use of flaps, grafts and Mohs' surgery, along with mention of lasers and photodynamic therapy, and of some basic cosmetic procedures.

Simple plastic repairs

Simple plastic repairs are carried out by the following:

- *Dog-ear excision*: dog-ears are redundant tissue at the end of an excision line. In sites of high elasticity or where tissue conservation is critical, circular excision of the lesion with appropriate margins is preferable to a predetermined ellipse excision. The redundant skin is lifted like a tent using a skin hook then excised each side ('dog ears'), and the extended wound is sutured (Fig. 53-1).
- *M-plasty*: the M-plasty is an excision that reduces the length of an ellipse where space is limited, e.g. on the face. The 'M' end of the ellipse is formed by imagining one tip of the ellipse is folded in.

Skin flaps

Side-to-side ('direct') closure of a surgical defect is often possible by undermining the edges of the wound using scissors to free the tissue but, when this is not possible, a skin graft or flap is considered. The simplest types of flap are advancement and rotation:

- *Advancement flap*: in this, the skin flap is advanced in one direction over the defect. The flap of skin is created by making excision lines away from the defect to be covered, undermining to free the pedicle, advancing it into the defect and then suturing it in place (Fig. 53-2).
- *Rotation flap*: a defect may be covered by rotating in skin from one or multiple sides. The configura-

tion creates curved incisions along the border of wound extended as arc whose length is depending on the area of the defect and the elasticity of the skin at the body site (the scalp and dorsal hand

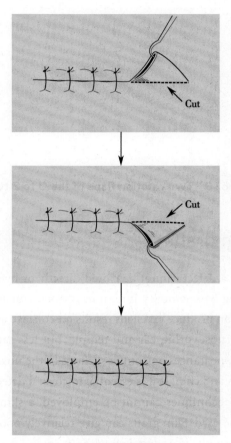

Fig. 53-1 **Dog-ear repair.**

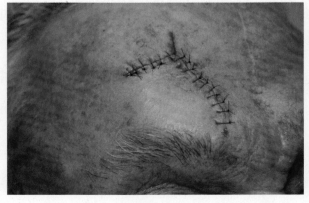

Fig. 53-2 **Advancement flap of the O to L type.**

are the least elastic). The pedicle is undermined, rotated in to the defect and sutured in place (Fig. 53-3).

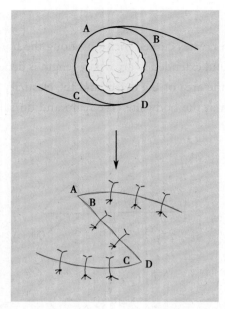

Fig. 53-3   **Two rotation flaps of the O to Z type.**

Skin grafts

When a defect cannot be closed directly or by a flap, healing by secondary intention is often considered. This can produce excellent results on concave aspects of the nose, orbit, ear and temple, but less satisfactory appearances on convex surfaces of the nose, lips, cheeks and chin. If it is essential to cover a defect and other techniques cannot be employed, a skin graft may be used. Skin grafts can give relatively poor cosmetic results if undertaken without careful planning and cause the added complication of creating two wounds. A graft is either full or split thickness:

- *Full thickness*: full-thickness skin is excised completely from the donor site, e.g. behind the ear, upper inner arm or abdomen, which is then sutured.
- *Split thickness*: in a spilt-thickness graft, the donor site skin is cut through the dermis leaving re-epithialization to occur from the epidermal cells of the hair follicles left behind. This method is usually used by plastic surgeons for covering large defects.

Mohs' micrographic surgery

Mohs' surgery describes an approach that maximizes tissue conservation by minimally excising skin cancers. Prior to skin closure, the narrowly excised tumour is examined microscopically. If the cancer is incompletely excised, the surgeon uses a mapping process to make further excisions until the margins are clear. It is indicated mostly for basal cell carcinomas that:

- are of the morphoeic type (clinical assessment of margins is unreliable)
- have recurred (scarring at site of previous excision can track tumour cells)
- have developed in embryonic folds, e.g. nasolabial site
- require tissue conservation as a priority (e.g. on the nose, around the eyes).

The bulk of the tumour is removed by curettage and then a saucer-like piece of skin is excised. This specimen is marked and flattened, and frozen sections are taken and read immediately by microscope, giving a 'map' that shows the extent of the tumour and the areas from which further excision is needed (Fig. 53-4). The defect is repaired conventionally, sometimes in collaboration with plastic surgeons. The cure rate is 98% for basal cell carcinoma.

Lasers and intense pulsed light (IPL)

The technology of *lasers* (*l*ight *a*mplification by *s*timulated *e*mission of *r*adiation) has advanced rapidly, and lasers can be used to treat vascular or pigmented lesions, tumours and tattoos and for hair removal. The variation in absorption of different wavelengths of light means that a range of different lasers is needed (Table 53-1). Laser therapy is carried out in specialized centres. Treatment is usually painful and several visits are often required. IPL treatment can be used for some conditions such as hair removal, and treatment is similar to laser but is a cheaper alternative. Fractional laser therapy refers to treatment of

Table 53-1 The application of commonly used lasers

Source type	Source	Wavelength peaks	Vascular lesions (red)	Pigmented lesions and tattoos	Hair removal	Wrinkles, facial scars, actinic damage	Benign lesion removal
Continuous wave	CO_2	10 600nm					Yes
Quasi-continuous wave	Potassium-titanyl-phosphate (KTP)	532nm	Yes				
	Copper vapour/bromide	510/578nm	Yes				
	Argon-pumped tunable dye (APTD)	577/585nm	Yes				
	Krypton	568nm	Yes				
Pulsed: long pulses or quality-switched (short pulses)	Pulsed dye laser (PDL)	585~595nm	Treatment of choice	Yellow, orange, red			
	Ruby	694nm			Yes		
	QS ruby	694nm		Black, blue-green			
	Alexandrite	755nm			Yes		
	QS alexandrite	755nm		Black, blue-green			
	Diode	810nm			Yes		
	QS neodymium (Nd): yttrium-aluminium-garnet (YAG)	1 064nm	Yes	Black, yellow, orange, red	Yes		
	Erbium:YAG	2 940nm				Yes	
	CO_2 (pulsed)	10 600nm				Yes	Yes
	Intense pulsed light	Non-laser			Yes		
Fractional (evolving field)	Erbium and others (non-ablative)	1 410~1 550nm				Yes	
	CO_2 and erbium:YAG (ablative)	2 940~10 600nm				Yes	

small zones within the target area patterned like the holes in a watering can rose.

Photodynamic therapy

Photodynamic therapy (PDT), in which the porphyrin precursor 5-amino-laevulinic acid is applied to a lesion that is then irradiated with visible or laser light, is very effective for extensive *in situ* squamous cell carcinoma, actinic keratoses and superficial basal cell carcinoma, and some other conditions.

Cosmetic procedures

Cosmetic procedures are part of the day-to-day practice of the average dermatologist in many countries, although not yet in the UK. Lasers are used extensively for telangiectasia or areas of pigmentation. Other procedures include botulinum toxins for wrinkles, dermabrasion, chemical peels, resurfacing and the use of fillers.

■ *Botulinum toxins*: injection of botulinum toxins into facial muscle paralyses the action of the mus-

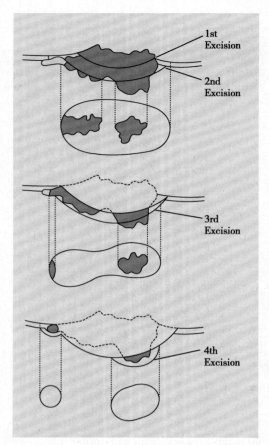

Fig. 53-4 **Mohs' micrographic surgery**. Microscopic examination of the removed saucer of skin shows where tumour is still present and indicates the sites at which further excision is required.

cle, thus reducing the prominence of frown lines. It is also used for axillary and sometimes palmar hyperhidrosis.

■ *Dermabrasion*: the technique of dermabrasion is used for the removal of pitted or depressed scars on the face. It involves abrasive planing in a sedated and prepared patient of the epidermis and superficial dermis using a high-speed rotary brush. Regeneration of the epidermis occurs rapidly due to abundant pilosebaceous structures.

■ *Laser resurfacing*: an erbium:YAG laser is used to remove the epidermis with minimal dermal damage, allowing regeneration of epidermis and the elimination of scars or photodamage.

■ *Chemical peels*: chemical peel is an alternative to dermabrasion to improve the appearance of photodamaged or wrinkled facial skin. Alpha-hydroxy acids or weak trichloroacetic acid solu-

tions are used.

■ *Fillers*: soft tissue defects, e.g. depressed scars or wrinkles, often on the face, may be corrected by the injection of biocompatible materials such as bovine collagen or hyaluronic acid derivatives.

■ *Body sculpturing*: removal of subcutaneous body fat by liposuction to produce a slimmer body shape has been widely used. However, newer approaches for lipotransfer and lipolysis by sub-cision, radiofrequency ablation and pharmaco-therapy are available.

■ *Hair transplant*: punch biopsies are taken from areas of normal hair density on the scalp. The hair follicles are dissected out one by one and inserted individually into areas of alopecia.

Advanced dermatological surgery

■ **Dog-ear excision** removes redundant tissue at the ends of an excision to give a better quality scar.
■ **Skin flaps** are used to repair a defect by the mobilization and advancement or rotation of skin.
■ **Skin grafts** are used to close a defect, but secondary intention healing may give a better cosmetic result.
■ **Mohs' surgery** describes the microscopically controlled serial excision of difficult-to-treat skin cancers, giving a high cure rate.
■ **Lasers** are used to treat vascular or pigmented skin lesions, tattoos, some skin cancers and for hair removal.
■ **Photodynamic therapy** is a very effective method of treating widespread *in situ* squamous cell carcinomas, actinic keratosis and condyloma acuminate.
■ **Cosmetic procedures** are increasingly seen as part of dermatological practice in many countries.

Web resource

http://www.bsds.org.uk/

Key words

Mohs' micrographic surgery　莫氏显微手术
photodynamic therapy　光动力治疗
skin grafts　皮肤移植
laser　激光
intense pulsed light (IPL)　强脉冲光
botulinum toxin　肉毒毒素
laser resurfacing　激光换肤

dermabrasion　皮肤磨削术
hair transplant　毛发移植

Review questions

1. What is the common application of Botulinum toxins in dermatology?

2. Which are the common sites where full thickness skin graft acquired?

(Xiuli Wang)

Chapter 54   New trends in dermatological treatment

Therapeutic advances have revolutionized the treatment of skin disease over the last 40 years. The 1960s saw the introduction of topical steroids, the 1970s the development of psoralen with ultraviolet A (PUVA), the 1980s retinoids, and the 1990s lasers and ciclosporin. The major advance of the 'noughties' was the biologics.

There have been changes in the delivery of care. Over the last two decades, the number of inpatient dermatology beds has fallen dramatically and in some places disappeared altogether. Patients who would have been admitted are now managed as outpatients with potent drugs. Nurse practitioners have a higher profile and run their own clinics, e.g. for patients with leg ulcers, eczema or psoriasis, prescribe treatments and perform surgical procedures.

Atopic eczema

The topical immunomodulators (calcineurin inhibitors) *tacrolimus* (Protopic) and *pimecrolimus* (Elidel) are alternatives to topical steroids and do not cause skin atrophy (Fig. 54-1). The systemic immunosuppressors may be beneficial in severe atopic eczema. Recently, biologics including monoclonal antibodies targeting IL-4, IL-13 and IL-31 have been shown to be promising treatments for atopic eczema.

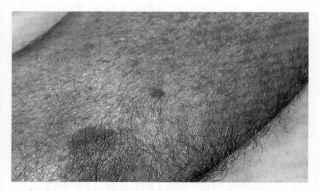

Fig. 54-1   **Skin atrophy with purpura due to excessive topical use of a potent steroid.**

Bullous diseases

Intravenous *immunoglobulin* is used for severe pemphigus or mucous membrane pemphigoid. The biologic *rituximab* has been used in resistant cases. Oral doxycycline may be effective in pemphigoid.

Cutaneous T cell lymphoma

The retinoid receptor agonist *bexarotene* (Targretin) is effective in some patients with cutaneous T cell lymphoma. *Photophoresis*, in which a lymphocyte-enriched blood fraction from the patient who has taken a psoralen is exposed to UVA outside the body and then re-infused, is sometimes effective, especially for the Sézary syndrome.

Erythema nodosum

Thalidomide can be considered in unresponsive cases. A pregnancy prevention programme is required in women of child-bearing age owing to the known teratogenic effects. Thalidomide may also be beneficial in Behçet's disease and recurrent erythema multiforme.

Fungal infections

Terbinafine (Lamisil) cream, applied once or twice daily for 1 week, cures tinea pedis (Fig. 54-2). Pulse treatment with oral *itraconazole* (Sporanox), *terbinafine* (Lamisil) or *fluconazole* (Diflucan) has given cure rates of 80% for fungal infection of the toenails. Three-weekly pulses of *terbinafine* (Lamisil) given over 8 weeks produce a 90% cure rate for childhood tinea capitis (Fig. 54-3).

Hand dermatitis

Alitretinoin (Toctino), an oral retinoid, was recently introduced as the first systemic treatment approved for use in severe chronic hand dermatitis unresponsive to potent topical steroid treatment, provided the

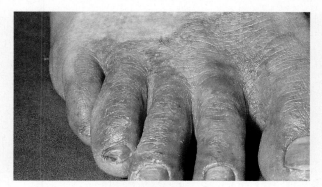

Fig. 54-2 **Tinea pedis.**

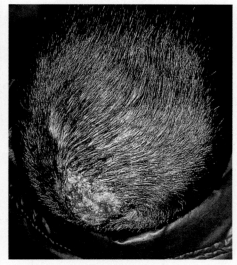

Fig. 54-3 **Kerion with associated alopecia.** The boggy pustular lesion results from a zoophilic fungal infection.

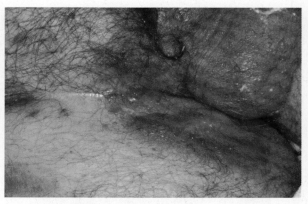

Fig. 54-4 **Hidradenitis suppurativa.** Multiple inflammatory nodules are evident. Scarring is common.

patient satisfies the criteria of severity and impaired quality of life (DLQI) score. In women of child-bearing potential, a pregnancy-prevention programme is followed as alitretinoin is teratogenic. The most common side-effect is headaches. Regular monitoring of blood lipids and thyroid function is required.

Hidradenitis suppurativa

Hidradenitis suppurativa is characterized by abscesses, sinuses and scars in the axillae and groin (Fig. 54-4) and is very difficult to treat. *Acitretin* is helpful in suitable patients, as can be the combination of the antibiotics *clindamycin* and *rifampicin*. Recently, *infliximab* infusion has been used with success.

Hyperhidrosis

The injection of *botulinum toxin A* into the axillary or palmar skin will control excessive sweating in these areas, but needs to be repeated every 9 months.

Leg ulcers

Larval therapy with sterile maggots (LarvE) can be used for managing sloughy leg ulcers. *Recombinant platelet-derived growth factor* is licensed for use in neuropathic ulcers, e.g. in diabetes. *Tissue-engineered skin equivalents*, e.g. Apligraf, can be effective in therapy-resistant wounds.

Psoriasis

The biologics have revolutionized the treatment of severe psoriasis. Other systemic approaches to consider in difficult to manage cases where biologics may be contraindicated or have failed include the fumaric acid esters and mycophenolate mofetil. Recently, small molecule inhibitors have been proven to be effective for psoriasis.

Scabies

Ivermectin, a drug used to treat onchocerciasis, may be effective for scabies, especially of the crusted (Norwegian) type and for use in institutional outbreaks.

Scleroderma

Topical *calcipotriene* (0.005%) has been shown to improve lesions of localized scleroderma (morphoea). Oral *methotrexate* is beneficial in certain types of morphoea, e.g. en coup de sabre. Systemic sclerosis (Fig. 54-5) can respond to *photophoresis* (see above) and *PUVA*.

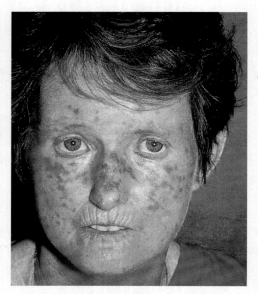

Fig. 54-5 **Systemic sclerosis of the face.** Telangiectasia and furrowing around the mouth are prominent changes.

Skin cancer

Topical use of the immunomodulator *imiquimod* and photodynamic therapy are effective for actinic keratosis, *in situ* squamous cell carcinoma and superficial basal cell carcinoma. 'Sentinel' lymph node biopsy is now becoming an accepted part of management of patients with malignant melanoma of greater than 1mm Breslow thickness. *Dacarbazine* and *interferon-* are used in the chemotherapy of metastatic malignant melanoma. The use of ipilimumab, a biologic that blocks cytotoxic T cell-associated antigen 4, is being studied in patients with metastatic malignant melanoma.

Toxic epidermal necrolysis

The use of high-dose intravenous *immunoglobulin* (1~2 g/kg daily for 34 days), started early, may be helpful in toxic epidermal necrolysis.

Vitiligo

The *Excimer 308-nm laser* (Fig. 54-6) is effective in the treatment of localized areas of vitiligo affecting the cosmetically sensitive sites, e.g. the face.

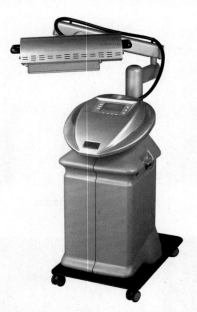

Fig. 54-6 **The Excimer 308-nm laser.** It can be used for treating localized areas of vitiligo, psoriasis or cutaneous T cell lymphoma.

Web resource

http://www.nice.org.uk/

Key words

psoralen 补骨脂素
ultraviolet 紫外线
retinoid 类视黄醇
laser 激光
cyclosporin 环孢素
biologics 生物制剂
immunomodulator 免疫调节剂
calcineurin inhibitor 钙调磷酸酶抑制药
immunoglobulin 免疫球蛋白
photophoresis 体外光化学疗法
thalidomide 沙利度胺
alitretinoin 阿利维甲酸
botulinum toxin A A型肉毒毒素
larval therapy 蛆虫疗法
recombinant platelet-derived growth factor 重组血小板衍生生长因子
tissue-engineered skin equivalents 组织工程皮肤类似物
Ivermectin 依维菌素
calcipotriene 卡泊三醇
methotrexate 氨甲蝶呤

New trends in dermatological treatment

Disease	Topical therapy	Systemic therapy
Atopic eczema	Pimecrolimus, tacrolimus	Mycophenolate, methotrexate, Biologics
Bullous disease	–	Immunoglobulin, rituximab, doxycycline
Cutaneous T cell lymphoma	–	Bexarotene, photophoresis
Erythema nodosum	–	Thalidomide
Fungal infection	Terbinafine	Pulse itraconazole, terbinafine, fluconazole
Hand dermatitis	–	Alitretinoin
Hidradenitis suppurativa	–	Acitretin, clindamycin/rifampicin, infliximab
Hyperhidrosis	Botulinum toxin (intralesional)	–
Leg ulcer	Sterile larvae, skin equivalent	–
Psoriasis	–	Biologics, fumaric acid esters, mycophenolate mofetil, small molecule inhibitors
Scabies	–	Ivermectin
Scleroderma	Calcipotriene	Methotrexate, photophoresis
Skin cancer	Imiquimod (superficial basal cell carcinoma)	Dacarbazine/interferon- (malignant melanoma)
Toxic epidermal necrolysis	–	Immunoglobulin
Vitiligo	–	Excimer laser

imiquimod　咪喹莫特

photodynamic therapy　光动力疗法

excimer laser　准分子激光器

Review questions

1. What are the new treatments for atopic eczema?

2. List the treatments for fungal infections.

3. Which drug has brought a great change of the treatment for severe psoriasis?

4. What diseases can be treated with retinoids?

(Yi Zhao)

Chapter 55 Paediatric dermatology

Some conditions are almost exclusive to childhood (e.g. napkin dermatitis and juvenile plantar dermatosis), and others are more common in children (e.g. atopic eczema or viral exanthems). The common childhood dermatoses not mentioned elsewhere are detailed here along with some rare but important disorders.

Childhood eczemas and related disorders

Forms of eczema found in childhood include:

- Napkin (diaper) dermatitis
- Infantile seborrhoeic dermatitis
- Candidiasis
- Juvenile plantar dermatosis
- Napkin psoriasis
- Atopic eczema
- Pityriasis alba

Napkin (diaper) dermatitis

Napkin dermatitis is the commonest type of napkin eruption. It is usually seen in infants who are only a few weeks old, and is rare after the age of 12 months. It is an irritant dermatitis due to the macerating effect of prolonged contact of the skin with faeces and urine. A glazed erythema is seen in the napkin area, sparing the skin folds. Erosions or ulceration may follow (Fig. 55-1), and hypopigmentation is a complication in pigmented skin. Secondary bacterial or *Candida albicans* infection is frequent, and the latter may account for the development of erythematous papules or pustules.

The *differential diagnosis* is from infantile seborrhoeic eczema and candidiasis, both of which tend to affect the flexures. The treatment of napkin dermatitis is aimed at keeping the area dry. The use of disposable super-absorbent nappies helps, as may more frequent changes. A bland white soft paraffin is used, with aqueous cream as a soap substitute, and

a silicone-based cream (e.g. Drapolene) may have a protective action. Topical 1% hydrocortisone, with an antifungal (e.g. Daktacort or Canesten-HC), is also effective.

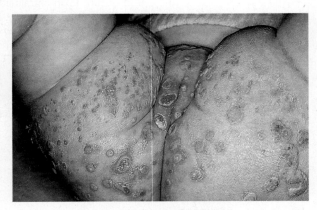

Fig. 55-1 **Napkin dermatitis.** A severe erosive variant is seen here.

Infantile seborrhoeic eczema

Infantile seborrhoeic eczema starts in the first few weeks of life and tends to affect the body folds, including the axillae, groin and neck, but it also may involve the face and scalp. Flexural lesions present as moist, shiny, well-demarcated scaly erythema (Fig. 55-2), but a yellowish crust is often found on the scalp. The condition can usually be differentiated from *napkin dermatitis* (which spares the flexures), *candidiasis* (which is usually pustular) and *atopic*

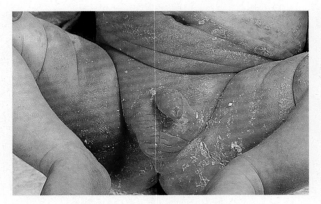

Fig. 55-2 **Infantile seborrhoeic eczema.** The condition involves the flexures.

eczema (which is more pruritic, although differentiation can be difficult in some cases). Infantile seborrhoeic eczema is treated by emollients and 1% hydrocortisone ointment, or with a hydrocortisone-antifungal combination. Scalp lesions respond to 2% ketoconazole shampoo. Olive oil will help to soften the scalp scales of cradle cap.

Candidiasis

Infection with *C. albicans* is relatively common in the neonatal period. The organism can also secondarily complicate infantile seborrhoeic eczema or napkin dermatitis. Erythema, scaling and pustules are seen, often involving the flexures, and there may be satellite lesions. Treatment is with a topical anticandidal agent, e.g. 2% ketoconazole cream, and 2% miconazole gel orally.

Juvenile plantar dermatosis

Juvenile plantar dermatosis, first recognized in 1968, presents with red, dry, fissured and glazed skin, principally over the forefeet but sometimes involving the whole sole (Fig. 55-3). It usually starts in the primary school years and resolves spontaneously in the early to mid teens. The condition is thought to be linked to the wearing of socks and shoes made from synthetic materials, although it may be a manifestation of atopy in some children. It is usual to advise cotton socks and less occlusive footwear, preferably made of leather. Topical steroids are ineffective but emollients help.

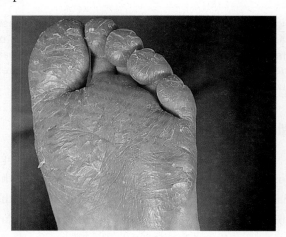

Fig. 55-3   **Juvenile plantar dermatosis.** The forefoot is mainly affected.

Other childhood dermatoses

Some uncommon but characteristic eruptions are found in childhood. These include:

- Urticaria pigmentosa
- Langerhans cell histiocytosis
- Kawasaki disease and other viral infections
- Ichthyosis
- Epidermolysis bullosa

Urticaria pigmentosa

Urticaria pigmentosa is characterized by multiple reddish-brown macules or papules on the trunk and limbs of an infant. The lesions may become red, swollen and itchy after a bath or when rubbed, and blistering may occur. Histologically, there are accumulations of mast cells in the dermis. The disorder normally resolves spontaneously before adolescence. There is a form with a later onset, usually beginning in adolescence or adult life, which rarely resolves and may involve internal organs - something that is rare in the childhood variety.

Langerhans cell histiocytosis (histiocytosis X)

Langerhans cell histiocytosis is a rare and serious condition that normally involves internal organs. The skin signs are common, variable and include a seborrhoeic-like dermatitis, papules or pustules on the trunk and ulceration, particularly of the flexures. The skin, abdominal organs, lungs and bones are infiltrated by clonal Langerhans cells, which may behave in a malignant fashion, although the condition is believed to be reactive and not a true malignancy. Skin biopsy is usually diagnostic. The prognosis is poorer when the onset is before 2 years of age.

Vascular naevi

Vascular naevi are common and are present at birth or develop soon after. Superficial lesions are due to capillary networks in the upper or mid dermis, but larger angiomas show multiple vascular channels in the lower dermis and subcutis.

Clinical presentation

There are four main clinical pictures, which are described below.

Salmon patch

This is the commonest vascular naevus, seen in 20%~ 60% of neonates. Patches at the upper eyelid fade quickly, but the 'stork mark' at the posterior neck persists in 20%~30% of cases. Parents should be reassured: no investigation or treatment is required.

Port wine stain

Present at birth, the port wine stain (or *naevus flammeus*) is an irregular red or purple macule that often affects one side of the face (Fig. 55-4), although other sites can be affected. Lesions vary from millimetres to centimetres in diameter. In middle age, it can darken and become lumpy. A port wine stain involving the ophthalmic division of the trigeminal nerve may have an associated intracranial vascular malformation (the *Sturge-Weber syndrome*). Port wine stains near the eye can be associated with glaucoma.

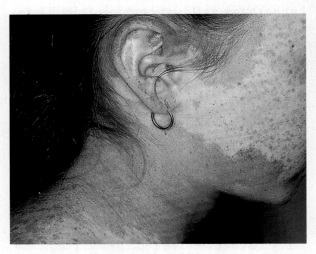

Fig. 55-4 **Port wine stain naevus.** These are often present at birth. Neurological and ophthalmological assessments may be needed. Early treatment with a flashlamp-pulsed dye laser is often recommended.

Arteriovenous malformation (AVM)

Aberrant vascular channels may occur in the skin, subcutis or deeper structures. Arteriovenous fistulae can be found, e.g. in a limb, and hypertrophy of the involved part sometimes is seen.

Infantile haemangioma

Infantile haemangiomas appear shortly after birth. Most occur on the head or neck and grow to reach a maximum in the first 12 months (Fig. 55-5). They remain static for the next 6~12 months and then involute. Most cases will have regressed by the age of 5~7 years, leaving an area of atrophy. Infantile haemangiomas are classified as superficial (e.g. strawberry naevus), deep or mixed, and can be localized or segmental. The deep type, e.g. cavernous haemangioma, is composed of larger and deeper vascular channels and presents as a nodular bluish swelling. The overlying skin may be normal or show a superficial vascular component (i.e. be mixed). Regression is not as complete as in the superficial type. Ulceration with bleeding and secondary infection can develop. Large haemangiomas may trap platelets and cause thrombocytopenia (the *Kasabach-Merritt syndrome*). In segmental haemangiomas, abnormalities in the underlying organs should be suspected.

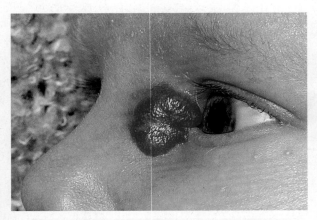

Fig. 55-5 **Strawberry naevus in an infant.** These haemangiomas develop during the first few weeks of life but often involute by the age of 5~7 years. Treatment is needed if they compromise vital structures such as the eye.

Management

Port wine stains may be covered with camouflage cosmetics, but treatment is now available with the flashlamp-pulsed dye laser, which obliterates the abnormal dermal vessels and improves the appearance. A child with a facial port wine stain needs neurological and ophthalmic assessment. An AVM

Paediatric dermatology

Disorder	Age at onset	Clinical features
Napkin dermatitis	First few weeks to 12 months	Glazed erythema that spares body folds
		Erosions may occur
Infantile seborrhoeic eczema	First few weeks	Moist scaly erythema
		Flexures and scalp affected
Candidiasis	Infancy	Erythema, with scaling and pustules
		Flexures affected
		Secondary infection found
Juvenile plantar dermatosis	School age to mid teens	Glazed red fissured skin on the forefeet and soles
Urticaria pigmentosa	Mostly at 3~9 months	Reddish-brown macules or papules on trunk, which urticate when rubbed
Langerhans cell histiocytosis	All ages (different types)	Seborrhoeic-like dermatitis, papules/pustules, ulceration
Vascular naevi	At birth, in first few weeks	Salmon patch on neck, port wine naevus (e.g. on face), strawberry naevus

requires the opinion of a vascular surgeon. Infantile haemagiomas should be allowed to involute unless they compromise vital structures such as the eye or airway. In this case, a short course of propranolol, prednisolone or even emergency surgery is needed. The Kasabach-Merritt syndrome is treated in a similar fashion. Haemangiomas at the lower back may have associated tethering of the spinal cord; a neurological assessment and imaging are indicated.

Web resource

http://www.emedicinehealth.com/skin_rashes_in_children/article_em.htm

Key words

napkin (diaper) dermatitis　尿布皮炎

infantile seborrhoeic dermatitis　婴幼儿脂溢性皮炎

candidiasis　念珠菌病

juvenile plantar dermatosis　青少年跖部皮病

napkin psoriasis　尿布区银屑病

atopic eczema　特应性湿疹

pityriasis alba　白色糠疹

urticaria pigmentosa　色素性荨麻疹

Langerhans cell histiocytosis　朗格罕斯细胞组织细胞增生症

Kawasaki disease　川崎病

ichthyosis　鱼鳞病

epidermolysis bullosa　大疱性表皮松解症

salmon patch　鲑鱼斑

port wine stain　鲜红斑痣

arteriovenous malformation　动静脉畸形

infantile haemangioma　婴幼儿血管瘤

thrombocytopenia　血小板减少

Review questions

1. Describe the features of napkin dermatitis.
2. What are the differential diagnoses for infantile seborrheic eczema?
3. What is the pathogen for candidiasis?
4. Describe the features of urticaria pigmentosa.
5. How to manage port-wine stains?

(Yi Zhao)

Chapter 56　The skin in old age

Poor nutrition, lack of self-care and general illness contribute to skin disease in the elderly. Few people die from old skin, but many suffer from it.

Intrinsic ageing of the skin

The changes in aged, sun-protected skin are more subtle than those of photoageing and consist of laxity, fine wrinkling and benign neoplasms. In addition, androgenetic alopecia and greying of the hair are age related.

Histologically, the epidermis is thinned with the loss of the rete ridge pattern and a reduction in the numbers of melanocytes and Langerhans cells. Individual epidermal cells are smaller. The dermis is thinned due, mainly, to loss of proteoglycans. Functionally, the skin is less elastic and has a reduced tensile strength. Resistance to injury, irritants and infection is reduced, and wound healing is slower.

Some inherited disorders, e.g. pseudoxanthoma elasticum, show features of aged skin. The misuse of potent topical steroids induces atrophy and purpura, signs also seen in old skin.

Dermatoses in the elderly

Few skin conditions are exclusive to old age, but some are seen more frequently (Table 56-1).

Dry skin and asteatotic eczema

Dryness with itching is common in elderly skin. It may be a mild roughness and scaling, or more severe, with fissuring and inflammation (asteatotic eczema). The changes often occur on the legs and are aggravated by low humidity, central heating and excessive washing. Emollients, sometimes with a mild or moderate potency topical steroid ointment, usually help.

Seborrhoeic dermatitis in the elderly (Fig. 56-1) may be flexural and resemble psoriasis, candidiasis or

Table 56-1	**Skin disorders common in the elderly**
The eczemas	Asteatotic/dry skin
	Seborrhoeic
	Contact
	Venous
Other eruptions	Psoriasis
	Drug eruption
	Erythema ab igne
Infections	Herpes zoster
	Candidiasis
	Onychomycosis
	Scabies
Ulceration	Leg ulcer
	Pressure ulcer
Autoimmune	Pemphigoid
Benign tumours	Seborrhoeic wart
	Cherry angioma
	Skin tag
	Chondrodermatitis nodularis
Photodamage	Photoageing
	Actinic elastosis
Premalignant	Actinic keratosis
	In situ squamous cell carcinoma
Cancers	Basal cell carcinoma
	Squamous cell carcinoma
	Lentigo malignant melanoma
	Cutaneous T cell lymphoma
Other	Senile pruritus

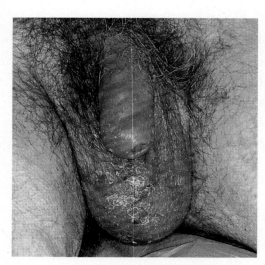

Fig. 56-1　**Flexural seborrhoeic dermatitis affecting the scrotum and penis.**

erythrasma. In old people, *allergic contact dermatitis* to allergens in topical medicaments or toiletries, e.g. lanolin, neomycin, fragrances and local anaesthetics, particularly needs to be considered.

Pruritus

Itch in old age can be severe and unrelenting. Examination will usually show asteatotic eczema, scabies, urticaria or the prebullous phase of pemphigoid, or investigations may reveal renal or liver disease or underlying malignancy. The small group of patients in whom no cause is found have 'senile pruritus'. Topical treatments and sedating antihistamines are often ineffective.

Psoriasis

Psoriasis has its peak onset in the teens with a second peak in the sixth decade. In the elderly patient, it is frequently flexural, but all patterns, except guttate, are seen. Methotrexate is used quite often and is mostly well tolerated.

Infections and infestations

Herpes zoster at some time affects 25% of people over 65. Post-herpetic neuralgia increases with age, occurring in 75% of shingles victims over 70. Early treatment with antivirals (e.g. aciclovir) together with amitriptyline or gabapentin makes neuralgia less likely.

Infection with *Candida albicans* is common in the flexures of obese elderly women. *Onychomycosis* is a frequent incidental finding in old people, especially men. Treatment is not always needed unless the nail produces pain.

Scabies epidemics are a problem in old people's homes and are difficult to control. Any itchy old person should be examined carefully, as burrows are easily missed. Elderly patients who are debilitated, paralysed, immunosuppressed or who cannot scratch may develop crusted 'Norwegian' scabies (Fig. 56-2), which is highly contagious due to the thousands of mites present.

Photodamage and skin tumours

Most benign and malignant skin tumours are more

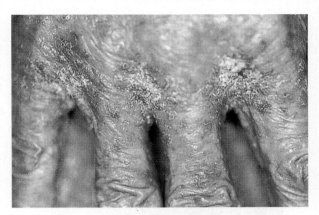

Fig. 56-2   **Crusted 'Norwegian' scabies.**

common in the elderly (Table 56-1). Many are related to sun exposure. Specific disorders of photodamage include:

- *Actinic (solar) keratoses*: these are single or multiple, discrete, scaly, hyperkeratotic, rough-surfaced areas, usually less than 1cm in diameter. They are seen on sun-exposed sites, especially the dorsal aspects of the hands, face and neck (Fig. 56-3). They are most common in those with a fair skin.

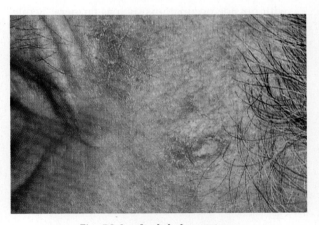

Fig. 56-3   **Actinic keratoses.**

Histologically, they show hyperkeratosis, abnormal keratinocytes with loss of maturation and dermal elastosis. Actinic keratoses may regress spontaneously. However, they can progress to squamous cell carcinoma, although this is relatively uncommon. Treatment is normally by cryosurgery, but certain lesions may be best treated with curettage, excision or by applying 5% fluorouracil cream (Efudix) once or twice daily for 3~4 weeks, 3% diclofenac gel (Solaraze) twice daily for 60~90 days or imiquimod (Aldara). Photodynamic therapy is a useful option in widespread ('field') actinic damage.

A *cutaneous horn* may occasionally develop in an actinic keratosis (Fig. 56-4). It is best treated by excision.

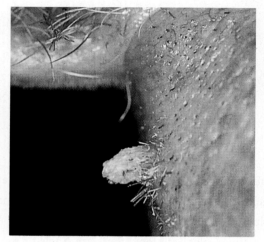

Fig. 56-4 **A cutaneous horn.**

■ *Actinic (solar) elastosis*: in solar elastosis, the sun-exposed skin is yellowed, thickened and wrinkled. On the neck, furrowed rhomboidal patterns are sometimes seen (Fig. 56-5), particularly in those with outside occupations such as farmers. 'Senile' comedones or thickened yellowish plaques may develop. Photodamage is worse in smokers.

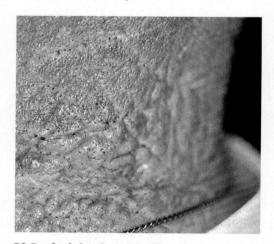

Fig. 56-5 **Actinic elastosis.** The characteristic rhomboid pattern is seen on the neck, associated with senile comedones. A history of chronic sun exposure, often occupational, is invariably obtained.

■ Damaged dermal collagen with inflammation in the dermis and cartilage is a feature of *chondrodermatitis nodularis* (Fig. 56-6). Treatment is by excision, although some early lesions can be halted by topical glucocorticoid treatment.

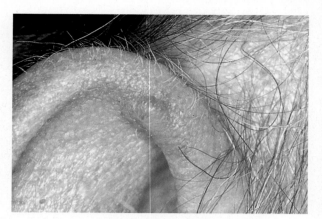

Fig. 56-6 **Chrondrodermatitis nodularis.**

■ *Actinic cheilitis*: excessive exposure to sun, often occupational, can induce inflammation and scaling of the lower lip. Treatment options are the same as for actinic keratoses. Diagnostic histology is recommended in thickened, tender or new lesions because squamous cell carcinoma can be missed.

Ulceration

■ *Leg ulcers*: venous ulcers often start in middle age but, because of their chronicity, are a problem in the elderly. Ischaemic ulcers become more common with advancing years.

■ *Pressure ulcers*: a pressure ulcer starts as an area of erythema and progresses to widespread necrosis of tissue with ulceration. Deep ulcers develop over the sacrum (Fig. 56-7), heels, ischia and greater trochanters. Secondary infection with *Pseudomonas aeruginosa* is common.

Pressure ulcers mainly occur in the elderly who are recumbent and immobile, e.g. due to a fractured femur, arthritis, unconsciousness or paraplegia. Malnutrition, reduced cutaneous sensation and arterial disease predispose to tissue breakdown.

Prevention is possible if at-risk patients are identified. Regular repositioning, the use of an anti-pressure mattress and attention to diet and to the patient's general condition help in prevention and treatment. A necrotic eschar separates by itself in 2~4 weeks. The resulting ulcer can be covered by a semi-permeable dressing, e.g. Opsite. Proteolytic enzymes (Varidase) may be used to debride heel lesions. Pain relief is vital. Surgical excision and flap repair are possible provided the patient's general condition is satisfactory.

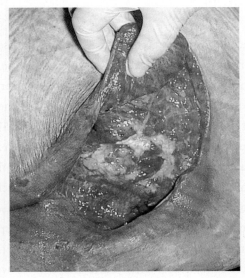

Fig. 56-7   **Pressure ulcer over the sacrum.**

> *The skin in old age*
> ■ **Asteatotic eczema** (also known as eczéma craquelé) is a dry, scaly, fissured eruption that commonly affects the elderly. Treatment is with emollients and mild topical steroids.
> ■ **Pruritus** in old people nearly always has a cause. Scabies, urticaria or prebullous pemphigoid are easily missed. Investigation for underlying systemic disease may be indicated.
> ■ **Herpes zoster** is common in old age. Aciclovir or famciclovir may make neuralgia less likely.
> ■ **Actinic keratoses** are roughened hyperkeratotic areas in sun-exposed sites. They are often treated by cryosurgery or the application of fluorouracil cream or diclofenac gel.
> ■ **Actinic elastosis** is a yellowed, thickened, wrinkled change in sun-exposed skin, e.g. on the neck, often seen in men who have had outdoor occupations.
> ■ **Pressure ulcers** result from reduced sensation, immobility, malnutrition and ischaemia. It is vital to identify at-risk patients and institute means to prevent these ulcers from developing.

Key words

intrinsic ageing   内源性老化

photoageing   光老化

asteatotic eczema   乏脂性湿疹

pruritus   瘙痒

actinic keratosis   光化性角化病

actinic elastosis   光线性弹性组织变性

pressure ulcer   压力性溃疡

benign tumour   良性肿瘤

cutaneous horn   皮角

cancer   肿瘤

Review questions

1. Please give examples of dermatoses in the elderly.
2. Please illustrate the clinical manifestation of actinic keratoses.

(Bingxue Bai)

Chapter 57 Genitourinary medicine

In the UK and Ireland, genitourinary medicine has traditionally been a separate specialty from dermatology, but the two are combined as 'dermatovenereology' in many countries. It has become increasingly important for those treating skin disease to know more about genitourinary disorders. Genitourinary diseases range as follows (see also Table 57-1): syphilis, gonorrhoea, human immunodeficiency virus (HIV) infection, chlamydial infection, pelvic inflammatory disease, vaginitis, chancroid viral warts, genital herpes simplex, hepatitis B and hepatitis C, vulval/perianal dermatoses, penile/scrotal dermatoses.

Syphilis (lues)

Syphilis is a chronic infectious disease due to *Treponema pallidum*. Skin signs are seen in all three stages.

Clinical presentation

T. pallidum may rarely be acquired congenitally or from a contaminated blood transfusion, but the normal mode of transmission is through sexual intercourse.

- *Primary chancre.* About 3 weeks after sexual contact, a primary chancre, a painless ulcerated button-like indurated papule, develops at the site of inoculation. This is usually genital (Fig. 57-1), but oral and anal chancres are seen in men who have sex with men. Regional lymphadenopathy is common. Without treatment, the chancre clears spontaneously in 3~10 weeks. Serology is not positive until 4 weeks after infection, but spirochaetes can be isolated from the chancre.

- *Secondary stage.* This phase starts 4~10 weeks after the onset of the chancre. It is characterized by a non-itchy pink or copper-coloured papular eruption on the trunk, limbs, palms and soles.

- *Tertiary stage.* About 30% of patients with untreated syphilis will develop late lesions, usually after a latent period of years. Painless nodules, sometimes with scaling, develop in annular or arcuate patterns on the face or back. Subcutaneous gran-

Table 57-1	**Other genitourinary infections**		
Condition	**Organisms**	**Clinical features**	**Therapy**
Non-gonococcal urethritis	*Chlamydia trachomatis Ureaplasma urealyticum Mycoplasma genitalium*	Males: dysuria, frequency, urethral discharge or asymptomatic	Single dose of azithromycin 1g orally or doxycycline 100mg twice daily for 7 days or eryrthromycin
Chlamydial muco-purulent cervicitis	*Chlamydia trachomatis* (exclude *Neisseria gonorrhoeae*)	Females: asymptomatic or yellow cervical exudate	Single dose of azithromycin 1g orally or doxycycline 100mg twice daily for 7 days or eryrthromycin
Pelvic inflammatory disease	*Chlamydia trachomatis Neisseria gonorrhoeae* Anaerobes *Gardnerella vaginalis Mycoplasma genitalium*	Acute abdominal pain and tenderness, fever, raised white blood cell count	Intramuscular ceftriaxone followed by oral doxycycline *plus* metronidazole or oral ofloxacin *plus* metronidazole for 14 days
Vaginitis	*Trichomonas vaginalis Gardnerella vaginalis Bacteroides C. albicans*	Asymptomatic or erythema, itch and discharge: male partners get urethritis and balanitis	Trichomonal/bacterial - oral metronidazole for 7 days; anticandidal topicals
Chancroid	*Haemophilus ducreyi*	Single or multiple tender, necrotic, erosive ulcers	Azithromycin (oral) or ceftriaxone (IM) or ciprofloxacin (oral) or erythromycin (oral)
Hepatitis B	Hepatitis B virus	Only one-third to one-half show symptoms of acute hepatitis	Vaccinate at-risk groups; interferon-α, lamivudine, adefovir and other antiviral agents

ulomatous gumma - usually on the face, neck or calf-, scar and never heal completely (Fig. 57-2). Cardiovascular syphilis and neurosyphilis may coexist.

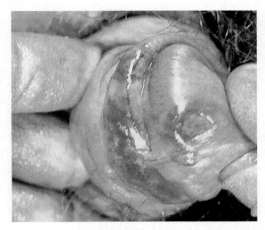

Fig. 57-1 **Primary chancre of syphilis.**

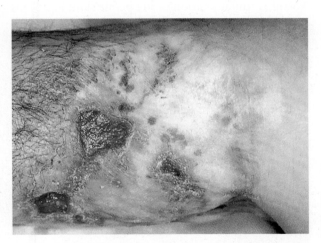

Fig. 57-2 **Gumma of tertiary syphilis.**

Management

Primary or secondary syphilis is treated with a single dose of benzathine penicillin G or procaine penicillin intramuscularly daily for 10 days as first-line therapy. Doxycycline, azithromycin and erythromycin are alternatives. Patients need contact tracing and assessment for other venereal diseases, and should be managed in a genitourinary medicine department.

Gonorrhoea

Gonorrhoea is caused by the Gram-negative diplococcus *Neisseria gonorrhoeae*. Infection may be symptomatic or asymptomatic.

Clinical presentation

Symptomatic males usually present with dysuria, frequency of micturition and a purulent urethral discharge. Females, when symptomatic, can have an abnormal vaginal discharge, dysuria, intermenstrual bleeding, menorrhagia or abdominal pain. Pharyngeal and anorectal infection may produce symptoms, or may be asymptomatic. The diagnosis relies on the microscopic identification of Gram-negative intracellular diplococci from urethral (males and females) or endocervical (females) smears, and culture for *N. gonorrhoeae*. Serological tests are unreliable. Women with untreated gonorrhoea are at risk of developing pelvic inflammatory disease and infertility. In men, complications include urethral stricture, infertility and epididymitis.

Gonococcaemia is rare but, when observed, results in fever, arthritis and pustules that are few in number and generally distributed on the hands, feet or near the large joints. This is a type of septic vasculitis which, like some other systemic infections (e.g. *Neisseria meningitidis*), may be purpuric.

Management

Uncomplicated acute gonorrhoea should be treated with single-dose cefixime (oral) or ceftriaxone (intramuscular) for pharyngeal infections. Single doses of ciprofloxacin or ofloxacin are alternatives as determined by microbiological sensitivities. Infection acquired abroad should be presumed to be multi-antibiotic resistant. Pharyngeal and rectal infection may be particularly difficult to eliminate. A repeated culture to test for a cure is made 4~7 days after treatment. Patients with gonorrhoea should be screened for coexisting sexually transmitted diseases, e.g. chlamydia. Management is most appropriate in a department of genitourinary medicine where contact tracing can be organized.

Vulval disorders

The vulva can be involved in many conditions, and itching (pruritus vulvae), often followed by secondary lichenification, is frequent. Commonly seen dermatoses include:

- lichen sclerosus
- eczemas including allergic contact dermatitis (Fig. 57-3) and seborrhoeic dermatitis
- psoriasis
- lichen planus

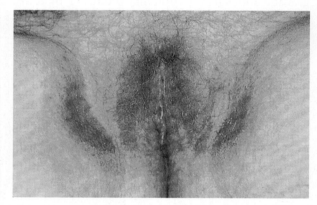

Fig. 57-3   **Contact dermatitis of the vulva.** This was caused by allergy to neomycin in a cream.

Herpes simplex, viral warts, candidiasis, venereal infections (see above) and extramammary Paget's disease also occur. Other specific disorders include the following:

- *Vulval intraepithelial neoplasia* (VIN): includes *in situ* squamous cell carcinoma and Bowenoid papulosis (Fig. 57-4). Cervical intraepithelial neoplasia can coexist and screening is required. Human papillomavirus infection may predispose to the precancerous change. There is a small risk of progression to invasive squamous cell carcinoma. Treatment is by cryosurgery or excision (for small areas), topical fluorouracil and laser therapy. Follow-up is needed.
- *Vulvodynia*: a chronic vulval discomfort, often with burning and soreness. It is sometimes due to erosive vulvitis, e.g. from lichen planus or VIN. Some patients have underlying psychological problems.
- *Genital ulceration*: may occur with pemphigoid or pemphigus, or acutely with erythema multiforme. It is also seen with Behçet's syndrome, a multisystem disorder in which recurrent oral aphthous ulceration and iridocyclitis also occur.

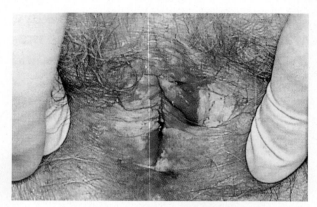

Fig. 57-4   **A hyperkeratotic variant of vulval intraepithelial neoplasia (VIN).** Reproduced courtesy of the editor of the British Journal of Dermatology and Dr E F Bernstein of Jefferson Medical College, Philadelphia, PA, USA.

Penile and scrotal eruptions

Balanitis (inflammation of the penile skin; Fig. 57-5) and scrotal eruptions can be caused by a similar list of conditions to those outlined above for vulval dermatoses. Specific disorders include:

- *circinate balanitis*, an eroded or crusted penile eruption seen in Reiter's syndrome
- *scrotal gangrene*, a necrotizing cellulitis of rapid onset, seen in diabetics. It has a mortality rate of 45%.

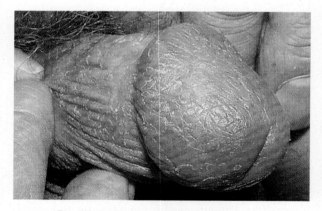

Fig. 57-5   **Eczema of the glans penis.**

Pruritus ani

The perianal skin is frequently involved in infective, inflammatory and occasionally neoplastic conditions, as for the genitalia. Pruritus ani is common in middle-aged men. Whatever the underlying derma-

Genitourinary medicine

Syphilis

- The primary chancre appears 3 weeks after sexual contact.
- The papular non-pruritic eruption of the secondary stage is seen 4~10 weeks following the chancre.
- Tertiary syphilis may be delayed several years.
- Treatment is with benzathine penicillin, procaine penicillin or doxycycline.
- Patients need contact tracing and should be screened for other venereal diseases.

Gonorrhoea

- Men present with dysuria, frequency and a urethral discharge.
- Women complain of a vaginal discharge, dysuria and abdominal pain.
- Infection may be asymptomatic.
- Late sequelae include pelvic inflammatory disease and infertility.
- Treatment is with a single oral dose of cefixime (or ciprofloxacin or ofloxacin dependent upon sensitivities).

Vulval disorders

- Common vulval disorders include lichen sclerosus, eczemas, psoriasis and vulvodynia.
- Vulval intraepithelial neoplasia requires long-term follow-up and cervical screening.
- Chronic ulceration may indicate a blistering disorder or Behçet's syndrome.
- Secondary contact dermatitis, e.g. due to medicament allergy, is common.

Pruritus ani

- Is common in middle-aged men.
- May be due to the irritant effects of faecal contamination on perianal skin.
- Anal carcinoma, anal fissure and haemorrhoids must be excluded.
- Local hygiene measures and a topical antiseptic or steroid are prescribed.
- Secondary allergic contact dermatitis is common.

---

tosis, faecal contamination of the perianal skin with bacteria, enzymes and allergens causes inflammation and itch. Persistent rubbing induces lichen simplex or maceration, and secondary infection with bacteria or fungi. A compounding contact dermatitis due to allergy to 'over-the-counter' creams is common. Anal carcinoma, fissure or haemorrhoids, and threadworm infestation in children, should be excluded.

Treatment requires attention to personal hygiene (daily baths are helpful but avoid the use of soap or hot water) and the topical application of an emollient, antiseptic or steroid preparation.

Web resource

http://www.bashh.org

Key words

syphilis   梅毒

chancre   硬下疳

gumma   树胶样肿

gonorrhea   淋病

vulvodynia   外阴痛

balanitis   阴茎头炎

pruritus ani   肛门瘙痒症

Review questions

1. What are the clinical stages of syphilis and the main clinical manifestation of each stage?
2. What are the serological tests for syphilis?
3. What is the etiological examination for gonorrhea?

(Yumin Xia)

Chapter 58   Racially pigmented skin

Common dermatoses may show variable manifestations in different races due to differences in pigmentation, hair or the response of skin to external stimuli. In addition, some conditions have a distinct racial predisposition. The response of darkly pigmented skin to injury and to certain therapeutic modalities needs to be taken into account when planning a programme of management.

Definition of race

The characteristics of our species, *Homo sapiens*, are continuously variable, and hence the division into 'races' is - to some extent - artificial. However, there are obvious differences between groups of humans, and these differences have an influence on the appearance of and susceptibility to disease. Most definitions of a '*race*' are unsatisfactory, but perhaps the best is 'a population that differs significantly from other populations in regard to the frequency of one or more of the genes that it possesses'. Obviously, this definition allows even rather small groups to be classified as a race!

It is generally assumed that changes in gene frequency result from mutation, natural selection and 'accidental' loss. Some changes are thought to be the result of adaptation to environmental conditions, although it is not always obvious what advantage is conferred. Racial classification has relied on physical characteristics, often skeletal, although hair form and skin colour are taken into account. The main divisions are the following:

- *Australoid*: e.g. Australian aborigines.
- *Capoid*: e.g. bushmen, hottentots.
- *Caucasoid*: Europeans, peoples of the Mediterranean, Middle East and most of the Indian subcontinent.
- *Mongoloid*: peoples of East Asia, Eskimos, American Indians.

- *Negroid*: e.g. black Africans.

Racial differences in normal skin

The most obvious difference is in pigmentation, but hair forms and colour also vary. Mongoloid hair is straight and has the largest diameter; black African hair is short, spiralled, drier and more brittle than that of other races; and caucasoid hair may be wavy, straight or helical. Hair colour is predominantly black in mongoloids and Africans, and black, blond or red in Caucasoids. Body hair is most profuse in Caucasoids. The black African stratum corneum differs from that of the caucasoid by showing greater intercellular adhesion and a higher lipid content.

Diseases that show racially dependent variations

In pigmented skin, eruptions that appear red or brown in white caucasoid skin may be black, grey or purple, and pigmentation can mask an erythematous reaction. Inflammation in pigmented skin often provokes a hyperpigmentary (Figs 58-1 and 58-2) or hypopigmentary (Table 58-1) reaction. Follicular, papular and annular patterns are more common in pigmented skin than in caucasoid. In addition, some skin disorders show an inter-racial variation in prevalence (Table 58-2).

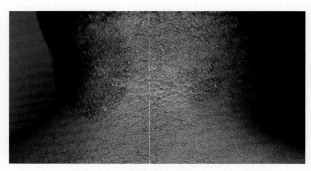

Fig. 58-1   **Lichen simplex chronicus showing hyperpigmentation and lichenification.**

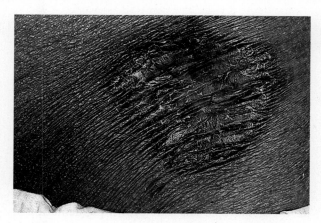

Fig. 58-2   **Lichen planus with hyperpigmentation.**

Table 58-1   **Causes of hypopigmentation in a pigmented skin**

Division	Disorder
Infections	Leprosy, onchocerciasis, pinta, pityriasis versicolor
Papulosquamous disorders	Pityriasis rosea, pityriasis alba, psoriasis (occasionally), seborrhoeic dermatitis
Physical and chemical agents	Burns, cryotherapy, hydroquinone, topical potent steroids
Post-inflammatory	Discoid lupus erythematosus, systemic sclerosis, sarcoidosis
Other	Albinism, vitiligo

Diseases with a distinct racial or ethnic predisposition

Hair disorders

Racially dependent hair conditions are most common in black Africans and include the following:

- *Folliculitis keloidalis* describes discrete follicular papules, often keloids, at the back of the neck in African males (Fig. 58-3). Intralesional steroids may help.
- *Pseudofolliculitis barbae* is a common disorder in black African men and is characterized by inflammatory papules and pustules in the beard area. It is thought to result from hairs growing back into the skin (Fig. 58-4). Treatment is difficult but includes attention to shaving technique and the topical use of antibiotics and steroids.
- *Traction alopecia* is mainly seen in black Africans because of the practice of plaiting or tightly braiding the hair (Fig. 58-5). Hairs are loosened from their follicles. The temples are often affected.
- *Hot-comb alopecia* is a traction alopecia caused by applying a hot comb to oiled hair in order to straighten it (curly black African hair is usually straightened by chemical methods).

Table 58-2   **Diseases with racially dependent variations**

Skin disorder	Caucasoid	Mongoloid	Black African
Acne	Most severe	Least common	Hyperpigmented lesions
Atopic eczema	Most common with western lifestyle	Lichenification is seen	Follicular and hyperpigmented lesions are found
Keloid	May occur	More frequent	More frequent
Lichen planus	Can show some pigmentation	Often hyperpigmented	Often hyperpigmented
Melanocytic naevi	Very common	A few may be present	Uncommon
Psoriasis	Common (2% prevalence)	Rare (0.3% prevalence but increasing)	East > West Africans: plaques bluish, leave hyper- or hypopigmentation
Sarcoidosis	Less common	Less common	In USA, 10 times more common than in Caucasoids
Skin cancer	Most common in northern Europeans	Intermediate prevalence	Uncommon
Vitiligo	Same prevalence, least obvious	Same prevalence, more obvious	Same prevalence, most obvious

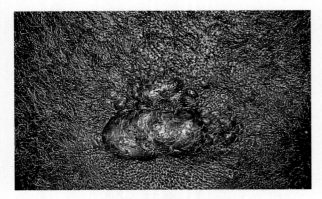

Fig. 58-3 **Folliculitis keloidalis.**

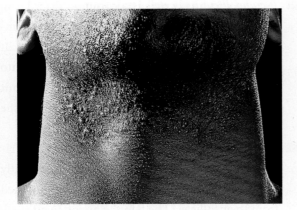

Fig. 58-4 **Pseudofolliculitis barbae.**

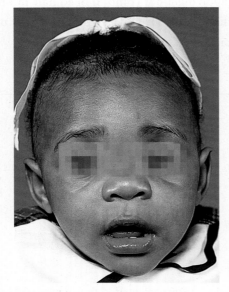

Fig. 58-5 **Traction alopecia.**

Pigmentary changes

Pigmentary abnormalities, as both a variation of 'normal' and otherwise, are also common. These include the following:

- *Dermatosis papulosa nigra* describes small, seborrhoeic wart-like papules often seen on the face in black Africans.
- *Lines of hypo- or hyperpigmentation*, often on the upper arms, are not infrequently found in black Africans.
- *Longitudinal nail pigmentation* and macular pigmentation of palms and soles occur mainly in black Africans.
- *Mongolian spot* is a slate-brown pigmentation at the sacral area in a baby and is found in 100% of mongoloids, 70% or more of Africans and 10% of Caucasoids. It usually fades by the age of 6 years.
- *Naevus of Ota* is a macular, slate-grey pigmentation in the upper trigeminal area, which may involve the sclera (Fig. 58-6). It is seen most frequently in mongoloids.

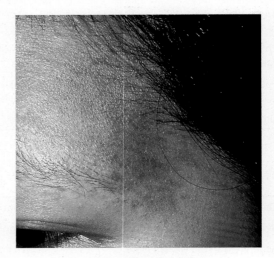

Fig. 58-6 **Naevus of Ota.**

Other conditions

A racial preponderance is also seen with the following conditions:

- *Sickle cell disease* occurs in black Africans. The main cutaneous findings are painful oedema of the hands and feet, caused by infarction in the small bones, and leg ulceration.
- *Vascular naevi*, such as the port wine stain naevus, and melanocytic naevi, are more common in Caucasoids.

Racially pigmented skin

- **A race** is a genetically defined group, although the characteristics of *Homo sapiens* are continuously variable.
- **The most numerous races** are mongoloids, black Africans and Caucasoids (the last include Middle East and Indian subcontinent peoples).
- **Eruptions that are red or brown** in caucasoid skin may appear *black*, *grey* or *purple* in people with pigmented skin.
- **Lichenification**: inflammatory dermatoses tend to become *lichenified* in mongoloids and may be *follicular* in black Africans.
- **Hypopigmentation** may follow from skin trauma, e.g. burns or from cryotherapy, topical steroids and some dermatoses, in pigmented skin.
- **Hair disorders**, e.g. pseudofolliculitis, keloidal change or traction alopecia, are common in black Africans.
- **Pigmentary lines** are frequently found on the limbs (e.g. the outer upper arm) or nails in black Africans and other races.
- **Sacral mongolian spots** are found in most mongoloid and black African babies, but in only a few caucasoid infants.
- **Vascular and melanocytic naevi** (e.g. port wine stain) are more common in Caucasoids than in other races.

Web resource

http://www.brownskin.net/conditions.html

Key words

pigmentation   色素沉着
folliculitis keloidalis   瘢痕性毛囊炎
pseudofolliculitis barbae   须部假性毛囊炎
traction alopecia   牵拉性脱发
naevus of Ota   太田痣
lichenification   苔藓样变

Review questions

1. What is the definition of race?
2. Describe the causes of hypopigmentation in a pigmented skin.
3. Describe the types of pigmentary changes of skin.

(XiaoYong Man)

Chapter 59   Occupation and the skin

Skin disorders, after stress and musculoskeletal problems, are the commonest reported cause of occupational disease and are responsible for much lost productivity. An occupational dermatosis is defined as a skin condition that is primarily due to components of the work environment and would not have occurred unless the individual were doing that job.

Diagnosis

Proving a work association can be difficult. The following give clues:

- Contact with a known noxious agent.
- Similar skin disease in other workers.
- Consistent exposure-to-onset time course.
- Attacks appear with exposure, improve on withdrawal.
- Site and type of eruption consistent with exposure.
- Corroboration by patch testing.

Contact dermatitis is the most common work-related skin disease and is more often irritant than allergic. Contact urticaria, particularly to latex, is now well recognized. Other occupational dermatoses are listed in Table 59-1. Certain infections, e.g. anthrax, orf and tinea corporis may be occupational. Heat, cold, ultraviolet radiation, vibration and X-rays can cause industrial disease.

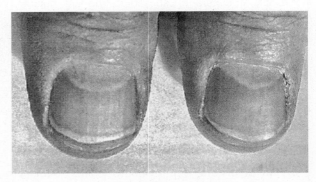

Fig. 59-1 **Blue discoloration of the nails due to argyria in a silver smelter.**

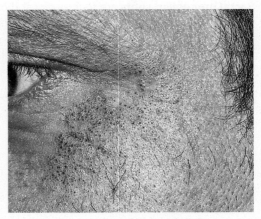

Fig. 59-2 **Chloracne showing comedones in a man exposed to dioxin contaminants.**

Table 59-1	**Rarer occupational skin disorders**	
Condition	**Presentation**	**Occupational exposure**
Argyria (Fig. 59-1)	Slate-grey pigmentation on face, hands, sclerae	Industrial processes, e.g. silver smelters
Chloracne (Fig. 59-2)	Multiple open and closed comedones on cheeks and behind ears	Halogenated aromatic hydrocarbons, e.g. contamination during manufacture
Occupational vitiligo	Symmetrical pigment loss on face and hands	Substituted phenols or catechols in oils, at coking plant
Tar keratoses (Fig. 59-3)	Small keratotic warts on face and hand, premalignant	Tar and pitch, e.g. road work or coking plant; UV is a co-carcinogen
Vibration white finger	Blanching and pain in digits, later swelling and impaired fine movement	Hand-held vibrating tools, as used by rock drillers or chainsaw operators

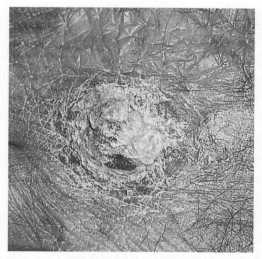

Fig. 59-3   **A tar keratosis in a coking plant worker.**

Contact dermatitis

It is often difficult to differentiate between allergic and irritant causes.

Aetiopathogenesis

Many industrial substances are irritants and some are allergens as well. Water, detergents, alkalis, coolant oils and solvents are important irritants. Common allergens include chromate, rubber chemicals, preservatives, nickel, fragrances, epoxy resins and phenol-formaldehyde resins (Table 59-2).

Irritant dermatitis frequently results from cumulative exposure to multiple types of irritant. An irritant dermatitis increases epidermal penetration by allergens and, because of this, it predisposes to superimposed contact sensitization. Similarly, allergic contact dermatitis renders skin vulnerable to attack by irritants.

Constitutional factors, especially atopic eczema, predispose to contact dermatitis. Environmental factors such as physical friction, occlusion, heat, cold, dry air from air conditioning or sudden swings in air temperature or humidity also have an effect.

Clinical presentation

The hands are affected, alone or with other sites, in 80%~90% of occupational cases. The arms can be involved if not covered, and the face and neck are affected if there is exposure to dust or fumes. Cement workers often have lower leg and foot dermatitis in addition to hand changes. Allergy to rubber chemicals can cause dermatitis from rubber gloves or boots. Some workers develop 'hardening', an adaptive tolerance to irritants or allergies.

Occupational dermatitis appears at any age, but peaks at each end of working life. In bakers and hairdressers, dermatitis appears early. In cement workers, chromate dermatitis requires a few years to develop. Cumulative irritant dermatitis appears after several years' exposure.

Table 59-2	**Contact dermatitis hazards in selected occupations**	
Occupation	**Irritants**	**Allergens**
Bakers	Flour, detergent, sugar, enzymes	Flavouring, oil, antioxidant
Building trade workers	Cement, glass wool, acid, preservatives	Cement (Cr, Co), rubber, resin, wood
Caterers, cooks	Meat, fish, fruit, vegetables, detergent, water	Vegetables/fruit, cutlery (Ni), rubber gloves, spice
Cleaners	Detergent, solvent, water, friction	Rubber gloves, nickel, fragrance
Dental personnel	Detergent, soap, acrylate, flux	Rubber, acrylate, fragrance, mercury
Electronics assemblers	Solder, solvent, fibreglass, acid	Cr, Co, Ni, acrylate, epoxy resin
Hairdressers	Shampoo, bleach, perm lotion, soap, water, friction	Para-phenylenediamine dye, rubber, fragrance, thioglycolate
Metal workers	Cutting fluid, cleanser, solvent	Preservative, Ni, Cr, Co, antioxidant
Office workers	Paper, fibreglass, dry atmosphere	Rubber, Ni, dye, glue, copying paper
Textile workers	Solvent, bleach, fibre, formaldehyde	Formaldehyde resin, dye, Ni
Veterinarians, farmers	Disinfectant, animal secretion	Rubber, antibiotics, plants, preservative

Case history 1

Hand dermatitis

A 17-year-old girl who had had childhood atopic eczema started as a hairdressing apprentice. Within 8 weeks, she developed hand dermatitis (Fig. 59-4) unresponsive to emollients and topical steroids. Patch testing was positive for ammonium thioglycolate (a permanent wave agent) and nickel. A diagnosis was made of contact dermatitis with irritant and allergic components, in an individual with underlying endogenous eczema. Her dermatitis cleared within weeks when she left hairdressing to work in an office.

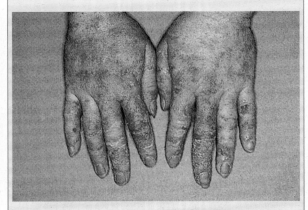

Fig.59-4 **Hand dermatitis in a hairdresser.**

Differential diagnosis

Contact dermatitis due to non-occupational exposure and endogenous eczemas need considering. Often, occupational dermatitis is multifactorial, with irritants, allergens, endogenous factors and secondary bacterial infection all causally involved.

Management

Patch testing is required if there is exposure to known allergens. A factory visit helps to ascertain the exact nature of irritant or allergen exposure.

Once recognized, occupational exposure to a causative agent can be minimized, but this does not always produce an improvement. Chromate allergy is particularly intransigent. Any dermatitis is treated along standard lines with special attention to hand care. Barrier creams are of dubious value.

Contact urticaria

Some proteins and chemicals provoke immediate urticaria. The release of mast cell histamine or other mediators may or may not be immunoglobulin (Ig) E mediated. Pruritus, erythema and whealing appear within minutes and last a few hours.

Occupational contacts include latex in rubber gloves, foods (e.g. fish, potato, eggs, flour, spices, meats and numerous fruits), *Myroxylon pereirae* (a perfume and flavouring agent) and animal saliva. Contact dermatitis may coexist.

Latex contact urticaria has been a problem in healthcare workers and other occupations. Anaphylaxis may occur if there is a massive latex exposure, e.g. in a patient exposed to surgeon's gloves during abdominal surgery.

Case history 2

Chromate dermatitis

A 30-year-old man had been employed for 3 years making pipes out of cement. This involved exposure to wet cement. Despite wearing gloves and overalls, he developed dermatitis on the hands (Fig. 59-5), arms and lower legs. Patch testing showed chromate allergy. He received compensation for having an industrial disease but, even when he changed his occupation to driving, he continued to have hand dermatitis.

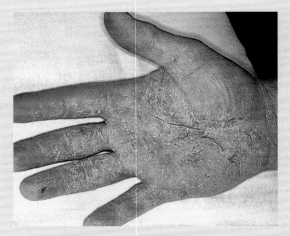

Fig. 59-5 **Hand dermatitis in a cement worker.**

Case history 3

Contact urticaria

A 40-year-old female nurse gave a 12-month history of itching, swelling and redness on her hands (Fig. 59-6), which developed within minutes of wearing disposable latex gloves. Patch testing was negative, but a prick test was positive for latex (confirmed by specific IgE test). Her symptoms resolved when she changed to nitrile gloves. Provision of latex-free disposable gloves to healthcare workers seems to have reduced the prevalence of latex allergy.

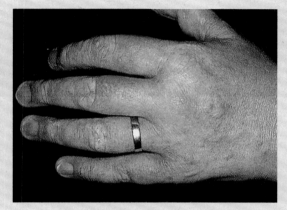

Fig. 59-6   Contact urticaria to latex.

Prevention

Reducing the contact time between the skin and noxious substances is the aim. It is achieved by:

- improved work practices, e.g. increased automation
- substituting an alternative, e.g. nitrile gloves instead of latex rubber
- provision of protective clothing
- taking better care of the skin.

Recognizing an occupational disease may highlight faulty work practices that can be corrected. Compensation may be due.

Occupation and the skin
- **Occurrence**: industrial skin disease is common, especially contact dermatitis.
- **Causation**: occupational contact dermatitis is caused more by irritants than by allergens but is often multifactorial, with endogenous factors frequently being involved in addition.
- **Predisposition**: previous atopic eczema predisposes to occupational contact dermatitis.
- **Patch testing**: can help identify an allergen, e.g. chromate or rubber chemicals.
- **Contact urticaria** to latex has been a risk in healthcare workers and other occupations, but appears less so now.
- **Prevention**: occupational skin disease is minimized by reducing the contact time of noxious agents with the skin and by increasing awareness of the problem.

Web resource

http://www.hse.gov.uk/

Key words

occupational dermatoses   职业性皮肤病

latex contact urticaria   乳胶接触性荨麻疹

chromate dermatitis   铬酸盐性皮炎

hairdresser   美发师

textile worker   纺织工人

veterinarians   兽医

chloracne   氯痤疮

argyria   银中毒

nitrile gloves   丁腈手套

Review questions

1. What's the main clinical presentation of occupational dermatosis?
2. How to prevent occupational dermatosis?

(Jianyun Lu)

Chapter 60   Immunological tests

Clinical and laboratory tests of an immunological nature are valuable in the diagnosis and management of certain skin diseases. Skin prick tests or serum immunoglobulin (Ig) E tests are sometimes of use in *atopic disease*, patch tests are helpful in the investigation of *contact dermatitis*, and immunofluorescent studies on biopsied skin (or with serum) are essential in the diagnosis of *bullous disorders* and in some other conditions such as connective tissue diseases (e.g. lupus erythematosus) or vasculitis.

Skin prick tests

Indications

Urticaria, atopic dermatitis, drug eruption and other allergic diseases related to *immediate (type I) hypersensitivity*.

Mechanism of action

The reaction is mediated by the antigen-triggered IgE-mediated release of vasoactive substances from skin mast cells.

Methodology

Small drops of commercially prepared antigen solutions are placed on marked areas on the forearm and lightly pricked into the skin using separate blunt lancets. The stratum corneum of the epidermis is punctured by gently pressing the blunt lancet perpendicular to the skin surface through the test solution. Food allergens are often tested by pricking the fresh food and then the skin (prick to prick testing). The sites are inspected at 20~30 min.

Interpretation

A positive result is regarded as one showing a wheal of 3mm or greater (Fig. 60-1).

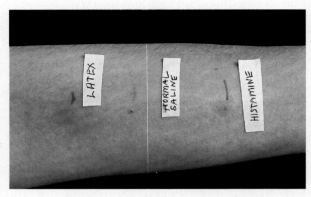

Fig. 60-1 **A positive prick test to latex is seen in a latex-allergic subject.** The wheal to histamine is shown as a positive control.

Notes

Patients should have stopped antihistamines 48h before the test. The risk of anaphylaxis is very small, but resuscitation facilities, including adrenaline (epinephrine) for intramuscular injection, antihistamines and oxygen are mandatory.

Patch testing

Indications

Contact dermatitis, occupational dermatitis, eczema and cosmetic dermatitis

Mechanism of action

The epicutaneous patch test detects cell-mediated (type IV) hypersensitivity.

Methodology

Commercially prepared allergens are available in the correct concentration for testing, usually in petrolatum (or sometimes water) as a diluent. Details of the procedure are shown in Fig. 60-2.

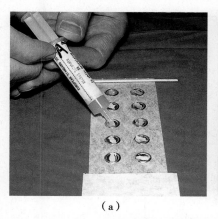
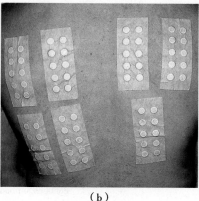
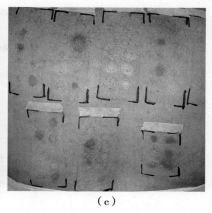

(a)   (b)   (c)

Fig. 60-2   **Patch testing methodology. (a)** Patch tests are prepared. Small amounts of the test substances are applied to the 8-mm-diameter aluminium discs on adhesive tape (Finn chambers) that are used for patch testing. The exact selection of test substances depends on the clinical problem, the location of the dermatitis, the environmental contacts and the patient's occupation. **(b)** Patch tests are applied. A 'standard series' of 38 substances is applied to every patient, with additional allergens if necessary. A record sheet is kept. The patches are fixed to the upper back, left on for 2 days and then removed after marking the top margin of each text strip with adhesive tape or with a marker pen. **(c)** Patch tests are read. Numerous allergic-positive patch test sites are shown. A positive allergic response is manifest by a localized eczema reaction, which is scored according to the following convention: ?+ doubtful: faint erythema only; + weak: erythema, maybe papules; ++ strong: vesicles, infiltration; +++ extreme: bullous; IR irritant (of various types, but often showing a glazed circumscribed area, frequently with increased skin markings). The test sites are read for a second time at 4 days, as positive reactions commonly do not appear until this time. The results are interpreted in the light of the clinical situation: a positive reaction is not always relevant to the current skin problem.

Notes

Patients should have stopped glucocorticoids 2 weeks and antihistamines 72h before the test.

Immunofluorescence

Immunofluorescence, either direct (on the patient's skin) or indirect (using the patient's serum reacted with an animal substrate) (Fig. 60-3), is helpful in making a diagnosis in the *autoimmune blistering diseases* (Table 60-1). Bullous disorders such as pemphigoid (Fig. 60-4) and pemphigus (Fig. 60-5) are characterized by the deposition of organ-specific autoantibodies (eg. IgG IgA, IgM and C3) in the skin and, less easily demonstrated, by the presence of these autoantibodies in the serum. Dermatitis herpetiformis (Fig. 60-6) and other conditions such as leucocytoclastic vasculitis or lupus erythematosus often show the deposition of immunoglobulin or complement components in the patient's skin (negative indirect immunofluorescence).

Table 60-1 **Immunofluorescence in bullous disease**		
Bullous disorder	**Direct immunofluorescence (skin)**	**Indirect immunofluorescence (serum)**
Bullous pemphigoid	Linear IgG/C3 at BMZ in 80%	Linear IgG at BMZ in 75% (IgA/IgM in 25%)
Pemphigus vulgaris	Intercellular epidermal IgG/C3 in 100% (IgA/IgM in 20%)	Intercellular IgG in 80% (the antibody titre reflects disease activity)
Dermatitis herpetiformis	Granular IgA deposition at dermal papilla (100%)	Absent
Linear IgA disease	Linear IgA at BMZ in 80% (IgG/IgM/C3 in 10%)	Linear IgA at BMZ found in some cases

BMZ, basement membrane zone.

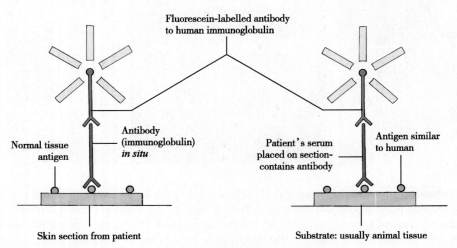

Direct immunofluorescence   Indirect immunofluorescence

Fig. 60-3 Immunofluorescence. In *direct immunofluorescence*, usually done on perilesional skin, the antibodies or complement components are detected by reacting the freshly cut skin sections with an antibody directed against the specific immunoglobulin or complement fraction and labelled with a fluorescent marker, which is visualized with a fluorescence microscope. The *indirect method* is a two-step procedure that involves the use of cut sections of an animal substrate (e.g. monkey oesophagus) or human skin. The patient's diluted serum (containing the putative antibody) is placed on this section, incubated for about an hour and then revealed using a fluorescein-tagged antihuman immunoglobulin antibody that is demonstrated by examining with ultraviolet radiation. Human skin, split at the dermoepidermal junction by saline incubation, may be used as a substrate to distinguish variants of pemphigoid, when deposition of the antibody on the epidermal or dermal side of the split can provide the references to the diagnosis.

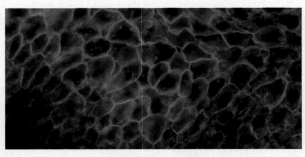

Fig. 60-5 Pemphigus vulgaris. Direct immunofluorescence demonstrates IgG antibodies, directed against desmoglein 3 (MW 130kDa), a desmosomal cadherin involved in mediating epidermal intercellular adhesion, showing up in a chicken-wire pattern throughout the epidermis.

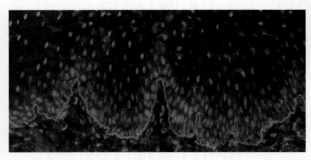

Fig. 60-4 Bullous pemphigoid. Indirect immunofluorescence demonstrates a linear band of IgG antibodies along the basement membrane zone (BMZ) using monkey oesophagus as substrate. These antibodies are directed against bullous pemphigoid antigens (MW 230 and 180kDa),. The two antigens are components of hemidesomosomes, which are adhesion complexes promoting epithial-stromal adhesion in stratified and other complex epithelia, such as the skin and mucous membrane.

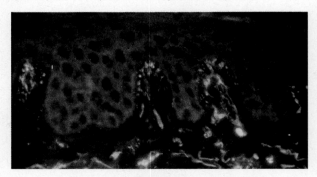

Fig. 60-6 Dermatitis herpetiformis. Direct immunofluorescence reveals the deposition of IgA in a granular pattern at the dermal papillae. This provide the references to the diagnosis of dermatitis herpetiformis, although the eruption is not solely due to the presence of this IgA.

Immunological tests

- **Prick tests** reveal type Ⅰ (IgE-mediated) hypersensitivity and can demonstrate airborne (e.g. house dust mite), food (e.g. hen's egg or peanut) and latex allergies.
- **Patch tests** detect type Ⅳ (cell-mediated) hypersensitivity and are helpful in investigating contact dermatitis, occupational dermatitis, hand eczema and cosmetic dermatitis.
- **Direct immunofluorescence** demonstrates immunoglobulin and complement deposition in the skin and is very useful in the diagnosis of bullous disorders, e.g. pemphigoid or pemphigus.
- **Indirect immunofluorescence** uses an animal substrate to detect antibodies in a patient's serum. It is often positive in pemphigus and pemphigoid, and sometimes in linear IgA disease, but is negative in dermatitis herpetiformis.
- **Autoantibodies in bullous pemphigoid (BP)** are against BP antigens of molecular weight (MW) 230 and 180kDa. and in pemphigus vulgaris against desmoglein 3 antigen (MW 130kDa). The autoantigen, if any, in dermatitis herpetiformis is not currently known.

Key Words

skin prick test   皮肤点刺试验

patch test   斑贴试验

direct immunofluorescence   直接免疫荧光

indirect immunofluorescence   间接免疫荧光

immunological test   免疫学检查

serum immunoglobulin (Ig) E test   血清 IgE 检查

basement membrane zone   基底膜带

desmoglein   桥粒芯蛋白

bullous pemphigoid   大疱性类天疱疮

pemphigus vulgaris   寻常型天疱疮

dermatitis herpetiformis   疱疹样皮炎

Review questions

1. What are the indications of the skin prick test, patch test, direct immunofluorescence and indirect immunofluorescence?
2. What is the mechanism of the skin prick test?
3. Please describe the methodology of the patch test.
4. How much do the autoantibodies in bullous pemphigoid weight?
5. Describe the features of direct immunofluorescence demonstrated in pemphigus vulgaris.

(Jinhua Xu)

Chapter 61   Dermatology and the Internet

The widespread availability of access to the Internet has had profound effects on dermatology. Doctors and students now have unlimited access to medical information, patients have readily available facts or opinions about their conditions, and both clinicians and patients have the possibility for remote consultation by 'teledermatology'. Teledermatology, first introduced into the literature in 1995 by Perednia and Brown, refers to the delivery of dermatologic care via information and communication technology for the purpose of reducing their isolation and increasing their knowledge of dermatology.

The Internet as a library

Databases

Searches can be made through databases such as PubMed (http://www.ncbi.nlm.nih.gov/sites/entrez) (Fig. 61-1) and online written information obtained through search engines. Another useful resource is McKusick's catalogue of inherited diseases (http://www.ncbi.nlm.nih.gov/sites/entrez?db=omim)

and up-to-data medical information (http://www.webmd.com/).

Organizations

All the major dermatological organizations have their own websites that give practical details for clinicians and patients, e.g. the British Association of Dermatologists (http://www.bad.org.uk/) (Fig. 61-2), the European Academy of Dermatology and Venereology (http://www.eadv.org/), the American Academy of Dermatology (http://www.aad.org/), the Chinese Society of Dermatology (http://csd.cma.org.cn/), and the Chinese Medical Doctor Association of Dermatology (http://cda.net.cn/cda/). Most large international institutions have their own websites, e.g. the World Health Organization (http://www.who.int/).

Education

There are websites specifically dedicated to education, such as emedicine (http://emedicine.medscape.com/dermatology), MedlinePlus (http://www.nlm.nih.gov/medlineplus/skinconditions.html) (Fig.

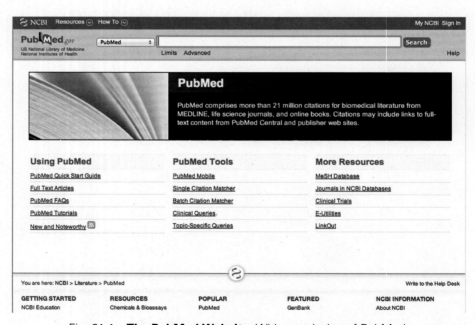

Fig. 61-1   **The PubMed Website.** With permission of PubMed.

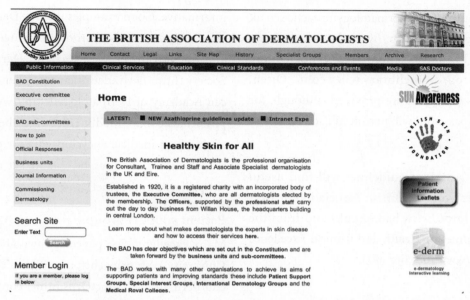

Fig. 61-2   **The website of the British Association of Dermatologists.** With permission of the British Association of Dermatologists.

61-3) and the New Zealand Dermatological Society (http://www.dermnet.org.nz/index.html).

Evidence-based medicine

In an age when the clinician is called upon to defend his or her practice, it is useful to know that there are Web pages dedicated to providing details and analysis on the true benefit or otherwise of many valuable therapies. The Cochrane Skin Group's Website (http://skin.cochrane.org/) and the National Library for Health (http://www.evidence.nhs.uk)

are invaluable resources.

Journals

Many journals are available online, often through a publisher's website; for example, Synergy (http://onlinelibrary.wiley.com/) provides the *British Journal of Dermatology*, and Nature (http://www.nature.com/jid/index.html) provides the *Journal of Investigative Dermatology*. JAMA Dermatology (formerly *Archives of Dermatology*) can be obtained at http://jamanetwork.com/journals/jamadermatology, *Dermatology*

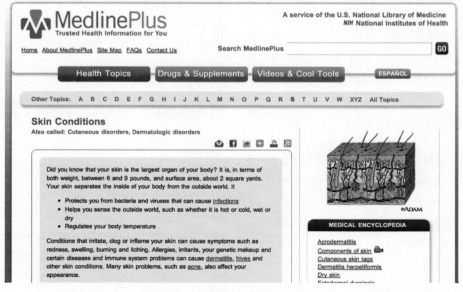

Fig. 61-3   **The MedlinePlus Web page.** With permission of MedlinePlus.

in Practice at http://www.dermatologyinpractice.co.uk and Elsevier journals at http://www.elsevier.com/wps/find/journal_browse.cws_home and Wiley Online Library at http://onlinelibrary.wiley.com/. Often, only abstracts of articles are provided, although, for subscribers, a password will permit full access.

Guidelines

Clinicians in search of guidelines will find useful the Web pages from the British Association of Dermatologists (http://www.bad.org.uk) and from the National Institute for Health and Clinical Excellence (NICE; http://www.nice.org.uk/).

Links

Some Web pages specialize in providing links to other resources, e.g. the Hardin Library (http://www.lib.uiowa.edu/hardin) and the British Association of Dermatologists (http://www.bad.org.uk).

Textbooks

Some reference textbooks now offer subscription to online access such as *Rook's Textbook of Dermatology* (http://www.rooksdermatology.com) and *Dermatology* (http://www.dermtext.com/).

Dermatology apps

The smartphone is likely to revolutionize the way we practise medicine, with rapid access to information on the move. There are many sites for downloading apps and those such as http://www.skyscape.com provide a dedicated library of dermatological apps for most platforms. Iagnosis, Dermatologists on Call are widely used in United States of American.

Resources for patients

Many patients are familiar with searching the Internet. Unfortunately, the Internet is not regulated, and some of the information posted is unreliable. It is therefore helpful to direct patients to reliable websites such as those listed here.

Patient websites

Web pages designed for use by patients can be very informative. Good examples include DermIS (http://www.dermis.net/dermisroot/en/home/index.htm), and ones from the New Zealand Dermatological Society (http://www.dermnetnz.org/) and the American Academy of Dermatology (http://www.skincarephysicians.com/). MedlinePlus (see above) also has an excellent medical encyclopaedia for patients, and reliable information can be obtained at Yahoo Health (http://health.yahoo.net).

Patient support groups

Many excellent Web pages are available. The Iowa University Web page (http://www.healthcare.uiowa.edu/dermatology/SuprtGrps.html) contains a comprehensive list including groups for rare conditions. Several sites give fact sheets about skin conditions and their treatment. Worth a particular mention are those from the Skin Care Campaign (http://www.skincarecampaign.org/), which gives a comprehensive list of patient support organizations, the UK National Eczema Society (http://www.eczema.org/) and the Psoriasis Association (http://www.psoriasis-association.org.uk/) Website (Fig. 61-4).

Handouts and patient information leaflets

The British Association of Dermatologists continues to update and expand its collection of patient information sheets which are invaluable when counselling patients about a disease or discussing the possibility of systemic therapy (http://www.bad.org.uk). Certain websites specifically produce handouts for patients, e.g. RxMed (http://www.rxmed.com/).

Teledermatology

Telemedicine is the practice of medicine remote from the patient using some form of electronic transfer via the Internet or a more secure computer network of clinical data for exchanging medical information for the purpose of diagnosis, consultation, treatment and teaching, such as a photograph. It is particularly suited to dermatology because of the visual nature of the specialty.

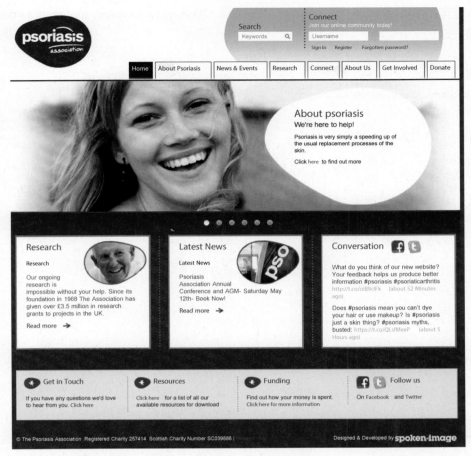

Fig. 61-4 **The Website of the UK Psoriasis Association.** With permission of the UK Psoriasis Association.

Electronic image

An accurate diagnosis and a suggested management plan obtained from the specialist examining an image on a computer is an attractive concept. Digitally captured still ('store and forward') or videoconference ('live') photographs can be transmitted electronically to a dermatologist hundreds or even thousands of miles away for an opinion. A good-quality image of high resolution is vital.

Accuracy

Teledermatology has been evaluated, mostly using the 'store and forward' method, for patients living in remote regions and has been found to be a useful adjunct to clinical medicine. It can be an accurate method for differentiating between benign and malignant skin lesions, but is not a substitute for face-to-face consultation, which should be available when indicated.

Dermatology and the Internet

- **Databases**, e.g. PubMed, are used to search for medical information.
- **Professional organizations**, e.g. the European Academy of Dermatology and Venereology, have Web pages for use by clinicians and patients.
- **Educational resources** for students include MedlinePlus and the Dermatology Image Atlas.
- **Evidence-based dermatology** is accessed via the Cochrane Skin Group's Web page.
- **Online journals** are obtained via the publishers' Websites.
- **Guidelines** can be viewed, e.g. from NICE or the British Association of Dermatologists.
- **Patient support groups** have numerous Web pages, e.g. Skin Care Campaign.
- **Teledermatology** may be of value for skin problems that occur in people who live in remote areas.

Key words

teledermatology   远程皮肤病学

communication ways   交流方式

organization　组织机构

database　数据库

Review questions

1. What is the teledermatology and the advantage?

2. What are the commonly used medicine databases?

(Xiaodong Li)

Index